Ian POPPLE   Otto W

SCUBA DIVE   SNORKEL   SURF
FLORIDA KEYS

Reef Smart team contributors: Ian Popple, Otto Wagner, Peter McDougall, Emil Stezar

Front cover photo Subphoto.com/Shutterstock
Back cover photo Worachat Sodsri/Shutterstock

For permission requests, please contact the publisher at:
Mango Publishing Group
2850 Douglas Road, 2nd Floor
Coral Gables, FL 33134 USA
info@mango.bz

For special orders, quantity sales, course adoptions and corporate sales, please email the publisher at sales@mango.bz. For trade and wholesale sales, please contact Ingram Publisher Services at customer.service@ingramcontent.com or +1.800.509.4887.

Florida Keys: Scuba Dive. Snorkel. Surf.
ISBN: (print) 978-1-68481-171-7, (ebook) 978-1-68481-172-4
Printed in the United States of America

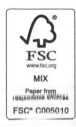

Acknowledgments

Reef Smart is indebted to numerous individuals and organizations who contributed their advice, knowledge and support in the production of this guidebook. We would particularly like to thank the following dive operators for their mapping support, including Captain's Corner, Horizon Divers, Islamorada Dive Center, Lost Reef Adventures, Rainbow Reef and Sail Fish Scuba, along with the many individuals who provided their input and lent us their expertise and support, including Alex Fogg, Rachel Bowman, Bradley Williams, Ernest Yale, Geneviève Déry, Matthew Lawrence and David Parkhurst. Thanks also to Kurt Tidd and Ben Edmonds for providing data on individual wreck sites and for giving us permission to use their images in this book. We also appreciate the support from Hannes Guggenberger and SCUBAJET, whose underwater propulsion vehicles allow us to collect vastly more data than would otherwise be possible in a single dive. In-kind support in the form of lodging was provided by 24 North Hotel Key West, Grassy Flats Resort & Beach Club and Bar Harbor Lodge & Coconut Bay Resort in conjunction with the Florida Keys and Key West Tourism.

Additional in-kind support provided by:

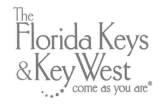

About Reef Smart:

Reef Smart creates detailed guides of the marine environment, particularly coral reefs and shipwrecks for recreational divers and snorkelers. Our products are available as printed guidebooks, waterproof cards, wall art, dive briefing charts, weatherproof beach signage and 3D interactive maps, which can be used on websites and as apps. Reef Smart also provides additional services to resorts that are dedicated to offering an environmentally aware experience for their guests; these include marine biology training for dive professionals and resort staff, implementation of reef monitoring and restoration programs, and the development of sustainable use practices that reduce the impact of operations on the natural environment.

www.reefsmartguides.com

Table of Contents

How to use this book

Objective

The main objective of this guidebook is to provide a resource for people, particularly divers and snorkelers, who are interested in exploring the underwater environment of the Florida Keys. This guide is designed to be used alongside Reef Smart waterproof cards, which can be taken into the water. This book will be most useful for watersports enthusiasts, but it also includes information that any visitor to the area will find useful.

Mapping

We have attempted to catalog as many of the region's dive and snorkel sites as we can, from the northeast to the southwest, starting in Key Largo and extending all the way down to Fort Jefferson in the Dry Tortugas – 70 miles west of Key West. We have presented these sites using Reef Smart's unique 3D-mapping technology. These maps provide useful information such as depths, expected currents and waves, suggested routes, potential hazards and unique attributes.

Disclaimer

Reef Smart guides are for recreational use only – they are not navigational charts and should not be used as such. We have attempted to provide accurate and up-to-date information for each site, as well as activities to enjoy in the surrounding areas. However, businesses close and new ones open, prices are adjusted, and change is inevitable in the marine environment.

DID YOU KNOW? ❓

The Florida Keys hosts the most extensive living coral reef in the United States. It is one of the largest living coral barrier reef systems in the world. As such, there are an almost unlimited number of potential dive and snorkel sites to explore. Our goal is to provide the information necessary to explore the main natural and artificial reef sites, including intentional and unintentional wreck sites – primarily those marked with mooring buoys. The reefs that make up the Florida Keys are under a great deal of pressure from both local and global factors, including diving pressure. Visitors can help alleviate some of these effects by practicing sustainable diving techniques, such as no touching of corals, ensuring proper buoyancy, and using sites with established mooring buoys .

The information contained in this guide i accurate only at the time of publication. The size and location of structures may vary. Depth and distances are approximated in both metric and imperial units, and the suggested rout is optional. Every diver should dive to thei certification and level of experience.

Reef Smart assumes no responsibility fo inaccuracies and omissions and assume no liability for the use of these maps. I you identify information that should be updated, please contact us at: info@reefsmartguides.com

Information boxes

Additional information for the featured sites i provided in the form of special information boxe that appear throughout the book:

DID YOU KNOW?

Interesting facts about the site or the surroundin area.

SAFETY TIP

Advice that aims to improve safety.

ECO TIP

Information that will help limit damage to th ecosystem or improve environmental awarenes

RELAX & RECHARGE

Information on where refreshments can t purchased, or where to unwind on land. N compensation was received in exchange f featuring these establishments.

SCIENTIFIC INSIGHT

Information of a scientific nature that can he you understand what you see and experience.

Map icons

 Scuba dive   Surf

 Snorkel   Kiteboard

 Wreck

 Access by boat   Wind surf

 Access by swim

 Access by car

 Access by walk

Species identification

The species listed for each location were chosen to represent the most unique or common organisms found at each site, as determined from personal observations, discussions with divers and snorkelers who have experienced these sites, and from scientific studies conducted in these areas. Many of the species described in this publication are mobile or cryptic (or both), and so may not always be found where indicated. However, we have attempted to place key species on maps in the locations where they are most commonly found.

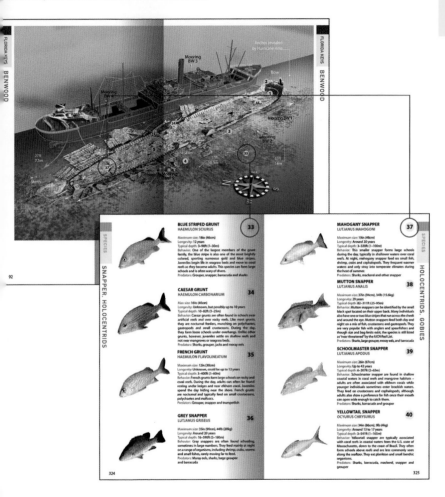

Species description

The species letters and numbers on various maps link to descriptions located at the back of the book on pages 308–341. Reef Smart uses the most frequently cited common name for a species. As common names vary from place to place, we have also provided the scientific name for each species, which remains the same worldwide. Scientific names are usually of Latin or Greek origin and consist of two words: a genus name followed by a species name. By definition, a species is typically a group of organisms that can reproduce together such that it results in fertile offspring; a genus is a group of closely related species.

The descriptions of each species are based on the scientific literature as it existed at the time of publication. Scientific knowledge often advances, however, and the authors welcome any information that helps improve or correct future editions of this guidebook. In-depth species profiles, including images and videos, are available for free on our website.

Visit: **Reefsmartguides.com.**

Our "blue planet"

Ocean

Water covers nearly three-quarters of our planet's surface and approximately 96 percent of this water is contained in the ocean. The ocean drives our planet's weather, regulates its climate and provides us with breathable air, which ultimately supports every living creature on Earth.

The ocean is also vital to our global economy. It produces the food that billions of people depend on for survival, while being a source of resources, including essential medicines that treat a wide range of ailments and diseases. The ocean also drives local and regional economies through tourism. Every year, millions of travelers are drawn to coastal regions around the world to enjoy activities above and below the water's surface. Considering how important the ocean is to our way of life, it is incredible how relatively little we know about what lies beneath its surface.

Coral reefs

The ocean includes a wide range of different ecosystems, but perhaps one of the most frequently visited marine ecosystems are coral reefs. Coral reefs are known as the "rainforests of the sea" for good reason – they are one of the most diverse ecosystems on the planet, supporting about a quarter of all known ocean species. This figure is even more astounding when you consider that coral reefs comprise just a fraction of one percent of the ocean floor. They are also particularly vulnerable to degradation, given they are only found in a narrow window of temperature, salinity and depth.

Humans have studied the biology and physiology of corals for decades, but the underwater environment remains largely foreign to many people. Fact is, we have more accurate maps of the surface of Mars than we do of the seafloor. And guides of the marine environment suitable for recreational users are almost non-existent.

Reef Smart aims to change this situation. Our detailed guides seek to educate snorkelers and divers alike. Our goal is to improve safety and enhance the marine experience by allowing users to discover the unique features and species that can be found at each site.

Preserve and protect

Hopefully our guidebooks, handheld waterproof cards and digital models will help you get to know the underwater environment in general, and reefs in particular. We believe that the more people that can come to appreciate the beauty of the underwater world, the more they will be willing to take steps to protect and preserve it.

The world is connected by a single ocean that is experiencing incredible pressures from all sides. Rising temperatures, increasing acidification and an astonishing volume of plastics that end up both in the water and in marine organisms are negatively impacting this precious system.

There are some big problems to overcome. But a better, more sustainable future is possible. Each and every one of us can make a difference in the choices we make and the actions we take. Together we can help make sure the coral reefs of this world are still around for future generations of snorkelers and divers to enjoy.

Sincerely, the Reef Smart team

ECO TIP

We hope this guide enhances your in-water experience. Share your passion for exploring the marine environment with others, because our ocean, and particularly coral reefs, need all the "likes" they can get. Coral reefs, as well as mangrove and seagrass ecosystems, are under serious pressure from a multitude of threats that include coastal development, pollution, over-fishing and global climate change. Some estimates put over half the world's remaining coral reefs at significant risk of being lost in the next 25 years; raising awareness can help protect them.

About the Florida Keys

Location and formation

The Florida Keys are a chain of islands stretching from the southern tip of Florida's mainland in an arc toward the southwest, where the Dry Tortugas Islands are located, 70 miles west of Key West. The Keys are limestone remnants of a time when sea levels were higher than they are now. The northern half of the island chain was once a series of ancient coral reefs that thrived during the Pleistocene Era, over 125,000 years ago. The islands in the southern half were originally ancient sand bars from the same era. When sea levels fell during the last Ice Age, around 100,000 years ago, both the reefs and sand bars were exposed to the air and underwent fossilization over the millennia that followed.

In total, the chain of islands stretches nearly 220 miles (355 kilometers) and encompasses over 137 square miles (356 square kilometers) of dry land. There are approximately 1,700 islands in the Florida Keys, although many of these are small and most remain uninhabited. In fact, only 43 of the islands are connected to one another via bridges.

The Florida Keys separates the Atlantic Ocean from Florida Bay, which is part of a geological formation called the Florida Plateau that dates back 530 million years. During the last Ice Age, when sea levels were at their lowest point, Florida Bay was a forest-covered plateau that stretched out into the Gulf of Mexico. The Bay flooded around 10,000 years ago and the waters remain shallow and generally turbid, leaving only the lands of the Keys poking above the modern-day sea level. In fact, the maximum elevation in the Keys is just 18 feet (5.5 meters) with many islands having an average elevation of just 4 feet (1.2 meters) above sea level.

The history of the Florida Keys

The Florida Keys were originally inhabited by the Calusa and Tequesta Indians – Native American tribes that played important roles in the early colonization of southwestern and southeastern Florida, respectively. Archaeologists date their presence in the Keys to around 800 CE. The Calusa were the dominant tribe in the Keys, fishing for their food instead of farming like the Tequesta. Their life on the coast enabled them to develop strong sailing and navigational skills. They fished the length of the southwest coast of Florida and down into the islands of the Keys in their Cypress dugout canoes. Some archaeologists believe they even ventured as far south as Cuba, although evidence of this feat is not definitive.

Official accounts hold that the first European to arrive in Florida was the Spanish explorer Ponce de León, who charted the Keys in 1513. However, an alternative historical view holds that the Italian explorer, Amerigo Vespucci and the Englishman John Cabot discovered the Keys before the Spaniard, as they sailed down the coast of North America in 1497, claiming the lands for King Henry VII of England.

Regardless of which European first set eyes on the islands, the Spanish gave them their first European name, "Los Martires" or the Martyrs. Accounts from early Spanish explorers describe

---

DID YOU KNOW?

Wrecking, or marine salvage was a very important economic driver for otherwise marginal coastal communities prior to the mid-1850s. Examples of wrecking (or wracking) economies exist all around the world, basically wherever trade routes passed near difficult-to-navigate hazards. Wrecking played a particularly important role in the early history of the Florida Keys. The Calusa undertook the practice as early as the 16th century, salvaging the many Spanish galleons that foundered as they passed along the coastline of the Keys. Spain had so many ships running aground that it began to station dedicated salvage vessels around the Caribbean manned by free divers

from Africa specialized in diving for pearls.

The laws of marine salvage varied from place to place and were often murky. Wrecking in the Keys was often undertaken from nearby Bahamas, who had laws specifying that salvaged goods needed to be landed in Nassau for auction. A portion of the proceeds went to the government, while a large share (anywhere from 30 to 60 percent by some accounts) went to the wreckers. Given the value of the cargo on some of these Spanish treasure ships, the industry was a boon for the small nation. However, it was dangerous work, and wreckers were often responsible for saving the lives of shipwrecked passengers and crew even as they risked their own.

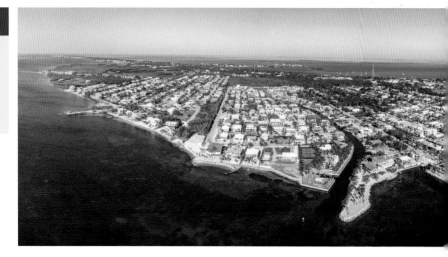

how the Calusa would paddle their canoes out to attack Spanish galleons that anchored too close to the shore of Los Martires. In fact, the Spanish provide the fullest exploration and accounting of what we now call the Keys, and many of the island's names and features still bear the mark of the Spanish language. The Calusa Indians also engaged in salvaging the many ships that fell prey to the treacherous reefs along the coastline here.

Shipwrecks along the Keys were common as the reefs are located miles from shore along the valuable trade route between the Caribbean and Europe. Storms also played an important role in the region, pushing entire fleets of ships up against the reef, as happened with the Spanish Plate Fleet in 1733 (see page 12 for more information). Thankfully the Spaniards kept meticulous navigational records, and those, along with the detailed charts from the salvage operations for the wrecked 1733 Fleet, provide the first clear picture of the Keys by the middle of the 18th century.

The Spanish never did much with their claim or the Keys, focused as they were on nearby Cuba The English assumed control of Florida in 176 following the Treaty of Paris, signed at the en of the Seven Years War in Europe. The Spanis took back control after the American Revolutio in 1783. Whether the islands of the Keys wer included in these transfers remained a point o ambiguity until representatives of the Unite States sailed down to Key West and planted th U.S. flag there in 1822.

Early settlers to the region included Bahamaniar who mostly settled in Key West with its natur deep-water port. They were drawn to the regic once the United States passed laws requirin that any salvage from American waters had to b landed at an American port. Salvaging was lucrativ business and Key West rapidly became a financi heavyweight. Many temporary camps cropped u and disappeared in the region, but permaner non-indigenous settlement of the Keys started

DID YOU KNOW?

The spirit of the Florida Keys has long been one of independence. Key West got its start as an anchorage and source of fresh water for mariners – pirates and privateers according to some. This spirit was taken to an extreme in 1982, when the mayor of Key West announced that Key West and the rest of the Keys were seceding from the United States due to a border patrol blockade and checkpoint at the junction between Key Largo and mainland Florida. Thus, the short-lived Conch Republic was born. At the time,

the Florida Keys was considered an entry point for drug smugglers and illegal aliens, and most locals would admit that there was a fair amount of lawlessness in the region in the 70s and 80s. The secession was short-lived, however, as the mayor surrendered to the U.S. Navy admiral stationed in Key West just one minute after declaring independence. The blockade came down soon after, and the Keys resumed their place within the Union However, the name Conch Republic can still be seen floating around Key West today, on the lips of locals and on the various shirts, towels and mugs sold in souvenir shops.

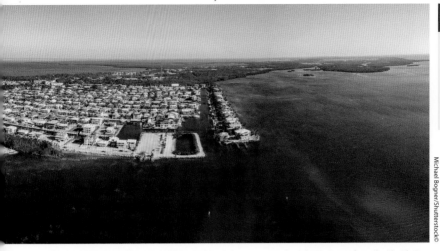

Key Largo is a narrow stretch of developed land that separates the Atlantic Ocean from the Florida Bay.

arnest after 1822. Even so the region remained argely isolated from the rest of the continental United States until the Overseas Railroad finally onnected Key West to the Florida mainland 1912. Built by Henry Flagler, the massive nfrastructure project included an engineering narvel dubbed the 8th Wonder of the World: the even Mile Bridge that spanned the open ocean etween the Middle and Lower Keys. While the ailroad itself was a financial boondoggle for Flagler, succeeded in transitioning transportation in the eys from marine to terrestrial and opened the egion up for development.

ecent history

erhaps not surprisingly, the development of the eys centered around the ocean, namely fishing nd tourism. The construction of lighthouses

along the coast greatly reduced the number of shipwrecks and all but ended the lucrative salvage trade, just as the Great Depression and a massive Category 5 hurricane dealt financial and physical blows to the economically sensitive region. The railroad was damaged in the 1935 storm, dubbed the Labor Day hurricane and the railroad spans were turned into a two-lane bridge for cars by 1938.

The birth of the Overseas Highway opened the region to car traffic and the population of the Keys grew following World War II and the Cuban Revolution. The Keys long held many cultural connections to the island nation that sits just 90 miles (145 kilometers) to its south – Key West is actually closer to Cuba than to Miami.

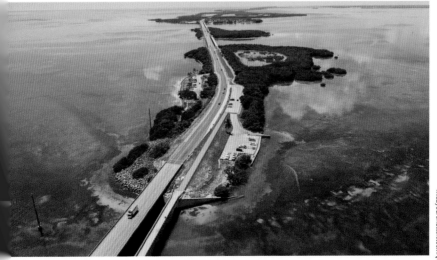

:le Duck Key sits at the southern end of Marathon and represents the border between the Lower and the Middle Keys.

The Spanish Fleet of 1733

Spain spent centuries transporting enormous riches from its American colonies back to Europe. The volume of goods flowing from the New World to the Old was such that the Spanish Crown established a convoy system where fleets of merchant vessels, guarded by armed galleons, would make their way from Havana, Cuba, along the coast of Florida and across the Atlantic to Europe. These convoys were first organized as far back as 1537, and were responsible for transporting gold and silver, porcelain from China, pearls, indigo and cochineal dyes, tobacco, vanilla and even chocolate. Separate fleets would gather the goods throughout the Caribbean before meeting in Havana ahead of the trans-Atlantic crossing. The system was relatively successful and lasted well over two centuries, until around 1800.

These convoys had to deal with the threat of piracy as well as the significant danger posed by navigation through the shallow reefs and shifting sand bars of the Keys. But perhaps the biggest threat was from the unpredictable weather. Hurricanes were virtually impossible to forecast – often a convoy's only warning came from observing cloud formations and abrupt changes in wind velocity and direction. Unless safe anchorage was available nearby, there was little a

ship could do except attempt to head into open water and outrun the storm. The worst place fo a ship to end up in a hurricane was to be caugh near shallow reefs with little room to maneuver This was the case for the Spanish Fleet of 1733.

On Friday July 13, 1733, the New Spain Flee consisting of four armed navios, 16 merchan vessels and two smaller ships departed Havana for Spain. The following day, shortly after sighting the Florida Keys, the wind direction suddenly shifted and increased markedly in strength – a clear indication that a hurricane was building The order to turn the convoy around and retur to Cuba was given, but it came too late. By the following day, the convoy was scattered across the reefs of the Florida Keys. Of the 22 vessels in the convoy, only four made it safely back to Cuba and one managed to run ahead of the storm to the north and returned to Spain safely.

By this time, Spain had developed an extensiv salvage operation throughout the Caribbean, an after the surviving crews were rescued, the ship that could not be refloated had their position carefully plotted on charts and were the burned to the waterline to hide their positio from looters and make future salvage easier. Th salvage operation took years and was remarkab effective. In fact, the final tally of salvaged goo

-	Populo	25° 21.850'N, 80° 09.690'W		H	El Terri (San Felipe)	24° 50.761'N, 80° 42.850'W
A	Infante	24° 56.556'N, 80° 28.531'W		I	San Francisco	24° 49.185'N, 80° 45.425'W
B	San José	24° 56.919'N, 80° 29.334'W		J	Almiranta	24° 48.633'N, 80° 45.932'W
C	Capitana (El Rubí)	24° 55.491'N, 80° 30.891'W		K	Nuestra Señora	
D	Chaves	24° 56.179'N, 80° 34.985'W			de las Angustias	24° 47.455'N, 80° 51.738'W
E	Tres Puentes	24° 53.612'N, 80° 35.012'W		L	Sueco de Arizón	24° 46.625'N, 80° 53.372'W ar
F	Herrera	24° 54.326'N, 80° 35.538'W				24° 46.728'N, 80° 53.480'W
G	San Pedro	24° 51.802'N, 80° 40.780'W				

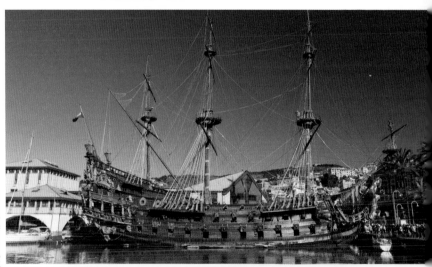

A replica Spanish Galleon, like those in the ill-fated 1733 Fleet, floats in the Port of Genoa, Italy.

from the fleet exceeded what was listed on the original cargo manifest for the convoy, which indicates the presence of smuggled cargo among the officially listed goods.

Today, the remains of the Spanish Fleet of 1733 offer a window into maritime history. Two of the wrecks, the *San Pedro* and the *Sueco de Arizón*, are described in greater detail among the dive and snorkel sites in this book (see pages 174 and 182). For more information on other wrecks of the 1733 Fleet, visit: **Info.flheritage.com/galleon-trail/**

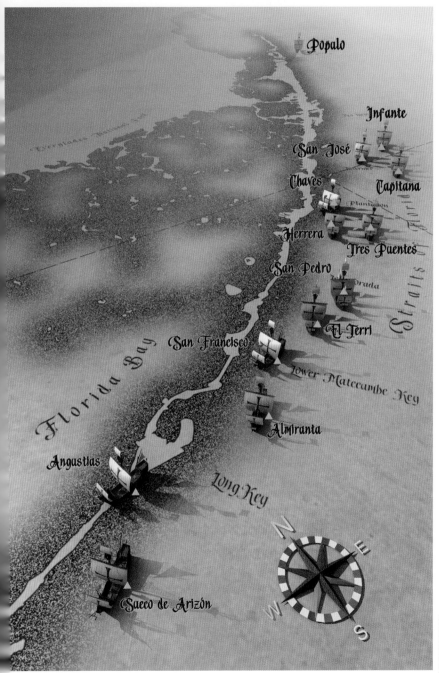

Popalo

Infante

San José

Chaves

Capitana

Herrera

Tres Puentes

San Pedro

El Terri

San Francisco

Florida Bay

Lower Matecumbe Key

Straits

Almiranta

Angustias

Long Key

Sueco de Arizón

Florida Keys today

Population

Today, the Florida Keys has a population of over 82,000 people. The Keys represents the bulk of the population of Monroe County, which extends from Key West to Key Largo and includes a large part of the Everglades National Park in the southwest corner of the Florida mainland. Key West, the county seat, is the largest population center in the Keys, accounting for nearly a quarter of all residents. Key Largo is the next largest population center after Key West.

The basics

English is the official language in the Florida Keys, as it is in the continental United States. The official currency is the U.S. dollar and there are plenty of bank branches and ATMs as well as foreign exchange counters in all the major towns.

The electricity in the Keys is the North American standard 110 volts / 60 hertz with flat-bladed plugs and a rounded grounding pin. WiFi is available at most hotels and in many coffee shops, eateries and other local businesses – sometimes free, sometimes paid. Tap water is safe to drink in Florida. The Florida Keys operates in the Eastern Standard Time (EST) zone and observes Daylight Savings Time (EDT) from March to November.

Visitors

There are over 5 million visitors to the Florida Keys each year, far surpassing the region's resident population. Nearly three-quarters of these are domestic visitors, while the rest are international. Visitors come for the warm climate, the beaches, the sport fishing opportunities and for the scuba diving and snorkeling.

Getting there and getting around

Getting there

There are no direct international flights to the Florida Keys, but the region's airports do connect to major American hubs. Many international travelers fly into nearby Miami (MIA) and then drive to the Keys from there. Airports in Key West (EYW) and Marathon (MTH) both serve the region, although Key West is the larger of the two and is serviced by more commercial carriers.

Getting around

Driving is the most common way of getting

around the Florida Keys. The Overseas Highway (U.S. Route 1) runs the entire length of the Keys and is either one lane or two lanes depending on the size of the island and the local population that it passes through. Most major car rental companies operate in the region, typically with rental counters in Key Largo, Marathon and Key West. Given there is only one road that provides access to the entire region, traffic can be a challenge during the morning and afternoon rush hours and when an accident has occurred.

Monroe County operates a shuttle bus that serves the Lower Keys from Key West to Marathon. Miami-Dade County operates another shuttle bus that goes from Florida City (the last population center on the mainland) to Marathon. For information on these two bus lines, visit **Monroecounty-fl. gov/1261/Bus-Routes.**

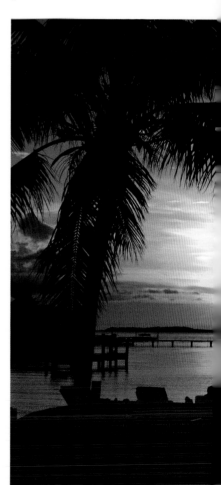

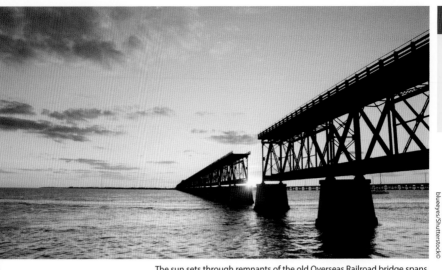

The sun sets through remnants of the old Overseas Railroad bridge spans.

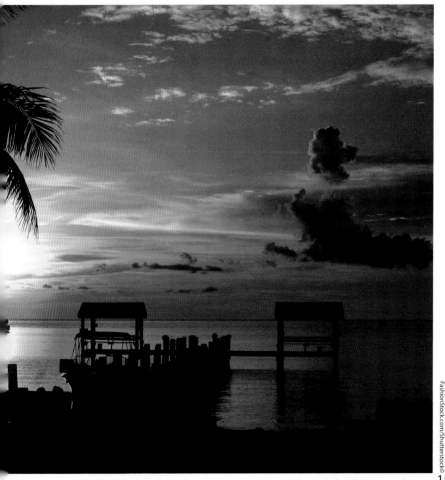

Most islands in the Keys boast spectacular sunrises and sunsets given how narrow they are.

Environment

Weather

The Florida Keys have a mild, tropical-maritime climate thanks to their subtropical location and proximity to the warm waters of the Gulf Stream. The winter season stretches from December to March with lows of 65°F to 69°F (18°C to 21°C), and highs of 75°F to 79°F (24°C to 26°C). The weather is pleasant the rest of the year, with highs of 80°F (27°C) and above. The winter season is characterized by high winds and large waves, which can make diving the outer reef line challenging if not impossible at times. The summer season is generally calmer except when large weather systems pass through. Wetsuits are often recommended in the winter, but they are generally not necessary during the rest of the year.

The Keys are prone to hurricanes, given their position extending out along the boundary between the Caribbean and the Gulf of Mexico. The official hurricane season stretches from June to November, with a peak in activity typically occurring between August and November. Hurricanes have caused a lot of damage to the low-lying islands of the Keys over the years, with high winds and flooding caused by storm surge.

Currents, tides and visibility

The Gulf Stream is the main driver of ocean currents along the coastline of the Keys. Currents typically move from the southwest to the northeast along the coastline, but when the Gulf Stream shifts away from the reef line, the current can double back and run in the opposite direction or even disappear. Currents in Hawk Channel, which runs the length of the Keys between the shoreline and the outer reef, are rarely strong, except when the tide is flowing out of Florida Bay through one of the many channels that separate the large clusters of Keys islands. The tidal cycle is not large in the region, varying less than 2 feet (0.6 meters) from high to low tide.

Visibility is related to the tide and weather. It is generally good along the outer reef tract where the Gulf Stream cycles water through the region. On good days it can reach 120 feet (36.5 meters) or more. But storm events can stir up the sediment in Hawk Channel and the sheltered spurs and grooves of the large reef tracts, reducing visibility in the process to 30 feet (9 meters) or less.

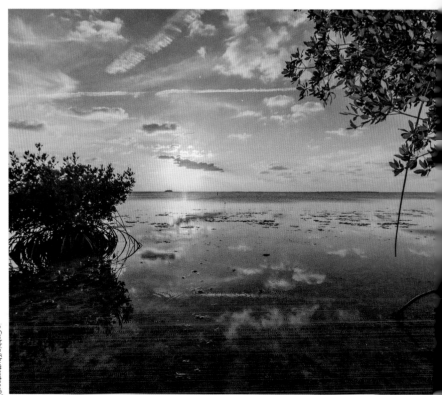

Mangroves line the edges of many islands in the Keys, creating important habitat for wildlife

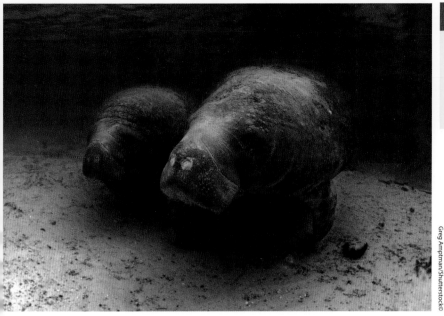

Manatees are often seen grazing on the seagrass beds that are common throughout the Keys.

Ecosystems

Coral reefs

Southeast Florida boasts the largest barrier reef system in the United States, and the third largest in the world behind the Great Barrier Reef in Australia and the Mesoamerican Reef along the coast of Mexico, Belize, Guatemala and Honduras. The coral reefs of the Keys boast a variety of hard and soft corals and sponges, including staghorn and elkhorn corals, brain corals and star corals, among others. In turn, the reefs support a variety of marine life including sharks, turtles, eels, snapper, grouper, jacks and all manner of fishes large and small. Unfortunately, disease, coastal development, eutrophication through runoff, invasive species, overfishing and climate change have all negatively impacted the coral reefs in the region, leading to a steady decline in coral health and density. Diving and snorkeling place additional pressures on the reef, which is why it is so important to adopt best practices, as well as taking care not to damage the reef when anchoring boats.

Seagrass beds

The Florida Keys are home to extensive seagrass beds that play an important role in the region's complex marine ecosystem. Seagrass beds of turtle grass, shoal grass and manatee grass support many species, including manatees, sea turtles and crustaceans, among others.

Many commercially important fish species rely on these ecosystems at some point in their development, including snapper and grouper. Seagrass beds help improve visibility by stabilizing the seabed and they are important contributors in the conversion of carbon dioxide to oxygen – they are often called the lungs of the sea. Pollution and eutrophication from runoff are negatively affecting seagrass beds throughout Florida and the Keys, which in turns has led to dramatic declines in manatee populations. Careless boating also leads to physical damage in seagrass beds, which further contributes to declines in this important ecosystem.

Mangroves

The Florida Keys also boasts extensive mangrove habitats. Large stands of primarily red, black and white mangroves line the waterways and highways up and down the Keys. These trees are incredibly important not just to the species that rely on the habitat for shelter and food, but also for the physical protection mangroves provide to coastlines. They build islands by trapping sand and sediments in their extensive root systems, and they buffer the shoreline from the high energy waves generated during storms, including hurricanes. Coastal development poses a risk to mangroves, which are cut down in favor of sandy beaches and unobstructed views.

17

National and state management

All the waters around the Florida Keys are protected by a national body, whether that is Everglades National Park, Florida Keys National Marine Sanctuary, Biscayne Bay National Park or Dry Tortugas National Park. In addition, there are state parks and wildlife parks in place that create a mosaic of different restrictions that help protect these marine ecosystems.

Biscayne National Park

Biscayne Bay and the reefs above North Key Largo fall under the jurisdiction of the Biscayne National Park. The park is 95 percent water, and there is no entrance fee required. Multiple historic wrecks can be found in the waters of the park, and fishing is allowed, although subject to regulations and a Florida fishing license. For more information, visit: **Nps.gov/bisc**

Florida Keys
National Marine Sanctuary

This marine sanctuary was established in 1990 and protects over 2,900 square nautical miles (9,946 square kilometers) of marine habitat. The Sanctuary boundary stretches from the waters north of Key Largo to the waters of the Florida Bay and Atlantic, stretching from Key Largo across to surround the Dry Tortugas National Park in the west. The Sanctuary designation came about as an effort to help protect the incredible coral reefs found along the Florida Keys.

The rules and regulations in place aim to balance the needs of the many stakeholders who enjoy these waters with the goal of protecting these natural resources for future generations. Across all waters of the Florida Keys National Marine Sanctuary, visitors must not touch, damage or remove coral (either living or dead) or damage, move or remove historical artifacts or resources. Specific zones within the Sanctuary provide additional protections. Currently there are five types of zones: ecological reserves (ERs), sanctuary preservation areas (SPAs), wildlife management areas (WMAs), existing management areas (EMAs) and special-use areas of which there are currently just Research-Only sites.

In general, ERs and SPAs prohibit fishing of all types (except catch-and-release trolling in just a small subset of sites). Research-Only sites represent areas that restrict access to everyone except for specifically permitted research and monitoring activities. WMAs are in place to help

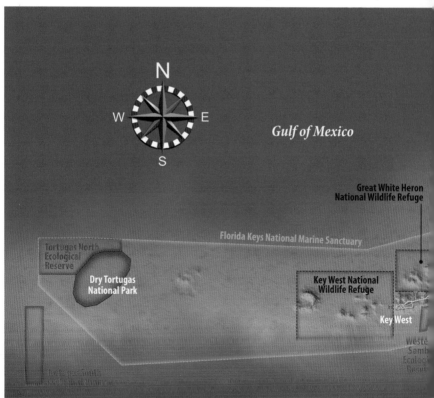

protect sensitive habitat, including bird nesting areas, and they often include buffer zones, closed zones and idle speed zones. There are a total of 27 WMAs in the Florida Keys, but most of them are located Bayside of the islands. Last of all are the six EMAs, which were in place before the Florida Keys National Marine Sanctuary zoning rules were established in 1997.

State regulations also apply, including the law that prohibits the damage or removal of archaeological resources on state submerged lands. It is a criminal offense to do so.

Rules and regulations can change as agencies shift their goals or as new information about the conditions and health of the ecosystem comes to light. Divers and snorkelers should check the current rules and restrictions for any site they plan to visit on their own while in the Keys – most operators keep current with regulations that relate to their regular trips. Moreover, the Florida Keys National Marine Sanctuary is in the process of revamping its regulatory and zoning structure, although no official timeline was available at the time of publication. In the meantime, you can visit the Florida Keys National Marine Sanctuary website to get the most up-to-date information on regulations: **Floridakeys.noaa.gov/regs/**

Dry Tortugas National Park

Officially established as a National Park in October 1992, the area gained National Monument status in 1935. A total of seven islands are protected inside the boundaries of the National Park, including Garden Key, which is the location of Fort Jefferson, and Loggerhead Key, which is the site of a lighthouse and popular shipwreck, the Windjammer. Fort Jefferson is one of the most popular snorkel sites in the Keys (see page 304 to learn about the snorkeling there). For more information about the park, visit:
Nps.gov/drto

John Pennekamp Coral Reef State Park

Established in 1963, this was the first undersea park in the United States. Its boundaries extend three miles from shore, helping to protect Turtle Rocks (page 42) in the northeast, down to Three Sisters (page 105) in the southwest. The park also features two shore-accessible snorkel sites (page 80). Spearfishing is prohibited inside the park boundaries, but hook-and-line fishing is allowed in accordance with Florida Law. For more information on the park,
visit: **Pennekamppark.com**

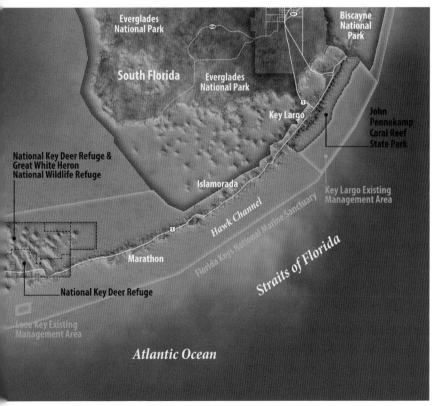

Everglades National Park

Biscayne National Park

South Florida

Everglades National Park

Key Largo

John Pennekamp Coral Reef State Park

National Key Deer Refuge & Great White Heron National Wildlife Refuge

Islamorada

Key Largo Existing Management Area

Hawk Channel

Florida Keys National Marine Sanctuary

Marathon

Straits of Florida

National Key Deer Refuge

Looe Key Existing Management Area

Atlantic Ocean

Conservation and education organizations

There are a host of not-for-profit educational organizations operating in the Keys region. These organizations play an important role in protecting the reefs and the marine life that rely on them, as well as educating the public about these incredible natural treasures. Below is information about just a few of the many organizations active in the region:

Reef Environmental Education Foundation (REEF)

Located in Key Largo but operating internationally, REEF actively engages and inspires the public through education, citizen science and partnerships with the scientific community. Part of their mission includes conducting volunteer fish surveys around the world. The data from these surveys is collected by recreational divers and snorkelers and is compiled into a master database that is accessible to the public. (Some of the species identified on the dive and snorkel sites covered in this book were cross-referenced with the REEF database.) Their other work touches on grouper, invasive species, and more general education and outreach efforts, as well as a nature center with self-guided interpretive exhibits that is open to the public at their Key Largo headquarters (98300 Overseas Highway). For more information on this non-profit organization, visit: **REEF.org**

Coral Restoration Foundation™

CRF™ was founded in 2007 and has been working to restore the coral reef system in the Florida Keys ever since. The reefs of the Florida Keys have lost around 98 percent of their original staghorn and elkhorn coral (*Acropora cervicornis* and *A. palmata*) cover dating back to the 1970s. The organization has developed a process to "farm" coral fragments of elkhorn and staghorn coral, growing them from lines anchored in the shallow, protected waters of the Keys until they reach a certain size, and then transplanting them on the reef just six to nine months later. As of the end of 2021, they had successfully restored more than 270,000 square feet (25,000 square meters) of the reef, including sites that are covered in greater detail in the pages of this guidebook. For more on this Key Largo-based organization, visit: **Coralrestoration.org**

MarineLab

The Marine Resources Development Foundation is based in Key Largo right on the Emerald Lagoon. The MarineLab Undersea Laboratory, which operated in the lagoon from

---

DID YOU KNOW?

Many of the dive and snorkel sites detailed in the pages of this guidebook are included in one of the different zones that regulate the types of activities that take place in the Florida Keys National Marine Sanctuary.

Ecological Reserves (ERs):
Western Sambo (page 250)
Tortugas (North and South) (page 304)

Sanctuary Preservation Areas (SPAs):
Carysfort Reef SPA (page 44)
Elbow Reef SPA (page 52)
Key Largo Dry Rocks SPA (page 68)
Grecian Rocks SPA (page 76)
French Reef SPA (page 98)
Molasses Reef SPA (page 108)
Conch Reef SPA (page 136)
Davis Reef SPA (page 140)
Hen and Chickens SPA (page 146)
Cheeca Rocks SPA (page 160)
Alligator Reef SPA (page 162)
Coffins Patch SPA (page 192)
Sombrero Key SPA (page 214)
Newfound Harbor Key SPA (page 230)

Looe Key SPA (page 232)
Eastern Dry Rocks SPA (page 282)
Rock Key SPA (page 286)
Sand Key SPA (page 288)

Research-Only Sites:
Conch Reef (SE deep section) (page 136)
Tennessee Reef (page 181)
Looe Key (NE patch reefs) (page 232)
Eastern Sambo (page 248)

Wildlife Management Areas (WMAs):
Pelican Shoal (page 246)
Cottrell Key (page 294)
Marquesas Keys (page 302)

Existing Management Areas (EMAs)
Key Largo (pages 40 through 134)
Looe Key Reef (page 232)
Key West National Wildlife Refuge (pages 292, 294, 301 and 302)

Not all of the different sanctuary zones are listed here. For a complete and up-to-date list of all marine zones visit:
Floridakeys.noaa.gov/zones/allzones.html

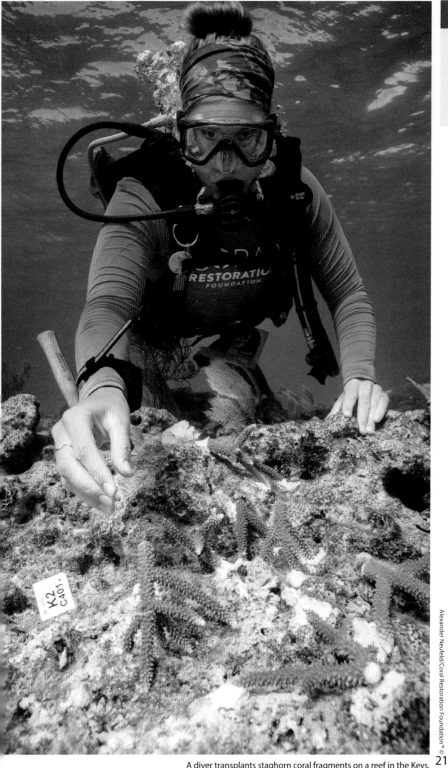

A diver transplants staghorn coral fragments on a reef in the Keys.

SCIENTIFIC INSIGHT

A big challenge facing coral reefs is a lack of awareness among the public (and policymakers) about how sensitive corals are and how much danger they face. Reefs suffer greatly from being out-of-sight, out-of-mind to most people who do not venture beneath the surface of the water. Passionate educators are looking to change that one STEM student at a time by developing STEM-based K through 12 learning initiatives, both in terms of extra-curricular activities and in supplementing in-class curricula. If your student is interested in learning more about the ocean in general, and coral reefs in particular, you can encourage that passion by getting in touch with some of the great education non-profits operating in the area, including **DiveN2Life** (Diven2life.org), **MarineLab** (Mrdf.org/marinelab-education), **Reef Relief** (Reefrelief.org) and many more.

1985 through 2018, is now sitting high and dry on shore as a museum. Visitors can experience what it was like to be one of the hundreds of aquanauts who stayed underwater overnight in the facility. Next to the lagoon is a small campus of dorm rooms, labs and classrooms for individuals and groups looking for everything from a single day to a full week of marine education experience. For more information visit: **Mrdf.org/marinelab-education**

History of Diving Museum

This small museum based in Islamorada is open daily from 10am to 5pm (82990 Overseas Highway near Mile Marker 83). Its mission is to preserve and interpret the history of diving, with a special focus on the contributions of divers and the dive industry in southern Florida and the Florida Keys. They offer exhibits that include a timeline of diving, deep sea diving and a treasure room featuring tools and genuine treasure recovered from wrecks located in the Florida Keys. To learn more visit: **Divingmuseum.org**

I.Care

This Islamorada-based organization is a community-based, grassroots effort that aims to restore the reefs of Islamorada, including Alligator Reef (page 162). The group engages in coral restoration, reef clean-ups and reef monitoring. To learn more, visit: **Icareaboutcoral.org**

Dolphin Research Center

The Dolphin Research Center is located on Grassy Key in Marathon (58901 Overseas Highway, Grassy Key). Its mission combines education, research and the rescue and rehabilitation of marine mammals. They participate in the U.S. Marine Mammal Stranding Network and are currently the only facility in the Keys licensed by the government to assist manatees in distress. The center also offers programs for visitors to interact with the dolphins along with an extensive educational program. For more information, visit: **Dolphins.org**

Turtle Hospital

Located in Marathon, the Turtle Hospital first opened its doors in 1986 with the goals of rehabilitating injured sea turtles, educating the public, assisting in turtle research, and supporting environmental legislation to make beaches and the ocean safer for sea turtles. The hospital is open to the public seven days a week, but this small non-profit (2396 Overseas Highway, Marathon) cannot host many visitors at the same time, so they strongly recommend calling ahead to make reservations if you wish to visit (Tel: 305-743-2552). For more information on this organization and to learn how you can help, visit: **Turtlehospital.org**

Pigeon Key Foundation and Marine Science Center

The Marine Science Center at Pigeon Key is dedicated to protecting the cultural history of the Florida Keys through marine science education. Located on Pigeon Key just south of Marathon, the island provides field trips and hands-on learning to visitors and school groups. For more information, visit: **Pigeonkey.net**

Reef Relief

This Key West-based non-profit focuses on educating the public and advocating for conservation with policymakers. Their work seeks to increase public awareness and increase scientific understanding of coral reef ecology. In addition to managing the Key West Marine Park on the southern edge

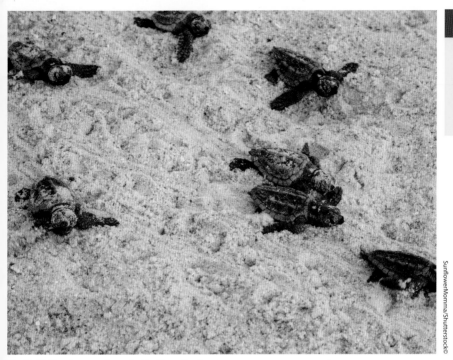

SunflowerMomma/Shutterstock©

The Florida Keys has many important turtle nesting beaches.

of downtown Key West (see page 278) they also have an environmental center located in the historic old town of Key West (631 Greene Street, Key West). Admission is free and visitors can watch daily movies on marine resource issues as well as learn about coral reefs and the challenges they face. For more information, visit: **Reefrelief.org**

Florida Keys Eco-Discovery Center

This interactive visitor center is based in Key West, just outside of Fort Zachary Taylor State Park (35 Quay Road, Key West). Operated by the Florida Keys National Marine Sanctuary, the exhibits include information about the maritime history, marine fauna and flora found

ECO TIP

If you discover a marine mammal or marine reptile in distress, call the Florida Fish and Wildlife Conservation Commission (FWC) at 1-888-404-FWCC (3922). The information you provide can help the FWC dispatch qualified personnel to assist as necessary.

in the Keys. Admission is free and the center is generally open from 9am to 4pm, Tuesday through Saturday. For more information, visit: **Floridakeys.noaa.gov/ecodiscovery/visit. html**

RELAX & RECHARGE

Habanos Oceanfront restaurant (73510 Overseas Highway, Islamorada) is located adjacent to Anne's Beach and is the place to go for genuine Cuban food. There is a range of options on the menu – they even have a Cuban-style pizza – but you cannot go wrong with their Cuban

sandwich, which will satisfy the healthiest of appetites. If you want to add a little more to your dish, however, consider a side of plantain and yuka fries and perhaps the conch fritters as an appetizer. The view is decent, the drinks are ice cold, and the prices are among the most reasonable you can find anywhere in the Florida Keys. Visit: **Habanosoceanfront.com.**

In case of emergency

There are many organisms that can put a damper on a visit to the Florida Keys, from jellyfish to stingrays to the invasive lionfish that have made the Keys their home. Many of these potentially dangerous marine creatures are listed in a special section toward the back of the book (see pages 314–317). We have included information in that section on the injuries these species can cause and some of the common treatments that might help. That said, this book is not intended as a substitute for professional medical help.

For visitors unlucky enough to become injured while enjoying their time at the southernmost point of the continental United States, there are many high-quality medical facilities they can visit to receive care. If an injury is not an emergency, consider visiting the nearest walk-in clinic or urgent care clinic during normal operating hours – most open at 8am – and there are a few larger hospitals with 24-hour emergency room access. The list provided in this guidebook does not constitute an endorsement, it is merely a reference should the need for medical attention arise while in the area. Visitors would do well to familiarize themselves with the nearest emergency resources to where they are staying.

Should the unthinkable happen, here are some important numbers and places for visitors to keep in mind if they need to seek help:

Emergency contacts

Police:	911
Fire:	911
Ambulance:	911
U.S. Coast Guard:	VHF 16

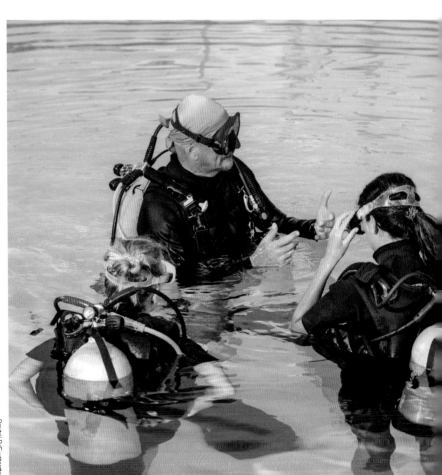

Dmitri D/Shutterstock©

Emergency and Urgent Care

Advanced Urgent Care
100460 Overseas Highway,
Key Largo
Tel: 305-294-0011
Urgentcarefloridakeys.com

Baptist Health
Mariners Hospital
(24hr ER)
91500 Overseas Highway,
Tavernier
Tel: 305-434-3000
Baptisthealth.net/services

Islamorada
Medical Center
90130 Old Highway, Tavernier
Tel: 305-852-9300
Islamoradamedicalcenter.com

Baptist Health Fishermen's
Community Hospital
(24hr ER)
3301 Overseas Highway, Marathon
Tel: 305-434-1000
Baptisthealth.net/locations/hospitals/
fishermens-community-hospital

Big Pine Medical & Minor Emergency
(24hr ER)
30 Cunningham Lane, Big Pine Key
Tel: 305-872-3321
Bigpinemedical.com

Advanced Urgent Care
1980 N Roosevelt Boulevard, Key West
Tel: 305-294-0011
Urgentcarefloridakeys.com

Key West Urgent Care
& Family Doctor
1501 Government Road, Key West
Tel: 305-295-7550
Keywesturgentcare.com

Lower Keys Medical Center
(24hr ER)
5900 College Road, Key West
Tel: 305-294-5531
Lkmc.com

Decompression / Hyperbaric Chambers

The only publicly-accessible hyperbaric chamber in the Keys available to treat divers is in Tavernier in the Upper Keys. The next closest chamber is in Miami.

Baptist Health Mariners Hospital
(Chamber available 24/7;
staff on call during off hours)
91500 Overseas Highway, Tavernier
ER Tel: 305-434-3600
Chamber Tel: 305-434-3603
Divers in distress should first present
themselves to the ER
Baptisthealth.net/services

Chambers are occasionally unavailable or offline for maintenance or repair. If you think you might be experiencing DCS, contact Divers Alert Network's emergency 24-hour number (919-684-9111) to identify the nearest available operational chamber to make sure you receive help as quickly as possible.

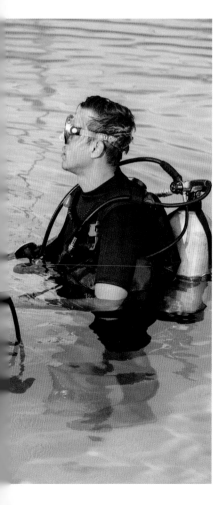

Divers discuss rescue training in the water.

Other activities

The Florida Keys offers visitors the chance to experience numerous beaches, many of them accessible to the public. We have provided additional details about the beaches offering diving and snorkeling opportunities later in this guidebook. Below is a list of beaches (from north to south) that may be worth visiting for other activities, such as kiteboarding, kayaking, swimming, hiking or simply to relax and unwind by the water.

Kiteboarding

The Florida Keys do not offer much in the way of surfing opportunities because most of the waves break along the outer reef line, many miles from shore. However, the steady easterly winds and miles of shallow calm water make the Keys perfect for kiteboarding, especially for beginners and those wanting to practice their skills before hitting more gnarly shores. The most consistent wind conditions are usually during the winter and through the spring. There are many kiteboarding launch spots in the Florida Keys, some are public, some are private, and some even lack an address and are known only by the closest mile marker (MM), which is mileage that counts up from MM 0 in Key West). It is always advisable to connect with a local kiteboarding shop beforehand for a little local knowledge and support.

Kayaking

There are some fantastic spots to kayak in the Florida Keys. The State Parks are usually the best places to visit and have established water trails that sometimes allows visitors to pass through the mangroves. John Pennekamp Coral Reef State Park and the Indian Key State Park are perhaps two of the most popular locations. Beyond these two examples, however, there are many unofficial places where kayaks can be launched from the side of the road to better explore the coastline of the Florida Keys. Just be aware that the current can be strong through these channels.

John Pennekamp Coral Reef State Park

102801 Overseas Highway, Key Largo (MM 102.5)
A popular State Park that covers 70 nautical square miles (240 square kilometers). Visitors often come here for the snorkeling (see page 80) and glass-bottom boat tours, but kayaking, fishing, hiking

and biking are also popular here. There is an entry fee and camping spots are also available.

Harry Harris Beach and Park

50 E Beach Road, Tavernier (MM 92.5)
This artificial beach in Tavernier offers fishing and swimming, has a children's playground, picnic areas, a softball field and basketball courts. An access fee is charged for non-county residents over the age of 16.

Founders Park Beach

87000 Overseas Highway, Islamorada (MM 86.5)
Founders Park Beach has something for everyone. There is a fee for access, but there are activities galore, including a marina, a skate park, an Olympic-sized swimming pool, picnic and BBQ areas, a playground for kids, various sports facilities and, of course, a beautiful sandy beach. The kiteboarding here is a little more challenging than at other locations and is therefore less suited to beginners.

Whale Harbor

83413 Overseas Highway, Islamorada (MM 83.5)
A private kiteboarding launch that charges a small fee for access. Many riders will find the cost well worth it for the onsite support offered by Seven Sports. There is plenty of parking as well as restrooms, showers and nearby food options.

Library Beach Park

84 Johnston Road, Islamorada (MM 81.5)
This is not your typical beach – this hidden gem is nestled in the mangroves and the water is actually a channel with a slight current. There is a mix of sand and grass to relax on, as well as a playground for kids, a covered BBQ area and restrooms.

Indian Key State Park

Islamorada near MM 77.5
This historic state park is a small island located about 0.6 miles (1 kilometer) south of the Overseas Highway just off the northern tip of

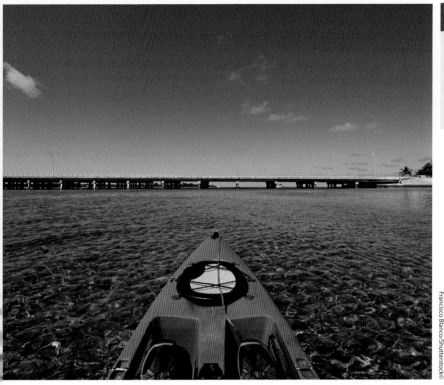

Francisco Blanco/Shutterstock©

Kayaking is popular in the shallow waters that surround many of the islands in the Keys.

Lower Matecumbe Key in Islamorada. The site charges an entry fee and is only accessible by boat or kayak. There are a couple of kayak rental locations on the shore close by and it is also a popular snorkeling spot (see page 172).

Anne's Beach

Islamorada near MM 73.5

This public beach located at the southern end of Lower Matecumbe Key is a great spot to explore and unwind. There are two parking lots,

restrooms, showers and several covered pavilions with picnic tables. The southern part of the beach serves as a great launch site for kiteboarders, particularly in winds that range from the south to the east.

Fiesta Key

70001 Overseas Highway, Islamorada (MM 70)

This small key is home to Fiesta Key RV Resort. Kiteboarders can launch from here and ride the waters north of the Overseas Highway. There is

SAFETY TIP

Florida law requires all divers and snorkelers use a dive flag when they are in the water unless in an area specifically designated for swimming. If diving or snorkeling from a boat, the boat may fly the official red and white dive flag so long as divers and snorkelers remain within 300 feet (91.5 meters) of the

dive boat – 100 feet (30.5 meters) when in an inlet or navigational channel. Snorkelers and divers must use a diver down flag when entering and exploring sites near the shore, typically towing a flag or diver-down buoy. Vessels operating in the area must stay more than 300 feet (91.5 meters) away from the buoy or flag, whether it is being towed by divers or flown from the dive boat.

no beach, but the resort's daily pass provides access to the pool and other amenities.

Long Key State Park

67400 Overseas Highway, Layton (MM 67.5)
Long Key is one of the more relaxed State Parks in the Florida Keys. It is a decent bird-watching spot and you can kayak and snorkel here as well (see page 180), or simply relax on the beach and enjoy the shoreline. Kayaks can be rented from the ranger station. As with the other state parks in the Keys, there is a fee for entry and camping spots are available.

Grassy Flats and Keys Cable

58182 and 59300 Overseas Highway, Marathon (MM 59)
Grassy Flats Resort provides access to Gull Key and Duck Key, which are ideal for kiteboarding regardless of the wind direction. Day passes must be purchased from the resort, but they also provide access to the resort's amenities. Lessons are also available. Keys Cable is only a few minutes up the road (to the north) if the wind dies and you still want to ride.

Curry Hammock State Park

56200 Overseas Highway, Marathon (MM 56)
This state park on Little Crawl Key charges an entry fee, but there is a boatload of amenities to enjoy for the price, including hiking and biking trails, kayaking and kiteboarding – watch out for the big sand bar to the east. You can also snorkel off the beaches (see page 190) and there is a campground if you want to make the most of your time here.

Coco Plum Beach

33050 Overseas Highway, Marathon (MM 54.5)
This is a natural beach where sea turtles nest in season. It runs along the south of Fat Deer Key, just over a mile (1.6 kilometers) south of Curry Hammock State Park. Restrooms and a covered pavilion are available.

Sunset Park

W Ocean Drive, Key Colony Beach (MM 53)
This small beach has amazing sunset views and is tucked away in the corner of the Key Colony

Beach community. The beach has multiple benches, picnic tables and restrooms available, and rarely gets busy.

Sombrero Beach

2130 Sombrero Beach Road, Marathon (MM 50)
Sombrero Beach is a popular sea turtle nesting beach that draws bathers from across the Keys. There are picnic pavilions, volleyball courts, restrooms and showers. Kiteboarding is often conducted from here, but it is suitable for only a limited range of wind conditions. The spot is also better suited to intermediate kiteboarders because of obstacles in the water. The beach is popular with snorkelers (see page 206).

Bahia Honda State Park

36850 Overseas Highway, Big Pine Key (MM 37)
Bahia Honda is another state park with an entrance fee and a decent mix of services, including hiking, swimming, fishing kayaking and camping (see page 224). It is one of the largest natural beaches in the Keys and it can get quite busy, even reaching capacity at times, so arrive early on weekends and holidays.

Horseshoe Beach

1969 Overseas Highway, Big Pine Key (MM 35)
Horseshoe Beach is immediately across the bridge to the west of Bahia Honda State Park. This stone and pebble beach is artificial and offers no amenities aside from parking. It is pretty much the only place in the Keys to kiteboard in a northern wind but watch out for submerged rocks. (For diving and snorkeling information, see page 226.)

Smathers Beach

2601 S Roosevelt Boulevard, Key West
This is a popular beach in Key West where big crowds can be expected. Kiteboarders launch at the eastern end of the beach (near the airport where there are fewer people. There are restrooms and showers here and a few beach vendors selling refreshments. The beach is free, but the parking is not. This location is rideable in most winds except northerly.

Clarence S. Higgs Memorial Beach Park

1000 Atlantic Boulevard, Key West (MM 0)
There is a lot to do at Higgs Beach, including swimming, snorkeling (see page 278), sunbathing, beach volleyball and tennis. There is also a playground for kids and a Civil War-era fort known as the West Martello, where free self-guided tours are available. Kayaks and paddleboards are available for rental but visitors must bring their own snorkel gear.

Fort Zachary Taylor Historic State Park

601 Howard England Way, Key West (MM 0)
This historic state park is worth spending the entire day exploring. Fort Taylor itself is a National Historic Monument that predates the Civil War. There is also a large beach, which is perfect for swimming and snorkeling (see page 280), as well as opportunities for kayaking and fishing. There is ample parking, along with picnic areas, food and drink options, and restrooms and showers. There is a fee to enter the park.

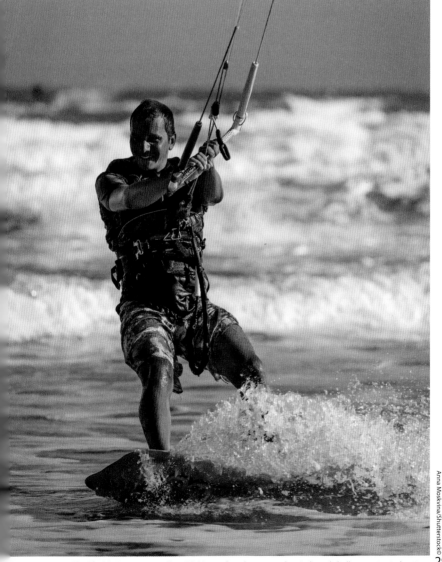

Anna Moskvina/Shutterstock©

The Florida Keys are popular with kite surfers due to steady winds and shallow, protected waters. 29

Diving and snorkeling

The Florida Keys offers an amazing array of diving and snorkeling experiences for visitors and locals alike – they do call themselves the dive capital of the world, after all. From shore-accessible snorkeling sites to incredible natural and artificial reefs, accessible to divers and snorkelers of all levels.

Most of the coral reefs in the Florida Keys are found along the outer reef line, located a few miles offshore. There are smaller patch reefs in the shallower waters in Hawk Channel, which runs parallel to shore inside the reef line. Historic shipwrecks pepper the large, shallow reefs up and down the Keys coastline. Meanwhile purposefully sunk artificial reefs are placed strategically in the deeper waters just off the reef. These artificial reefs are generally more accessible to advanced divers due to their depth.

We have highlighted 102 of the region's most popular dive and snorkel sites in this guidebook, some of which are accessible from shore. The Florida Keys Reef Tract is the only living coral barrier reef in the continental United States. It is so long that it would be impossible to cover every potential dive and snorkel site in the Keys in a reasonably sized guidebook. Instead, we have focused our mapping efforts on the official sites as well as some popular-but-unofficial sites in the region. The official sites are ones that include one or more Florida Keys National

Marine Sanctuary mooring buoys, so there is no need to anchor on sensitive habitat. Be sure to tie up your boat properly, leaving plenty of rope between the boat and the buoy.

For each site described in detail, we provide the history of the reef (if available) to give divers some interesting context during their visit. Our three-star rating system offers insight into the difficulty level, strength of the current, depth and the quality of the reef and fauna that divers and snorkelers are likely to encounter. We offer a suggested route, where applicable, and point out some of the key information to enhance the in water experience, such as what species to look for and what key features to observe. When coupled with our detailed 3D renderings of reefs and wrecks, this constitutes the most comprehensive dive and snorkel guidebook to the Florida Keys. Divers and snorkelers will know what to expect before they venture into the water.

The underwater environment is dynamic and constantly changing. Management of these remarkable resources must evolve to protect them. This guidebook is accurate as of its publication date, and divers and snorkelers should check with local dive operators and the Florida Keys National Marine Sanctuary to see what new and exciting sites there are to visit or if any previously popular sites have been closed. We will continue to revise and expand our guidebook in the future to help ensure we offer the most up-to-date information possible.

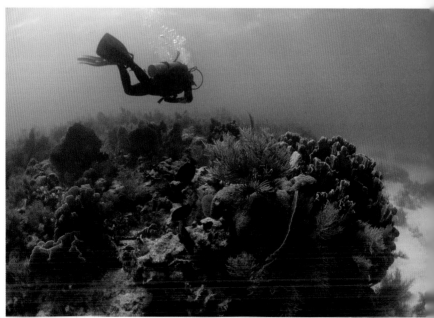

The shallow coral reefs of the Florida Keys are dominated by hard and soft corals as well as spong

Diving and snorkeling activities

There are literally dozens of dive shops, charters and snorkel tour operators in the Florida Keys. Many of them are dedicated to education and habitat conservation through the Florida Keys National Marine Sanctuary's Blue Star program. This voluntary program recognizes operators who promote sustainable and responsible practices. The Blue Star operators are indicated in the list of dive and snorkel services below by the official Blue Star Operator icon seen here. The dives shops are presented in alphabetical order by region. For more about Blue Star Operators, visit: **Floridakeys.noaa.gov/onthewater/bluestar.html**

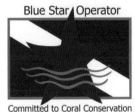

Blue Star Operator

Committed to Coral Conservation

Key Largo

Amoray Dive Resort
104250 Overseas Highway, Key Largo
Tel: 1-800-4-AMORAY
Tel: 305-451-3595
Email: divecenter@amoraywatersports.com
Amoray.com

BlueWater Divers
1 Garden Cove, Key Largo
Tel: 305-453-9600
Email: info@bluewaterdiver.net
Bluewaterdiver.net

Horizon Divers
105800 Overseas Highway, Key Largo
Tel: 305-453-3535
Email: info@horizondivers.com
Horizondivers.com

Island Ventures
513 Ocean Bay Drive, Key Largo
Tel: 305-451-4957
Email: dive@islandventure.com
Islandventure.com

John Pennekamp Dive Shop
(Inside John Pennekamp Coral Reef State Park)
102601 Overseas Highway, Key Largo
Tel: 305-451-6300
Email: info@pennekamppark.com
Pennekamppark.com

Jules Undersea Lodge
51 Shoreland Drive, Key Largo
Tel: 305-451-2353
Email: info@jul.com
Jul.com

Key Largo Dive Center
100670 Overseas Highway, Key Largo
Tel: 305-451-5844
Email: scuba@keylargodivecenter.com
Keylargodivecenter.com

Keys Diver & Snorkel Tours
99696 Overseas Highway, Unit 1, Key Largo
Tel: 305-451-1177
Email: info@KeysDiver.com
Keysdiver.com

Lucky Fish
21 Garden Cove Drive, Key Largo
Tel: 305-766-2166
Email: info@luckyfishscuba.com
Luckyfishscuba.com

Pirates Cove Watersports
103800 Overseas Highway, Key Largo
Tel: 305-453-9881
Email: pcwatersports@gmail.com
Pcwatersports.com

Quiescence Diving Services
103680 Overseas Highway, Key Largo
Tel: 305-451-2440
Email: info@keylargodiving.com
Keylargodiving.com

31

Rainbow Reef Dive Center
Retail: 100800 Overseas Highway, Key Largo
Dive Center: 100 Ocean Drive, Key Largo
Tel: 1-800-457-4354 (305-451-7171)
Rainbowreef.com

 ### Sail Fish Scuba
103100 Overseas Highway, Suite 33, Key Largo
Tel: 305-453-3446
Email: info@sailfishscuba.com
Sailfishscuba.com

Scuba Tech Key Largo
99101 Overseas Highway, Key Largo
Phone: 305-900-0855
Email: info@scubatechkeylargo.com
Scubatechkeylargo.com

 ### Scuba-Fun Dive Center
99222 Overseas Highway, Key Largo
Tel: 305-394-5046
Email: info@scubafunflorida.com
Scubafunflorida.com

 ### Sea Dwellers Dive Center
105 Laguna Avenue, Key Largo
Tel: 1-800-451-3640
Tel: 305-451-3640
Email: info@seadwellers.com
Seadwellers.com

 ### Silent World Dive Center
51 Garden Cove Drive, Key Largo
Tel: 305-451-3252
Email: silentworlddivecenter@gmail.com
Silentworld.com

Sun Sports Charter and Scuba
1313 Ocean Bay Drive, Key Largo
Tel: 305-906-1206
Email: info@sunsportscharter.com
Sunsportscharter.com

Sundiver Snorkel Tours
102840 Overseas Highway, Key Largo
Tel: 305-451-2220
Snorkelingisfun.com

Divers prepare to explore a Key Largo Reef with Sailfish Scuba.

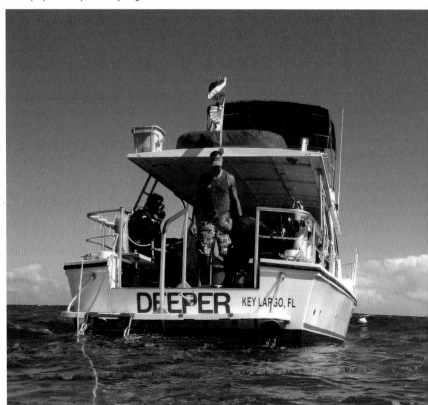

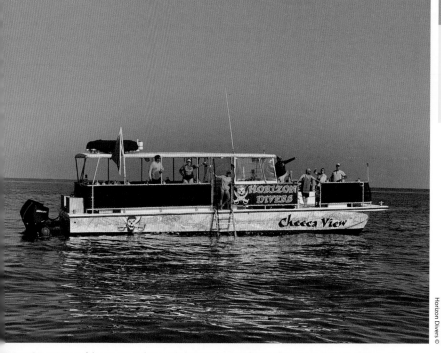

Horizon Divers ©

orizon Divers is one of the operators that regularly visits the Carysfort Reef sites located north of Key Largo.

 The Dive Shop at Ocean Reef
9 Fishing Village Drive, Key Largo
el: 305-367-3051
mail: info@thediveshoporc.com
hediveshoporc.com

avernier

aptain Slate's Scuba Adventures
)791 Old Highway, Unit 1, Tavernier
el: 305-451-3020
mail: captainslate@captainslate.com
aptainslate.com

 Conch Republic Divers
)800 Overseas Highway, Suite 9, Tavernier
el: 1-800-274-DIVE (305-852-1655)
mail: dive@conchrepublicdivers.com
onchrepublicdivers.com

Keys Unique Diving (SNUBA)
6 Arctic Avenue, Tavernier
: 305-942-4643
mail: tomscaribbean@gmail.com
keysuniquediving.com

 Florida Keys Dive Center
90451 Old Highway, Tavernier
Tel: 305-852-4599
Email: info@flkdc.com
Floridakeysdivecenter.com

Islamorada

 Forever Young Charter Company
80460 Overseas Highway, Islamorada
Tel: 305-680-8879
Email: tony@diveyoung.com
Diveyoung.com

 Islamorada Dive Center
84001 Overseas Highway, Islamorada
Tel: 305-664-3483
Email: info@islamoradadivecenter.com
Islamoradadivecenter.com

Jake's Offshore Adventures
(at the World Wide Sportsman)
81576 Overseas Highway, Islamorada
Tel: 508-280-6034
Email: contact@jakesoffshoreadventures.com
Jakesoffshoreadventures.com

33

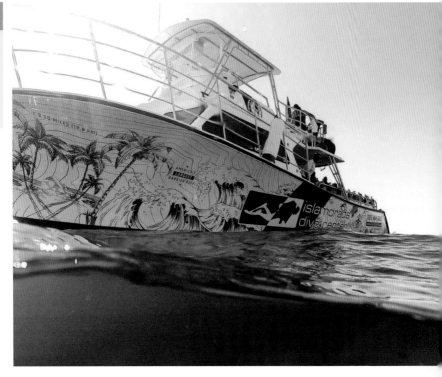

Most dive operators in the Keys provide spacious dive boats, like *Aquatic Freedom* with Islamorada Dive Center

 ### Key Dives

79851 Overseas Highway,
Islamorada
Tel: 1-800-344-7352 , Tel: 305-664-2211
Email: info@keydives.com
Keydives.com

 ### KeyZ Charters

77522 Overseas Highway,
Islamorada
Tel: 305-393-1394
Email: info@keyzcharters.com
Keyzcharters.com

Tropic Scuba

Tel: 305-205-7829
Email: ed@tropicscuba.com
Tropicscuba.com

Sea Monkeys Divers

80461 Overseas Highway,
Islamorada
Tel: 305-664-4555
Email: seamonkeyspadivers@gmail.com
Seamonkeydivers.com

Marathon

A Deep Blue Dive Center

13205 Overseas Highway, Marathon
Tel: 305-743-2421
Email: adeepbluedive@aol.com
Adeepbluedive.com

Better than Most Watersports

4590 Overseas Highway, Marathon
Tel: 305-432-1214
Email: betterthanmostwatersports@gmail.com
Betterthanmostwatersports.com

 ### Captain Hooks Marathon

11833 Overseas Highway, Marathon
Tel: 305-743-2444
Email: captainhooks@gmail.com
Captainhooks.com

Captain Pip's/Spirit Snorkeling

1480 Overseas Highway,
Marathon
Tel: 305-289-0614
Email: captpips@aol.com
Captainpips.com/snorkeling

Dive Isla Bella
1 Knights Key Boulevard, Marathon
Tel: 786-638-8047
Email: diveislabella@gmail.com
Diveislabella.com

Starfish Marathon Snorkeling
1248 Overseas Highway, Marathon
Tel: 305-481-0407
Email: starfishsnorkeling@gmail.com
Starfishsnorkeling.com

Formula Freediving
2940 Overseas Highway, Marathon
Tel: 386-235-2713
Email: andrew@formulafreediving.com
Formulafreediving.com

 Tilden's Scuba Center
4650 Overseas Highway,
Marathon
Tel: 305-743-7255
Email: tildensscubacenter@gmail.com
Tildensscubacenter.com

Capt. Bradley Williams helms the Key Dives dive boat with the iconic Alligator Lighthouse in the background.

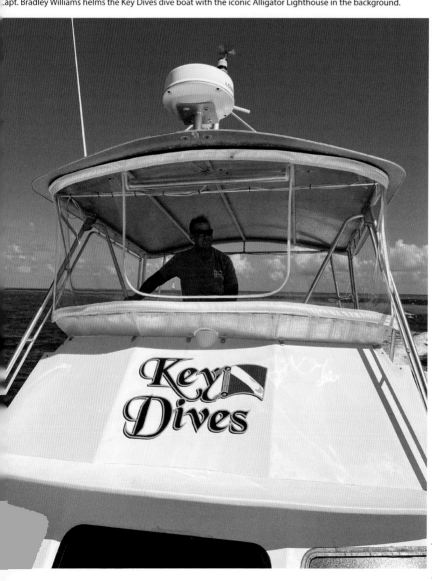

Big Pine Key

Bahia Honda Shop
(Inside Bahia Honda State Park)
36850 Overseas Highway, Big Pine Key
Tel: 305-872-3210
Email: info@bahiahondapark.com
Bahiahondapark.com

Captain Hooks Big Pine Key
29675 Overseas Highway, Big Pine Key
Tel: 305-872-9863
Email: bookhooks@captainhooks.com
Captainhooks.com

Keys Boat Tours
Big Pine Key Resort
33000 Overseas Highway, Big Pine Key
Tel: 305-699-7166
Email: info@keysboattours.com
Keysboattours.com

Ramrod/Summerland Keys

Looe Key Reef and Dive Center
27340 Overseas Highway, Ramrod Key
Tel: 305-872-2215
Email: info@looekeyreefresort.com
Looekeyreefresort.com

Scuba Steve's Dive Service
24326 Overseas Highway, Summerland Key
Tel: 407-698-4456
Email: zach@scubastevesdiveservice.com
Scubastevesdiveservice.com

Key West

Adventure Watersport Charters
6000 Peninsular Avenue, Key West
Tel: 305-453-6070
Email: adventurewatersportcharters@gmail.com
Adventurewatersportcharters.com

Captain's Corner Dive Center
125 Ann Street, Key West
Tel: 305-296-8865
Email: info@captainscorner.com
Captainscorner.com

Captain Hook's Dive Key West
3128 N Roosevelt Boulevard, Key West
Tel: 305-296-3823

Email: bookhooks@divekeywest.com
Divekeywest.com

Finz Dive Center
5130 Overseas Highway, Key West
Tel: 305-395-0880
Email: Info@Finzdivecenter.com
Finzdivecenter.com

Divemaster Key West
3218 N Roosevelt Boulevard, Key West
Tel: 305-292-4616
Email: Info@divemasterkeywest.com
Divemasterkeywest.com

FURY Water Adventures
Loc#1: 241 Front Street, Opal Key Marina
Loc#3: 631 Greene Street,
Key West Bight
Tel: 1-855-831-5997
(305-930-81610)
Email: info@furykeywest.com
Furycat.com

Lost Reef Adventures
261 Margaret Street, Key West
Tel: 305-296-9737
Email: info@lostreefadventures.com
Lostreefadventures.com

Sea, Key West
720B Caroline Street, Key West
Tel: 305-741-7490
Email: john@seakeywestlocal.com
Seakeywestlocal.com

SNUBA Key West
711 Eisenhower Drive, Slip 7,
Key West
Tel: 305-292-4616
Email: info@snubakeywest.com
Snubakeywest.com

Southpoint Divers
606 Front Street., Key West
Tel: 305-292-9778
Email: diving@southpointdivers.com
Southpointdivers.com

Try Scuba Diving Key West
6010 Front Street,
Key West
Tel: 305-330-3375
Email: keywest@tryscubadiving.com
Tryscubadiving.com/key-west

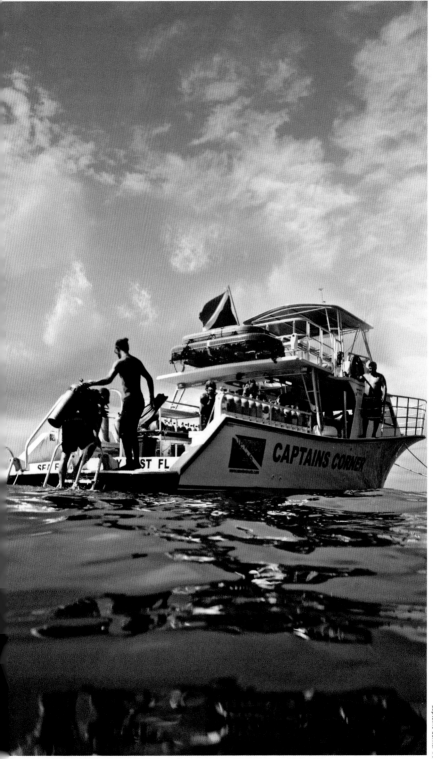

ers return after exploring the wreck of the *Vandenberg* with Captain's Corner Dive Center.

UPPER KEYS DIVE SITES
Key Largo, Tavernier and Islamorada

Key Largo acts as the proverbial gateway to the Florida Keys. Visitors who drive down U.S. Route 1 from the Florida mainland arrive first in Key Largo, a census-designated region with over 8,000 residents and dozens of dive shops and snorkel tour operators. The narrow spit of land that makes up Key Largo runs roughly northeast to southwest and is bordered by the Atlantic Ocean to the east and the Florida Bay and Everglades National Park to the west. Located just south of Key Largo is the unincorporated community of Tavernier, with its own complement of operators. South of that is the town of Islamorada, which straddles both the Upper and Lower Matecumbe Keys. This region is often called the Upper Keys,

and it hosts some of the most incredible diving in the entire state of Florida.

The Upper Keys boasts large reef tracts with defined spur and groove formations, such as Molasses Reef and Elbow Reef. Each of these reefs includes their own complement of historical wrecks that have accumulated over centuries of shipping in these waters. The natural sites have been supplemented with artificial reefs over the decades, including the famous *Spiegel Grove* that sits just off the coast of Key Largo, and the *Eagle*, which sits offshore of Islamorada. Almost half the dive sites covered in this guidebook are in the Upper Keys region.

Dive and snorkel sites

1	North Patch	
2	Northeast Patch	
3	Turtle Reef (aka Turtle Rocks)	
4	Carysfort Trench	
5	North Carysfort Reef	
6	South Carysfort Reef	
7	Elbow Reef	
	• *City of Washington*	
	• *Hannah M. Bell* (aka *Mike's Wreck*)	
8	Horseshoe Reef	
9	North North Dry Rocks	
10	North Dry Rocks	
11	Dry Rocks	
	• Christ of the Abyss	
12	Emerald Lagoon	
	(Jules Undersea Lodge)	
13	Grecian Rocks	
14	John Pennekamp State Park	
15	*Spiegel Grove*	
16	*Benwood*	
17	French Reef	
	• Christmas Tree Cave	
18	White Banks	
19	Three Sisters	
20	Wolfe Reef	
21	Sand Island	
22	Molasses Reef	
	• Winch Hole	
23	*Bibb*	
24	*Duane*	
25	Pickles Reef	
26	Snapper Ledge	

27	Conch Reef	
28	Conch Wall	
29	Little Conch Reef	
A	*El Infante*	
B	*San Jose*	
30	Davis Reef	
C	*Capitana* (aka *El Rubi*)	
31	Davey Crocker Reef	
32	Crocker Reef	
33	Hen & Chickens	
D	*Chaves*	
34	Victory	
35	Islamorada Fingers	
36	Rocky Top	
E	*Herrera*	
37	Morada	
F	*Tres Puentes*	
38	*Eagle*	
39	*Alexander Barge*	
40	Cheeca Rocks (aka The Rocks)	
41	Alligator Reef	
	• Alligator Wreck	
42	Alligator Canyon/Deep	
43	*Cannabis Cruiser* (aka *Pot Wreck*)	
44	Indian Key Historic State Park	
45/G	*San Pedro*	
H	*El Terri* (aka *San Felipe*)	
46	Caloosa Rocks	
I	*San Francisco*	
J	*Almiranta*	

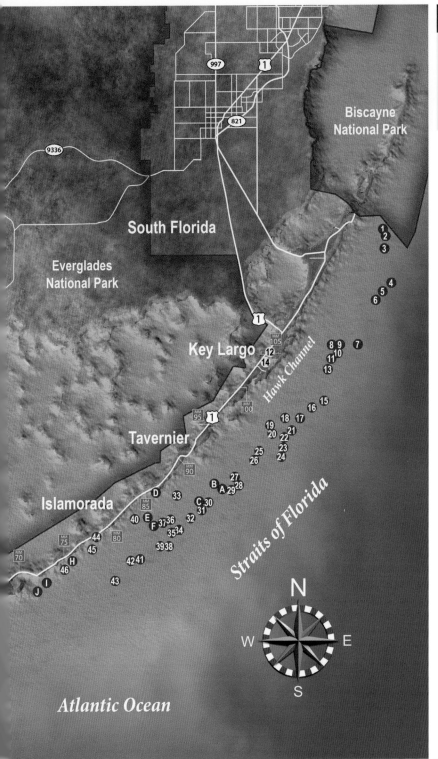

NORTH PATCH & NORTHEAST PATCH

Difficulty ● ○ ○
Current ● ○ ○
Depth ● ○ ○
Reef ★★☆
Fauna ★★☆

Access 🚤 25mi (40km) from Key Largo

Level Open Water

Location North Key Largo
GPS   NP1 25° 18.671'N, 80° 11.979'W
         NP2 25° 18.820'N, 80° 11.931'W
         NP3 25° 18.777'N, 80° 11.883'W

         NEP1 25° 18.400'N, 80° 12.106'W
         NEP2 25° 18.434'N, 80° 12.051'W
         NEP3 25° 18.503'N, 80° 12.034'W

Getting there

North Patch and Northeast Patch are two medium-sized patch reefs located on the border between the Florida Keys National Marine Sanctuary to the south and Biscayne

National Park to the north. They sit just ‹ miles (6.5 kilometers) offshore from Nort⊦ Key Largo. At more than an hour by boat fron Key Largo, they are out of the range of mos‹ Key Largo-based dive shops, meaning mos‹ visitors must get there on their own.

Access

These reefs are only accessible by boat given the distance from shore. They are suitable for diver and snorkelers of all levels as they are typicall‹ sheltered from the strongest currents given the location slightly shoreward of the outer reef lin‹ To access the site, boats should tie up to one ⊂ the three anchored buoys.

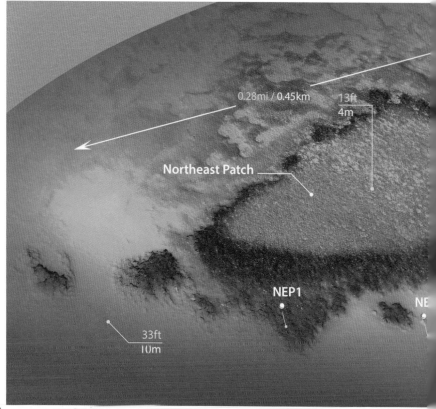

0.28mi / 0.45km   13ft / 4m

Northeast Patch

NEP1

NE

33ft / 10m

Description

These two shallow patch reefs are surrounded by a scattering of small coral heads and patch reefs spread across a sand bottom ranging from 24 to 33 feet (7.5 to 10 meters). The tops of the reefs reach up to just 13 feet (4 meters) below the surface of the water. North Patch is the smaller of the two reefs, measuring roughly 650 feet (200 meters) in length. In an example of unimaginative site naming, North Patch is located just to the north of Northeast Patch. The latter reef is nearly 1,500 feet (450 meters) in length. Like many of the other shallow reefs in the Keys, North and Northeast Patches are dominated by sea fans and other soft corals. They shelter a variety of reef creatures commonly found in shallow reef habitat, such as damselfish, hamlets, surgeonfish, grunts and wrasses.

ECO TIP

When possible, help protect the marine ecosystem by choosing to visit sites with permanent mooring buoys. This system was established in the Florida Keys in 1981 to help protect the fragile coral reef ecosystem from anchor damage. Keys mooring buoys are 18 inches (0.5 meters) in diameter and are generally white with a blue stripe. In total, there are approximately 500 mooring buoys located across the Keys, which are installed and maintained by the Florida Keys National Marine Sanctuary. Mooring buoys are available on a first-come, first-served basis at no cost. If a mooring buoy is unavailable, boat operators are permitted to anchor in sand so long as they are outside of a no-anchor zone. Anchoring on living coral within the sanctuary is prohibited in waters less than 40 feet (12 meters) and when the bottom is visible. If you notice a damaged or missing line or buoy, please call the appropriate sanctuary office. From Key Largo to Marathon, call 305-852-7717. For Marathon through Key West and the Tortugas, call 305-809-4700.

NORTH PATCH & NORTHEAST PATCH

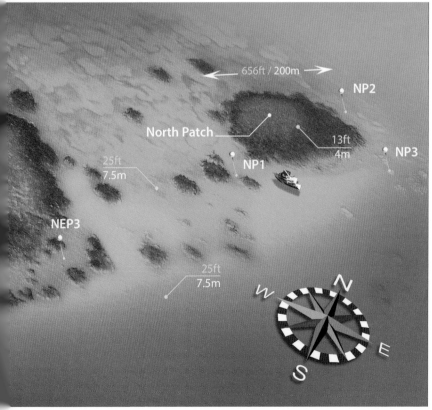

656ft / 200m

NP2

North Patch

13ft
4m

NP3

25ft
7.5m

NP1

NEP3

25ft
7.5m

N
W
E
S

TURTLE REEF (TURTLE ROCKS)

Difficulty ● ○ ○
Current ● ● ○
Depth ● ○ ○
Reef ★★☆
Fauna ★★☆

Access 🛥 23mi (37km) from Key Largo

Level Open Water

Location North Key Largo
GPS TR1 25° 16.529'N, 80° 12.492'W
TR2 25° 16.747'N, 80° 12.449'W
TR3 25° 16.824'N, 80° 12.419'W
TR4 25° 16.956'N, 80° 12.417'W
TR5 25° 17.022'N, 80° 12.382'W
TR6 25° 17.105'N, 80° 12.378'W
TR7 25° 18.000'N, 80° 12.908'W
TR8 25° 18.090'N, 80° 13.034'W
TR9 25° 17.746'N, 80° 13.042'W
TR10 25° 17.662'N, 80° 13.148'W
TR11 25° 17.590'N, 80° 13.251'W
TR12 25° 16.647'N, 80° 13.613'W
TR13 25° 16.533'N, 80° 13.462'W
TR14 25° 16.443'N, 80° 13.718'W

Getting there

Turtle Reef consists of a series of reef ledge located on the border between the Florida Key National Marine Sanctuary and Biscayne Nation Park. They sit just 4 miles (6.5 kilometers) offshor from North Key Largo. At nearly an hour's tri from Key Largo by boat, they are out of the rang of most Key Largo-based dive shops, meanin most visitors must get there on their own.

Access

These reefs are only accessible by boat given the distance from shore. They can be explored by dive and snorkelers of all levels although the main ledg is sometimes exposed to the stronger currents the outer reef line. To access the site, boats shou tie up to one of the mooring buoys.

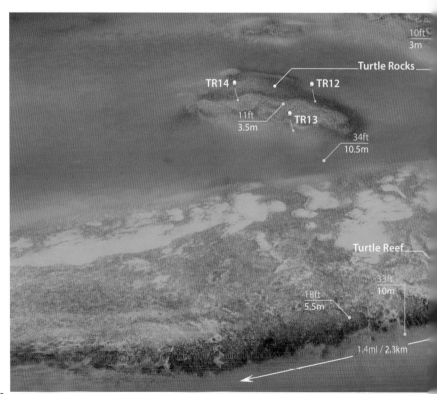

Description

Turtle Reef, also called Turtle Rocks, consists of two shallow reef ledges and a smaller patch reef that sits in between. The primary ledge runs for nearly 1.5 miles (over 2 kilometers), from south to north, with the edge of the ledge topping out at around 13 feet (4 meters) before dropping to a rubble and sand bottom at around 30 feet (9.5 meters). The second ledge is set back nearly a mile (1.5 kilometer) from the first and positioned just to the north. This latter ledge is more often associated with the name Turtle Rocks and sits inside the boundary of the John Pennekamp Coral Reef State Park. It is a no-lobstering zone.

The remains of Totten Beacon "K" can be found on the shoreward edge of the main reef ledge, sitting in just 8 feet (2.5 meters) of water. This beacon

was once an important navigational marker to the safe anchorage site called Turtle Harbor – hence the name of the reef. Turtle Harbor was the intended destination of the *Thiorva* when she ran aground on Turtle Reef back in 1894, the wreckage of which is still located here.

Visitors to Turtle Reef will be able to see plenty of marine life at these sites, including rough and smooth starlet coral and brain corals; gorgonians are also common. Bluehead, yellowhead, and clown wrasses are abundant, as are yellowtail snapper, French grunts, bicolor damselfish and sergeant majors. Divers and snorkelers may also spot a hawksbill or loggerhead sea turtle, as they have been known to visit the reef from time to time.

DID YOU KNOW?

Thiorva was a Norwegian sailing bark (often misidentified as a schooner) built in 1876 in Canada. She ran aground near Turtle Reef while transporting a shipment of timber from Pensacola, FL, to Germany. After colliding with the reef, she was deemed a complete loss and soon broke up in the shallow water. Her debris field is scattered across numerous parts of the reef and the adjacent sandy area. There are no mooring buoys located near the *Thiorva*, and boaters should anchor in the sand well clear of the reef to avoid damaging the sensitive habitat or disturbing the shipwreck.

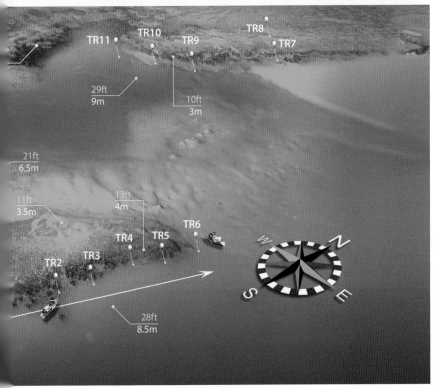

FLORIDA KEYS

CARYSFORT TRENCH, NORTH & SOUTH

Difficulty ● ● ○
Current ● ● ○
Depth ● ● ○
Reef ★★☆
Fauna ★★☆

Access 🚤 16mi (26km) from Key Largo

Level Open Water

Location Key Largo
GPS   CT1 25° 13.970'N, 80° 11.897'W
         CT2 25° 14.026'N, 80° 11.870'W

         CR1 25° 13.178'N, 80° 12.652'W
         CR2 25° 13.205'N, 80° 12.627'W
         CR3 25° 13.274'N, 80° 12.595'W
         CR4 25° 13.297'N, 80° 12.591'W
         CR5 25° 13.321'N, 80° 12.589'W
         CR6 25° 13.350'N, 80° 12.528'W
         CR7 25° 13.488'N, 80° 12.679'W
         CR8 25° 13.468'N, 80° 12.697'W
         CR9 25° 13.433'N, 80° 12.718'W
         CR10 25° 13.384'N, 80° 12.711'W
         CR11 25° 13.321'N, 80° 12.757'W

CR12 25° 13.287'N, 80° 12.780'W
CR13 25° 13.241'N, 80° 12.773'W

CS1 25° 12.405'N, 80° 13.253'W
CS2 25° 12.495'N, 80° 13.160'W
CS3 25° 12.567'N, 80° 13.093'W
CS4 25° 12.707'N, 80° 13.052'W
CS5 25° 12.666'N, 80° 13.188'W
CS6 25° 12.594'N, 80° 13.248'W
CS7 25° 12.538'N, 80° 13.325'W
CS8 25° 12.434'N, 80° 13.356'W

Getting there

The Carysfort Reefs and Trench are th
northernmost dive sites regularly visited by Ke
Largo dive operators. The three separate regior
sit nearly 6.5 miles (10.5 kilometers) offshore (

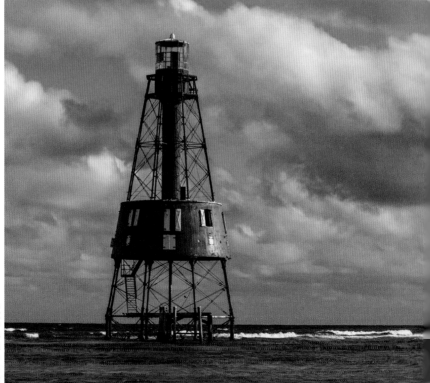

Ralph Krugler/Shutterstock©

44

The iconic Carysfort Reef Lighthouse towers above the waves breaking on North Carysfort r

DID YOU KNOW?

The reefs of the Florida Keys are more treacherous for ships heading south than they are for vessels heading north. The Gulf Stream current can be powerful as it passes through the narrow straits between Florida, Cuba and the Bahamas. While this phenomenon means that ships sailing north can make excellent time on their voyage, it also means vessels sailing south need to hug the shoreline as close as they can to avoid fighting against the powerful current. Carysfort Reef juts out into the ocean relative to the reefs located farther north, making it a particularly challenging navigational hazard when traveling south. According to some records, 20 percent of the 324 vessels wrecked on Florida reefs between 1833 and 1841 were lost on Carysfort. The reef was first marked with the help of a lightship – which ironically ran aground on another reef to the north during its maiden voyage south from New York in 1825. After a string of replacement lightships took their turn marking the reef, a permanent lighthouse was finally built on the reef and officially opened in 1852 after many years of construction. The lighthouse was deactivated in 2014 after navigational signaling duties were taken over by a nearby 40-foot (12-meter) lighted marker.

North Key Largo in a line running roughly south to north on the outer reef. It takes around 45 minutes to get there by boat from Key Largo.

Access

These reefs are only accessible by boat given their distance from shore. They are suitable for divers and snorkelers of all levels, although the mooring buoys anchored on the shallower side of the reef offer more protection from the currents and surge. Access is relatively easy by tying up to one of the nearly two dozen mooring buoys across all three sites. There are two buoys on Carysfort Trench, while Carysfort North boasts six buoys on the ocean side and seven on the inland side. For its part, Carysfort South offers four buoys on each side of the reef.

Description

The Carysfort Reef system gets its name from the HMS Carysfort, a British Royal Navy frigate that ran aground on the reef on its way to Jamaica in 1770. The ship survived the grounding and was able to continue her journey, but the reef now bears her name.

There are two main sections of reef located half a mile (0.9 kilometers) apart. These two reefs are protected as one of the Sanctuary Preservation Areas (SPA). Carysfort Trench, which is predominantly a diver-only site, is located just to the north of Carysfort North, and just outside the boundary of the SPA. At nearly 1.5 square nautical miles, the Carysfort Reef SPA is the largest SPA in the Florida Keys National Marine Sanctuary. Included in the SPA are both the main reefs and the rare double reef that sits in deeper waters, just across the sand channel that runs roughly southwest to northeast. As with other SPAs, there is no fishing by any means allowed within the boundaries, which include Carysfort North and South.

Carysfort Trench (also called Carysfort Wall) is a relatively deep sand channel that runs along the center of the deeper double reef system, nearly splitting it in two for a short stretch. The channel is widest in the middle, measuring almost 300 feet (90 meters) at its widest point, although it tapers significantly at its northern end. The sand bottom of the channel reaches a depth of almost 70 feet (21 meters) along the eastern edge, where the buoys are anchored, but is just 57 feet (17.5 meters) deep along the western edge. The slope

DID YOU KNOW?

The remains of a historic wreck lie just south of Carysfort Reef South. The wreck of the HMS Winchester lies just inside the southern Carysfort SPA boundary line. A British Man-of-War built in 1693, she ran aground just south of Carysfort Reef as she traveled north from Jamaica on her way back home to England. She was discovered by a local fisherman in the late 1930s and was extensively salvaged over the intervening years. Some of her cannons currently "guard" the aptly named Cannon Beach inside the boundaries of the John Pennekamp Coral Reef State Park (see page 80). Very little of the original shipwreck remains at the site of the original grounding, and the debris that does remain has since become fully incorporated into the reef. The site is very shallow and there are no mooring buoys present in the area; as such, visiting the site is very difficult and not recommended.

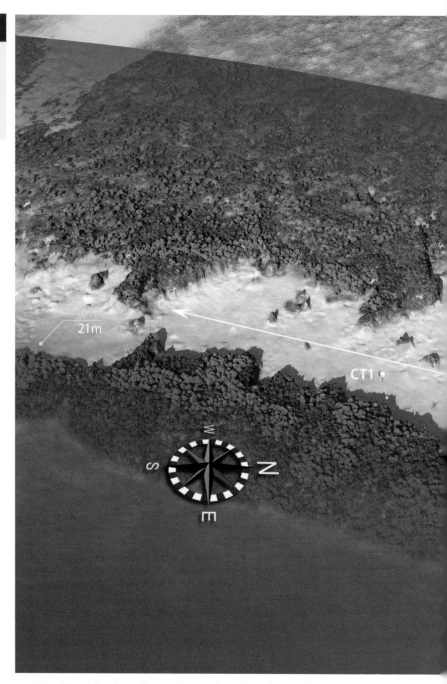

on either side of the channel is predominantly older, fossilized reef with shallow sand channels running through it. The reef is scattered with staghorn and brain corals, as well as numerous soft corals that host a wide variety of other marine organisms.

The reef at Carysfort North becomes very shallow around the lighthouse and along the narrow section of its crest. The reef even breaks the surface of the water at low tide and in the trough of large waves. Seaward from the reef crest is relatively shallow region of tall coral towers and irregular spurs and grooves. The line of buoy

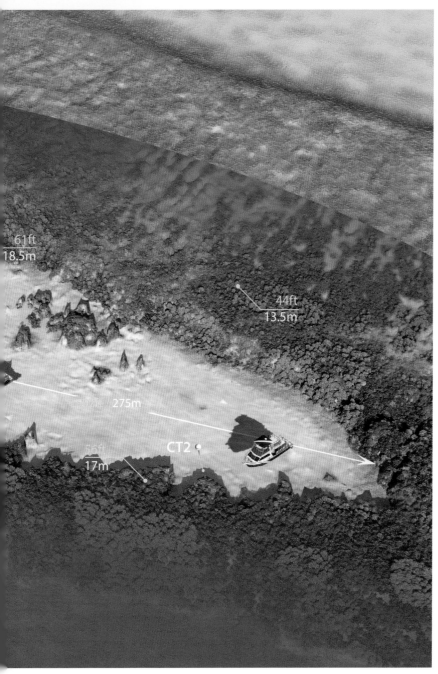

61ft
18.5m

44ft
13.5m

275m

CT2

17m

marks the transition from this structured region to a relatively flatter area dominated by turf algae and interspersed with occasional coral heads and patch reefs. The reef drops off at a ledge that measures as high as 20 feet (6 meters) in some areas, before giving way to a wide sand channel that measures nearly 250 feet (75 meters) across.

Carysfort South has a much better-defined system of spurs and grooves than Carysfort North. These features extend from the reef crest down to the sand channel located on the seaward side or southeastern edge of the reef. Hard and soft corals line rubble- and sand-bottomed grooves that run roughly along a west

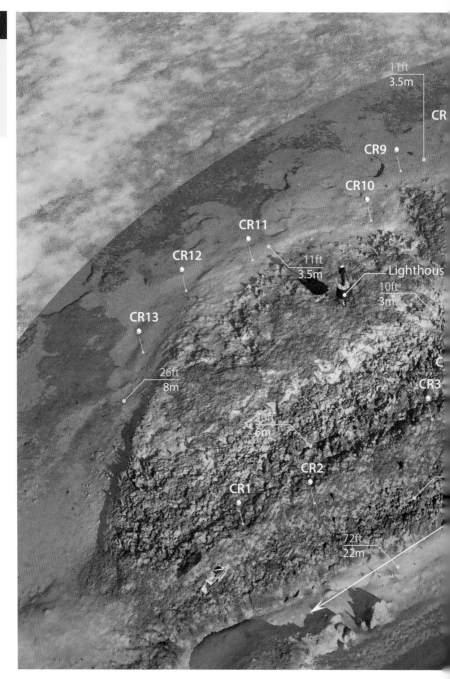

11ft
3.5m

CR

CR9

CR10

CR11

CR12

11ft
3.5m

Lighthous

10ft
3m

CR13

26ft
8m

C

CR3

6m

CR2

CR1

72ft
22m

to east axis. Toward the southern end of the reef, a flatter slope dominated by turf algae extends out into the sand channel, much as it does on Carysfort North.

Across all three sites, divers and snorkelers will encounter a wide variety of reef fish species, including stoplight and redband parrotfish, yellowtail and schoolmaster snapper, black an red grouper and even goliath grouper in th deeper sections of the reefs. Nurse sharks a common here, while reef sharks are occasionall seen patrolling the deeper sand channel Elkhorn and staghorn coral stands are scattere

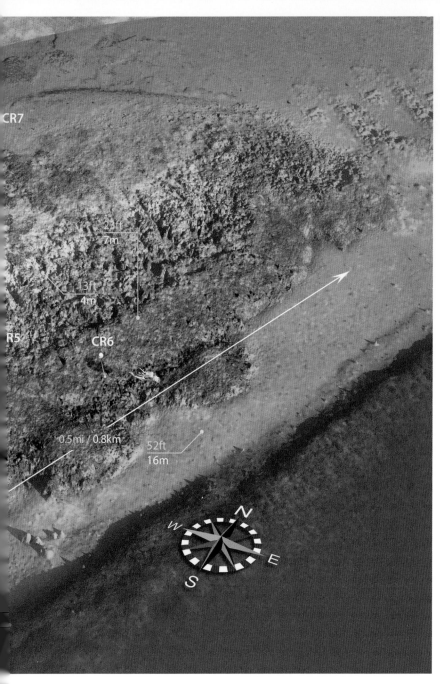

throughout the area, providing complex reef structure that supports a healthy ecosystem.

Route

The best route to follow will depend on the mooring buoy used. There are many named dives on Carysfort Reefs, which vary between dive operators. As one of the best developed reefs in the Keys, however, there is always something to explore no matter where divers begin. For example, divers on Carysfort Trench may want to head down the reef slope to start, finishing their dive by exploring the reef ledge.

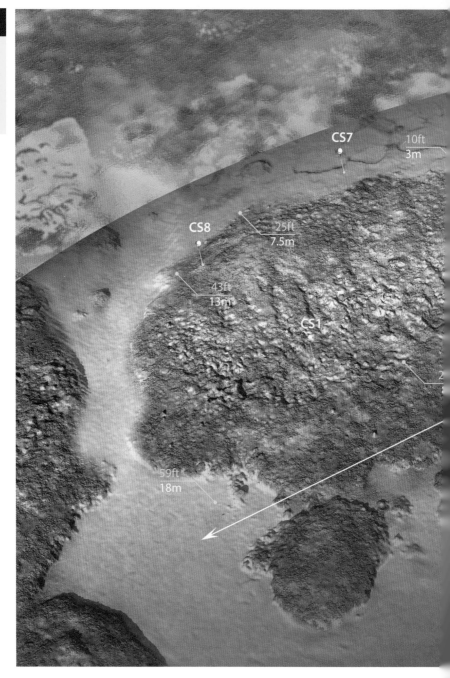

CS7

10ft
3m

CS8

25ft
7.5m

43ft
13m

CS1

59ft
18m

For the sites on North and South Carysfort Reefs, snorkelers typically stay in the area between the reef crest and the buoy lines. Divers, meanwhile, often prefer to head outward from their respective mooring buoy. Along the deeper buoy lines of the two reef sites, divers can head east into deeper water to explore along the tall ledge next to the sand channel. They can either swim out and back along the ledge, following the same route, or choose a square pattern to return up the reef slope. For either route, consider leaving some bottom time to explore the shallower structure area near the buoys.

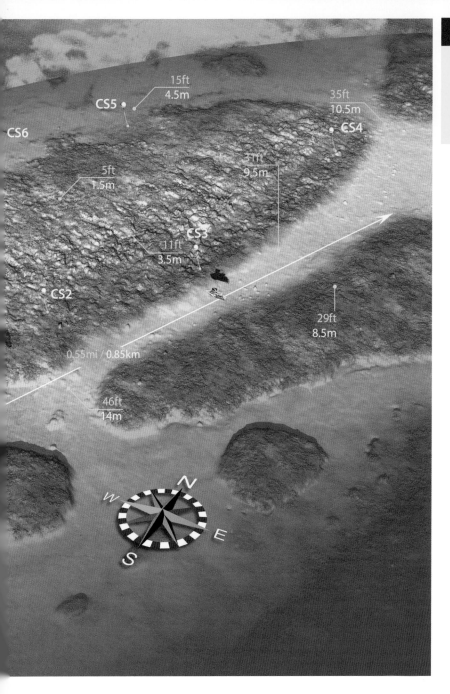

CS5
15ft
4.5m

CS6

35ft
10.5m
CS4

5ft
1.5m

31ft
9.5m

CS3

11ft
3.5m

CS2

29ft
8.5m

0.55mi / 0.85km

46ft
14m

N
W   E
S

ELBOW REEF & WRECKS

Difficulty ● ○ ○
Current ● ● ○
Depth ● ○ ○
Reef ★★★
Fauna ★★☆

Access 🚤 10mi (16km) from Key Largo

Level Open Water

Location Key Largo
GPS   E1 25° 08.169'N, 80° 15.559'W
       E2 25° 08.387'N, 80° 15.567'W
       E3 25° 08.449'N, 80° 15.545'W
       E4 25° 08.520'N, 80° 15.505'W
       E5 25° 08.566'N, 80° 15.478'W
       E6 25° 08.617'N, 80° 15.433'W
       E7 25° 08.682'N, 80° 15.416'W
       E8 25° 08.725'N, 80° 15.374'W
       E9 25° 08.776'N, 80° 15.359'W
       E10 25° 08.830'N, 80° 15.329'W
       E11 25° 08.893'N, 80° 15.141'W

Getting there

Elbow Reef is a well-developed reef system along the outer edge of the Keys reef line. It sits 7 miles (11 kilometers) offshore of the northern end of Key Largo. It is regularly visited by many Key Largo dive operators, and it can take around 30 minutes to get there from Key Largo.

Access

Elbow Reef and the many wrecks located there are only accessible by boat given their distance from shore. They are suitable for divers and snorkelers of all levels, although the reef's position, which juts out from the reef line, makes it susceptible to stronger currents. Access to these sites is relatively easy thanks to the 11 mooring buoys that stretch in a rough line from south to north. The reef here is part of a Sanctuary Preservation Area (SPA) and there is no fishing of any kind permitted inside the boundaries of this SPA.

Description

Elbow Reef is another Keys reef that has proved treacherous to vessels over the years. The reef gets its name from its position projecting out from the rest of the reef line – much like an elbow. The many historical wrecks that can be found scattered among the spurs and grooves of the reef can attest to the real dangers of getting too close to the shallow reef here.

The reef itself is a wonder of well-defined

coral spurs interspersed with rubble and sand-bottomed grooves. The reef is shallow, making it a prime site for both snorkelers and divers. The tops of the spurs reach as shallow as 13 feet (4 meters) deep in many places, putting the waving sea fans and other gorgonians that top the spurs well within sight of snorkelers at the surface. The bottom of the sand and rubble grooves reach a maximum depth of between 25 and 30 feet (7.5 to 9 meters) along the main stretch of nine buoys (E2 through E10) that represent the core of the reef sites. Many of the buoys are named after specific features found in the surrounding reef area. For instance, buoy E4 is often called Train Wheels Reef (or Train Wreck or Train Wheels Wreck) because of the train wheels that were once cargo onboard a ship that either sank there or foundered long enough for them to fall overboard – the story varies. Nearby, buoy E5 is named for the length of anchor chain that is still visible even after being incorporated in the reef. Other site names include, Mid Reef (E6), South Ledges or Sand Highway (E2), and Elbow Wall (E1).

A broad sand and rubble channel runs parallel to shore and separates the spurs and grooves from the reef area that gently slopes out to sea. The channel narrows in the middle section of the reef but at its southern end, it forms what is known as Sand Highway. The edge of the reef slope supports its own complement of hard and soft corals along with its associated reef creatures. But this area is less commonly visited by divers and snorkelers from the main line of buoys as it takes a long time to kick out to the reef line and back.

Among the spurs and grooves lie the remains of three historic wrecks, with a fourth found on the sandy north side of the reef in shallow water. The latter wreck was referred to by locals as the Civil War Wreck until it was positively identified as the *SS Tonawanda*. Built in 1863 and originally named the *SS Arkansas*, she was a sail and steam powered transport vessel used by the Union Navy for naval blockades during the Civil War. She was decommissioned in 1865, and eventually sold into service in the merchant fleet under the new *SS Tonawanda*. She ran aground on Elbow Reef in

RELAX & RECHARGE

Backyard Café at Key Largo Fisheries (1313 Ocean Bay Dr. Suite A, Key Largo) is a waterfront café set in the backyard of Key Largo Fisheries, which is the source of much of the fresh seafood they serve. There is a wonderful range of fish sandwiches, including hogfish, snapper, grouper and mahi mahi, not to mention the popular lobster BLT. But the extensive menu, which offers nearly one hundred separate items, also includes a range of soups, salads, ceviche, tacos and desserts. The café is open from 11am to 7pm (6pm on Sundays) and often has live music. With their great food and stunning views over the Marina, this relaxed spot has been a favorite of locals since 1972.
Visit: **Keylargofisheries.com/cafe**

1866 on her way to Cuba from Boston, and her wooden frame was quickly broken down by the ocean. Most of her debris now lies hidden in the sand. There is little to see at this site now, and without a buoy to tie into, there is significant risk of damaging what little is left of the debris or the surrounding coral when anchoring.

One of the most popular wrecks on Elbow Reef lies to the east of *Tonawanda* amidst the spurs and grooves found between buoys E9 and E10. *SS City of Washington* offers divers far more structure to explore than the *Tonawanda*, even though all that remains of the former is mostly the lower bilge area and a few stretches of vertical hull plating. The site stretches 325 feet (99 meters) in length with a visible engine mount and pedestal in the aft portion of the wreck. Originally an iron-

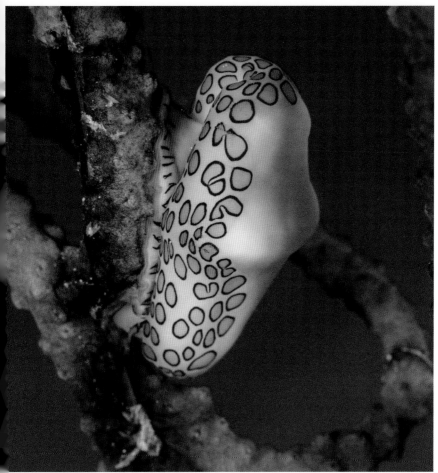

lamingo tongues are often found on sea fans like the ones that dominate the shallow waters of Elbow Reef.

ELBOW REEF & WRECKS

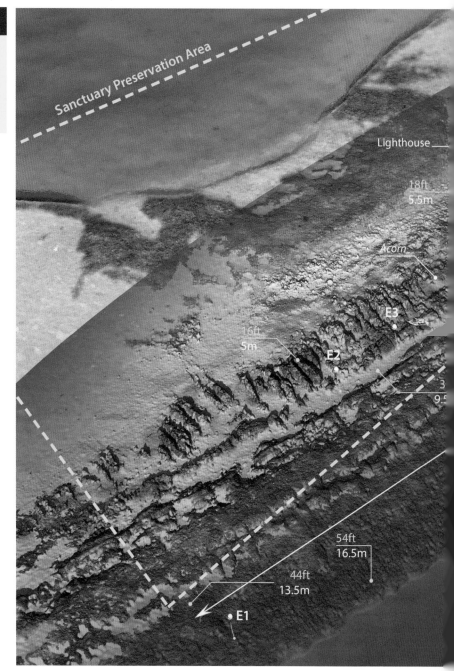

Sanctuary Preservation Area

Lighthouse

18ft
5.5m

Acorn

E3

16ft
5m

E2

3
9.5

54ft
16.5m

44ft
13.5m

E1

hulled steamship, she was built in Pennsylvania in 1877 and used as a passenger and cargo transport ship between New York, Cuba and Mexico. She was moored next to the *USS Maine* in Havana Harbor when the latter ship was blown up at the start of the Spanish-American War in 1898. *City of Washington* took damage in the explosion but managed to participate in the rescue of the *Maine*'s crew. By 1911, she wa bought and cut down to a barge to transpor coal. She foundered on Elbow Reef in 1917 on he way south carrying coal to Gulfport, Mississippi She is one of nine wrecks on the Florida Key National Marine Sanctuary Shipwreck Trail, and

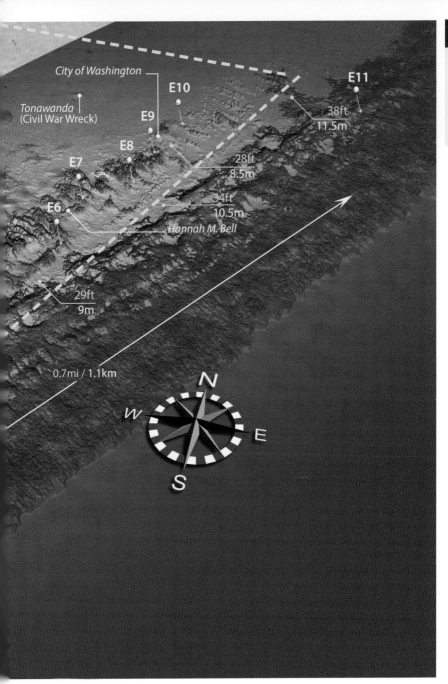

City of Washington

Tonawanda
(Civil War Wreck)

E10

E9

E8

E7

E6

E11

38ft
11.5m

28ft
8.5m

34ft
10.5m

Hannah M. Bell

29ft
9m

0.7mi / 1.1km

N

W   E

S

one of the easiest to access.

ust south of *City of Washington* lies a second historical wreck. Long referred to as *Mike's Wreck* by locals after the diver who discovered her, it was positively identified as the *SS Hannah M. Bell* in 2012. The 315-foot (96-meter) steamship was

headed south with a cargo of coal bound for Vera Cruz when she ran aground on Elbow Reef in 1911. She foundered before the salvage tugs could reach her, although the local papers at the time reported that all her crew remained safe. The resulting wreck site is an impressive stretch of intact hull plates and surrounding debris that

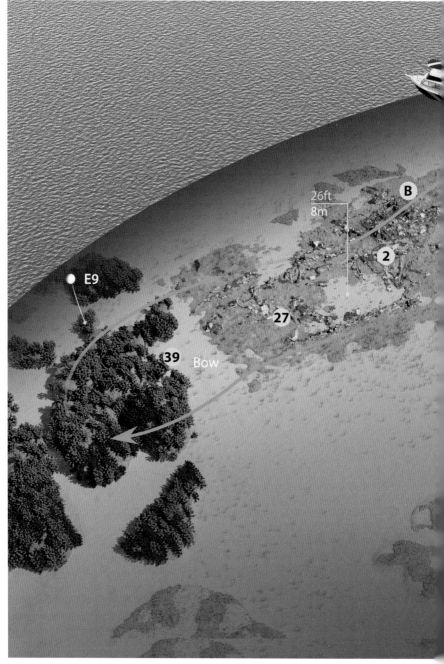

26ft
8m

B

2

E9

27

39   Bow

extends to either side of buoy E7. Portions of the hull rise 15 feet (4.5 meters) above the sand and rubble seafloor and, given that she rests partially on top of a set of coral spurs, the wreckage has not been covered over. Her bow points to the south and her stern is located at the northern end of the site. The wreck and surrounding reef offer some interesting relief and shelter a wide variety of marine life, including elkhorn coral on the reef spur immediately adjacent to the bow. The *Hannah M. Bell* is one of the most popular dive sites on Elbow Reef because of the incredible complexity of the site.

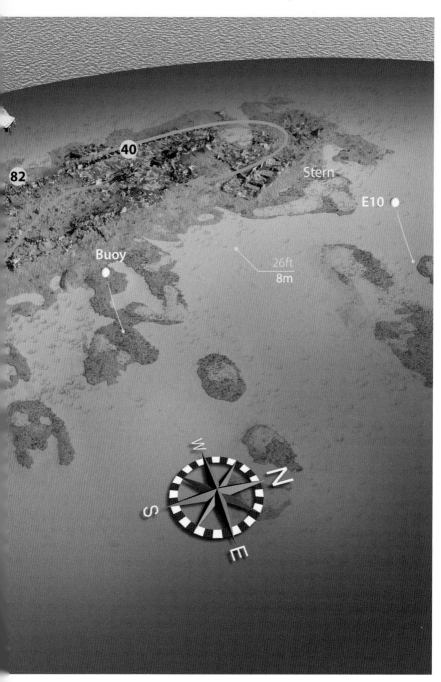

82

40

Stern

E10

Buoy

26ft
8m

arther south on buoy E4 lie the scattered
emains of the *SS Acorn*. Built in 1881 in Scotland,
his 165-foot (50-meter) steamship collided with
bow Reef on February 8, 1885 – a mere four
ears after her launch. Not much remains of the
reck, although what debris is visible has been
ushed up against coral spurs along the eastern

edge of the sand and rubble channel to the west
of the buoy.

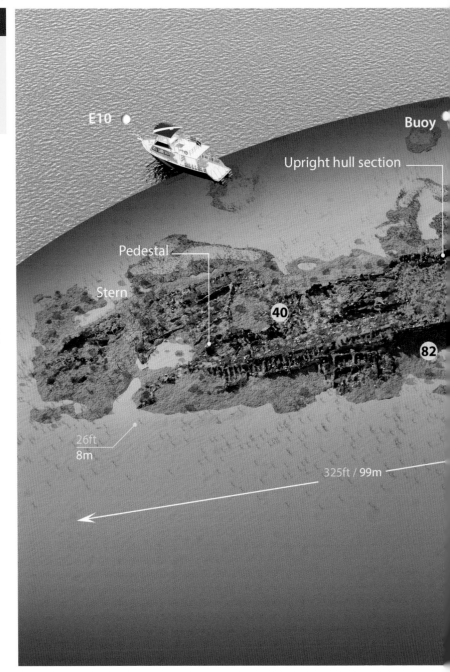

E10

Buoy

Upright hull section

Pedestal

Stern

40

82

26ft
8m

325ft / 99m

Route

The best route for a diver to take while exploring Elbow Reef and its many wrecks will depend on the specific buoy that serves as the starting point. The reef is far too large to explore in a single visit, so divers and snorkelers should consider each buoy to be a separate site. The current on

Elbow Reef typically runs roughly south to north parallel to the shore, but it can reverse directio under the right conditions. Most dive operator will tie up to the buoy that is down current of th target site so that divers and snorkelers can begi their exploration by swimming into the current. The wrecks offer an incredible sight for dive

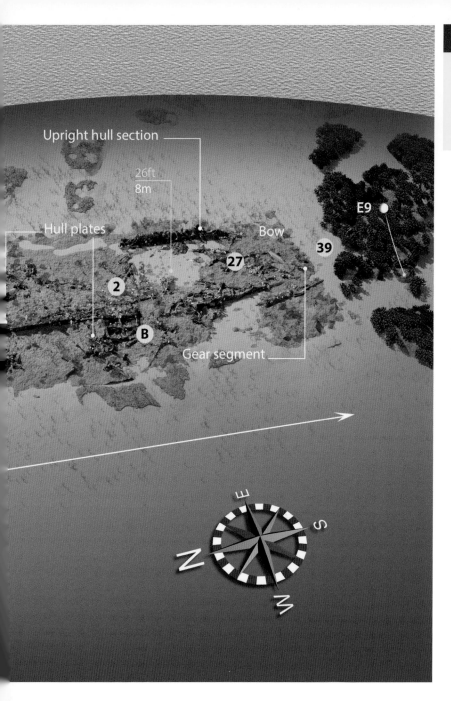

Upright hull section

26ft
8m

Hull plates

Bow

27

2

39

E9

B

Gear segment

ame:	*SS City of Washington*	Chester, PA, 1877
ype:	Cargo steamer	**Last owner:** Luckenback SS Co. Inc
revious names:	n/a	**Sunk:** Oct. 7, 1917
ength:	325ft (99m)	
onnage:	2,600 grt	
onstruction:	John Roach & Sons,	

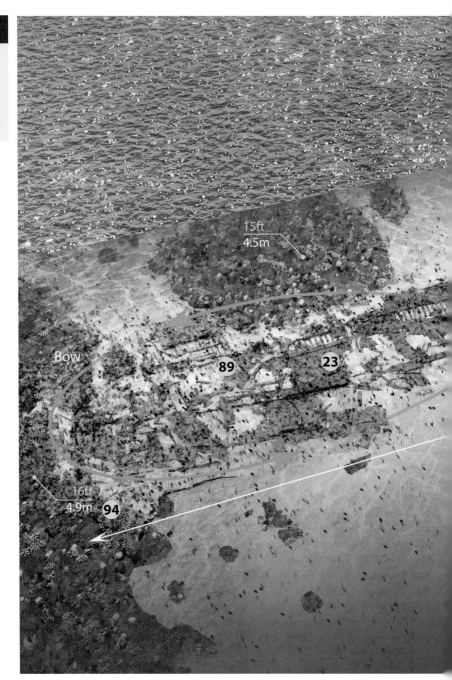

15ft
4.5m

Bow

89

23

16ft
4.9m 94

and snorkelers alike, but the surrounding coral spurs are equally interesting to explore. With a maximum depth of just 30 feet (9 meters) bottom time for divers is generally limited only to air supply. This makes Elbow Reef and its many wrecks worth savoring one buoy at a time. As a bonus, the position of the reef projecting out into the ocean beyond the reef line means tha visibility is often better here than at surroundin reefs. Great visibility, plenty of marine life and lo of bottom time make this a favorite reef amor macro photographers as well.

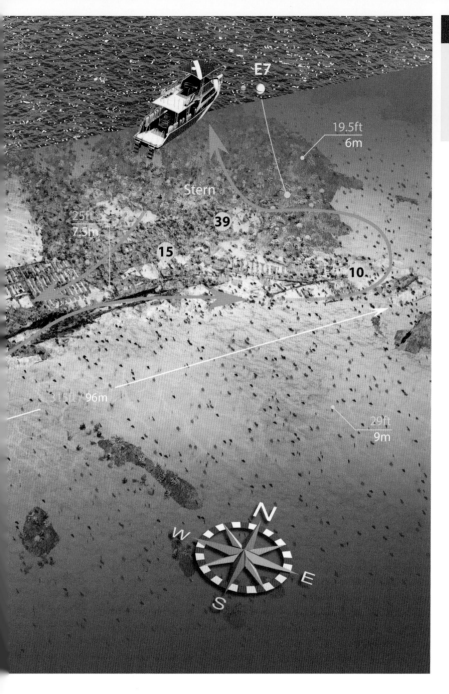

E7

19.5ft
6m

25ft
7.5m

Stern

39

15

10.

15ft / 96m

29ft
9m

N

W

S

E

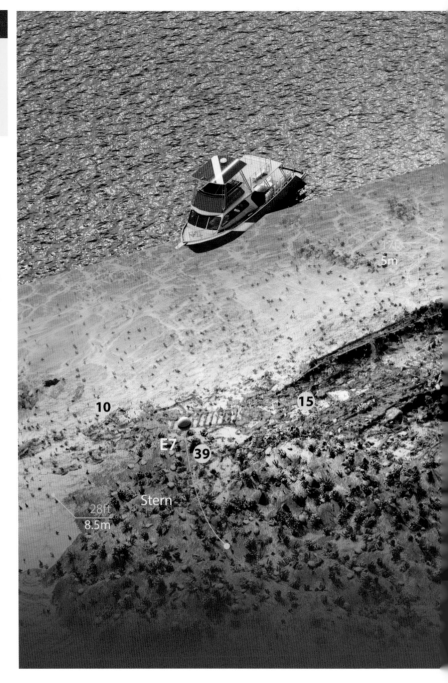

HANNAH M BELL

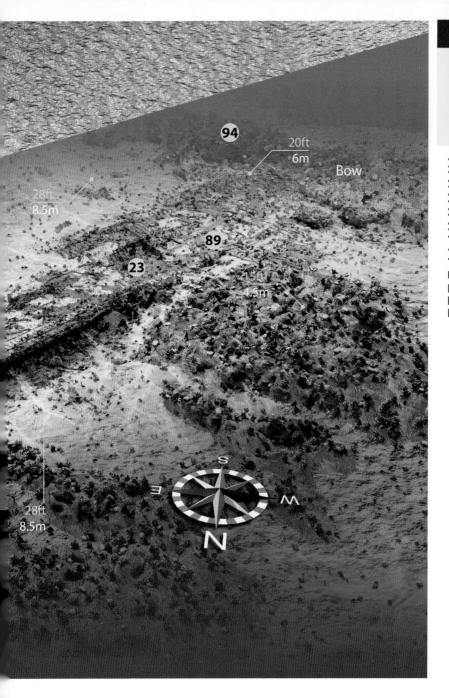

94

20ft
6m

Bow

28ft
8.5m

89

23

15ft
4.5m

28ft
8.5m

me:	SS Hannah M Bell		Stockton, UK, 1893
pe:	Cargo steamer	**Last owner:**	Crosby, Magee & Co.
evious names:	n/a	**Sunk:**	April 4, 1911
ngth:	315ft (96m)		
nnage:	2,998 grt		
nstruction:	Ropner & Sons, Ltd,		

HORSESHOE REEF

Difficulty ● ○ ○
Current ● ○ ○
Depth ● ○ ○
Reef ★★☆
Fauna ★★☆

Access 8mi (13km) from Key Largo

Level Open Water

Location Key Largo
GPS   HR1 25° 08.313'N, 80° 17.690'W
       HR2 25° 08.383'N, 80° 17.644'W

Getting there

Horseshoe Reef is a large patch reef located due west of Elbow Reef, and just northwest of nearby North North Dry Rocks. The reef is just a 25-minute boat ride from Key Largo.

Access

Horseshoe Reef is only accessible by boat given its distance from shore. This site is suitable fo divers and snorkelers of all levels and is sheltere from most currents by Elbow Reef. Boats tie up to either of the two buoys on the site to avoi damaging the bottom.

Description

Horseshoe Reef is a popular site for snorkeler as it boasts a maximum depth of just 25 feet (meters), which puts the entire site generall within view of the surface. The site boast colorful corals, including large stands of elkhor coral and an abundance of sea fans and othe soft corals. The colors really pop at this site du to its shallow nature, making it popular wit

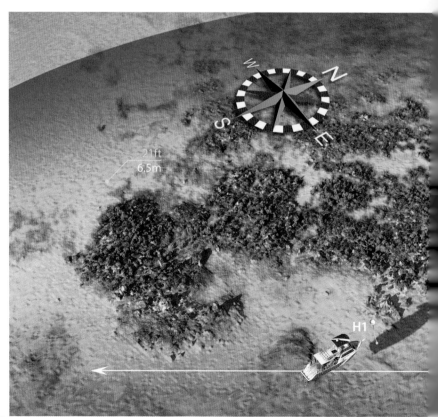

21ft
6.5m

H1

underwater photographers. Visibility can be poor when the weather picks up and waves stir up the sediment. But after a few days of calm, the water at this shallow site can become crystal clear.

Despite the shallowness, the reef offers a great deal of complexity and is widely considered one of the best shallow sites in the Keys. Scuba divers and more adventurous snorkelers can explore the site's many swim-throughs and crevices that shelter schools of silversides. These small fish attract larger predatory fishes, making this site a great place to see a wide range of fish species, including goliath grouper.

One explanation for the site's name is that Horseshoe Reef is rumored to have caused a vessel carrying golden horseshoes to run aground. The rumor is false, but it has still led many divers to search for these artifacts in the past, often leaving their mark on the reef and surrounding seabed. Please remember to maintain neutral buoyancy during your visit to this reef and leave anything you find on the substrate.

ECO TIP

It is illegal to disturb a site or recover artifacts located within a National Marine Sanctuary without a permit. Even if you see what you think might be garbage on the reef, do not pick it up or otherwise bring it to the surface. Staff at Blue Star dive operators in the Keys are specifically trained to identify what is a piece of debris and what is a natural or protected object that should not be disturbed. You can point out debris to your dive master to ask whether it can or should be removed from the reef. When in doubt, leave it where it is. If you are interested in helping clean up the reef, many operators conduct Dive Against Debris trips throughout the year, which often includes volunteers. Please dive responsibly to protect these precious underwater resources for future generations to enjoy.

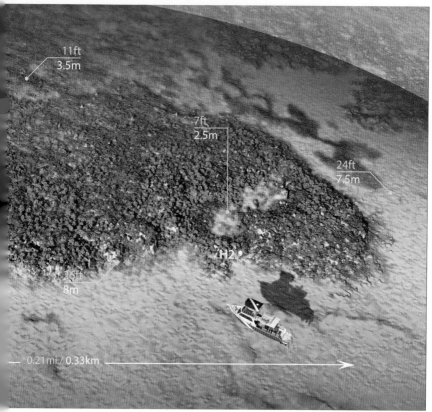

NORTH NORTH DRY ROCKS & NORTH DRY ROCKS

Difficulty ● ○ ○
Current ● ○ ○
Depth ● ○ ○
Reef ★★★☆
Fauna ★☆☆

Access 🚤 7mi (11km) from Key Largo

Level Open Water

Location Key Largo
GPS   NNDR1 25° 08.170'N, 80° 17.392'W
         NNDR2 25° 08.185'N, 80° 17.361'W
         NNDR3 25° 08.210'N, 80° 17.331'W

         NDR1 25° 07.755'N, 80° 17.613'W
         NDR2 25° 07.799'N, 80° 17.613'W
         NDR3 25° 07.835'N, 80° 17.655'W

Getting there
North North Dry Rocks (sometimes called Double North) and North Dry Rocks are two adjacent patch reefs that sit just north of the more famous Dry Rocks Reef. The reef is just a 25-minute boat ride from Key Largo.

Access
These reefs are only accessible by boat given their distance from shore. They are suitable for divers

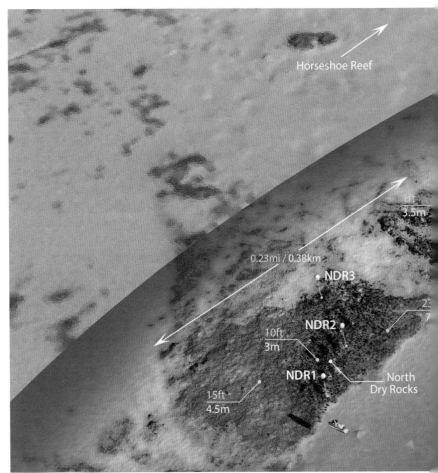

and snorkelers of all levels and are sheltered from most currents by Elbow Reef. Boats should tie up to the designated mooring buoys that are present along both sites to avoid damaging the reef.

Description

These creatively named adjacent patch reefs form a mile-long (1.5-kilometer) stretch of coral reef in the more sheltered inner reef line found in Hawk Channel, which runs between the Key Largo shoreline and the outer reef line. Situated to the west of Elbow Reef, North North Dry Rocks and North Dry Rocks have less current but can be subjected to reduced visibility given the shallowness of the water and the potential for sandy sediments to get stirred up during high wind and wave events.

Patch reefs in this area are often called "middle ground" reefs by local operators, as they are located in the shallow area between the exposed outer reef line and the more protected Hawk Channel. The maximum depth along the line of reefs at these two sites is a fairly consistent 20 feet (6 meters) among the coral reef and rubble areas. However, the seabed can get down to as deep as 34 feet (10.5 meters) in areas that are farther away from the reef.

These two adjacent sites are popular with less experienced divers because of their shallowness. Snorkelers like visiting these sites as marine life typically congregates around the shallow corals, which makes them easy to observe from the surface. Benthic reef fish are the most common species spotted by divers and snorkelers at these sites, including blue tangs, sergeant majors, gray, Queen and French angelfish and a variety of grunt species, most commonly bluestriped and French. Barracudas have been known to cruise the reef, while stingrays are sometimes spotted in sandy areas.

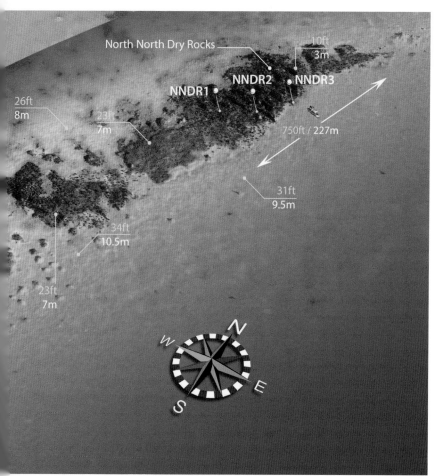

DRY ROCKS & CHRIST OF THE ABYSS

Difficulty ● ○ ○
Current ● ○ ○
Depth ● ○ ○
Reef ★★★☆
Fauna ★★☆

Access 🛥 7mi (11km) from Key Largo

Level Open Water

Location Key Largo

GPS	
DR1	25° 07.328'N, 80° 17.882'W
DR2	25° 07.333'N, 80° 17.858'W
DR3	25° 07.345'N, 80° 17.840'W
DR4	25° 07.365'N, 80° 17.829'W
DR5	25° 07.378'N, 80° 17.824'W
DR6	25° 07.405'N, 80° 17.817'W
DR7	25° 07.432'N, 80° 17.819'W
DR8	25° 07.452'N, 80° 17.833'W
DR9	25° 07.471'N, 80° 17.843'W
DR10	25° 07.498'N, 80° 17.864'W
DR11	25° 07.499'N, 80° 17.911'W
DR12	25° 07.476'N, 80° 17.945'W
DR13	25° 07.426'N, 80° 17.959'W
DR14	25° 07.368'N, 80° 17.935'W
DR15	25° 07.342'N, 80° 17.915'W

Getting there

Dry Rocks Reef is also called Key Largo Dry Rocks to differentiate it from the popular East and West Dry Rocks located near Key West. This large palm shaped reef sits on the inner reef line just slightly to the north of another popular reef site near Key Largo named Grecian Rocks. The reef is located just a 25-minute boat ride from Key Largo.

Access

Dry Rocks Reef is only accessible by boat given its distance from shore. The site is suitable for divers and snorkelers of all levels and is sheltered from strong currents by the shelf that extends seaward to the outer reef line. Boats generally tie up to one of the 15 mooring buoys that encircle the reef and vessels should not attempt to transit the reef as it is shallow enough to pose a serious grounding risk. There is no fishing of any kind allowed at the Key Largo Dry Rocks, as it is protected by a Sanctuary Preservation Area (SPA).

Description

Dry Rocks gets its name from the shallowness of the reef. It rises to about sea level in some places, thus leaving "dry rocks" visible during low tide. The reef measures just over 0.2 miles

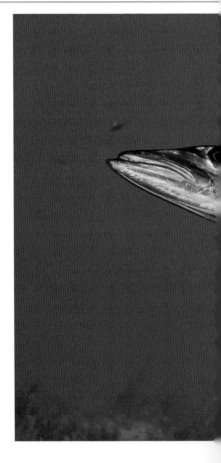

(300 meters) from north to south and feature pronounced spurs that extend seaward, li the fingers of a hand, with sand and rubbl bottomed grooves between. A dense covering corals and sea fans along the tops of the shallc spurs makes this one of the most popular ree in the Key Largo area and interesting to explc for both divers and snorkelers. In fact, the si is particularly well known for its healthy bra corals. The main attraction of the Key Largo C Rocks, however, is without question, the Chr of the Abyss statue located at the southern e of the reef.

The statue is nestled in a rubble-bottomed groove that is open to the sand in between buoys DR3 and DR4. Many published GPS coordinates place the statue in the northern part of the reef, often out in the sand. However, the correct placement is 25° 07.359'N, 80° 17.857'W, and the statue is usually marked by a pencil buoy.

The 400-pound (181-kilogram) bronze statue has a square, three-tiered, multi-ton concrete base that anchors it to the seabed at a depth of around 23 feet (7 meters). The statue stands 8.5 feet (2.5 meters) tall and depicts Jesus Christ standing with his arms outstretched toward the surface and his head tilted back slightly. It is a copy of the original bronze statue "Il Christo Degli Abissi" (Italian for Christ of the Abyss) created by the artist Guido Galletti, which sits off the coast of Italy near Portofino in the Mediterranean Sea. The original marks the

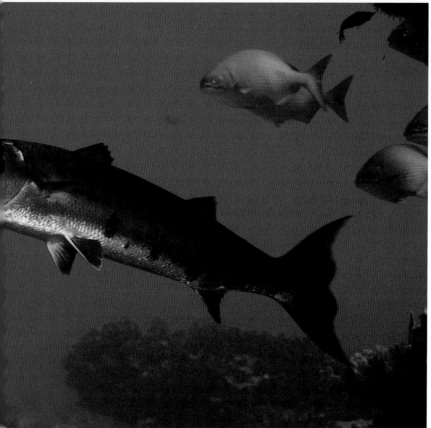

Image Source Trading Ltd/Shutterstock©

 Barracuda often hang out near the statue of the Christ of the Abyss.

DID YOU KNOW? ❓

The second casting of the Christ of the Abyss statue sits in St. George's Harbor in Grenada. It was placed there to commemorate the survivors of the Italian passenger ship *Bianca C* that caught fire in 1961 while anchored in the Grenada port. Local fishermen were able to rescue all 700 passengers and most of the crew. Only one crew member died and that was during the initial engine-room explosions that set the ship on fire. Fortunately, a nearby British frigate was able to tow the burning wreck away from the mouth of the harbor to her current resting place in the Bay just off the popular Grand Anse Beach. The fire burned through the tow lines before the wreck could be moved to a safer place, but the efforts still prevented the massive liner from blocking the entrance to the island's main harbor.

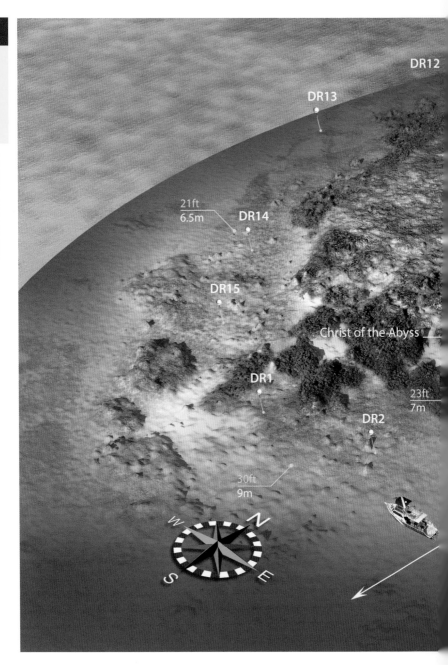

DR12

DR13

21ft
6.5m

DR14

DR15

Christ of the Abyss

DR1

23ft
7m

DR2

30ft
9m

spot where Dario Gonzatti, a diving pioneer in Italy, died in 1947. The Key Largo statue is the third statue to be cast from the original mold, and it was commissioned in 1961 by the dive equipment manufacturer Egidi Cressi. He gifted the statue to the Underwater Society of America, and it has rested at Dry Rocks Reef ever since it was placed there in August 1965.

The statue has become heavily encrusted corals over the many decades spent underwa including patches of fire coral that can st unprotected skin. In a way the statue mirr the health of the surrounding reef, which covered extensively by hard and soft corals. complex structure supports a variety of species, including snapper, hogfish, damself

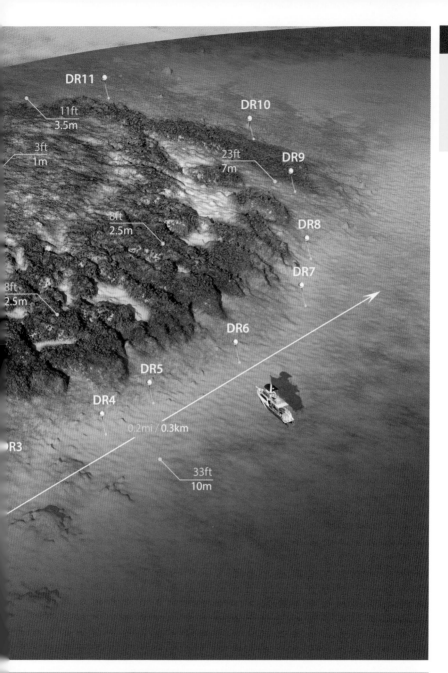

DR11
11ft
3.5m

DR10

3ft
1m

23ft
7m

DR9

8ft
2.5m

DR8

DR7

8ft
2.5m

DR6

DR5

DR4

0.2mi / 0.3km

R3

33ft
10m

ECO TIP

It is popular to try to swim down to touch the statue's outstretched hands. Not only is this not advised as the statue is covered in fire coral that can sting unprotected skin, but it can also damage the delicate corals that have colonized the surface of the statue. Be sure to keep a safe distance from both natural and artificial reefs – this not only keeps the benthic marine life healthy, but also allows everyone a chance to experience the statue for themselves.

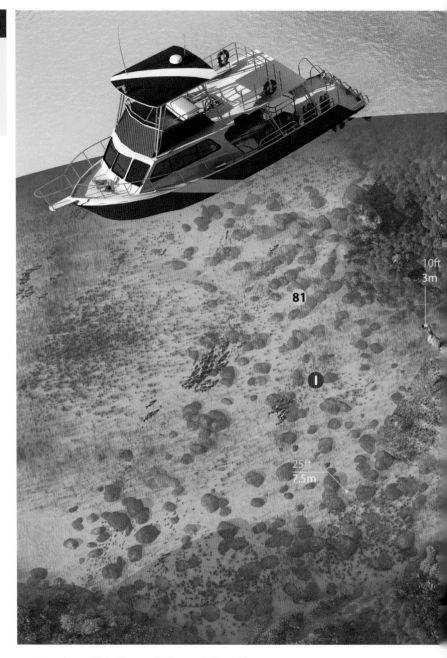

81

10ft
3m

25ft
7.5m

grunts and angelfish. Barracuda frequent the site, and divers and snorkelers often describe a particularly "friendly" individual that visits the statue on a regular basis. Butterflyfish and parrotfish can be found along the edges of the spurs while stingrays may be spotted hiding in the sandy bottoms of some of the grooves.

Route

The best route will depend on which buoy t dive boat ties up to. Snorkelers will want head toward the middle of the reef where t water is shallower, while divers should consid exploring the deeper grooves. Althou not generally subject to a lot of current, t shallow nature of the reef along the tops of t

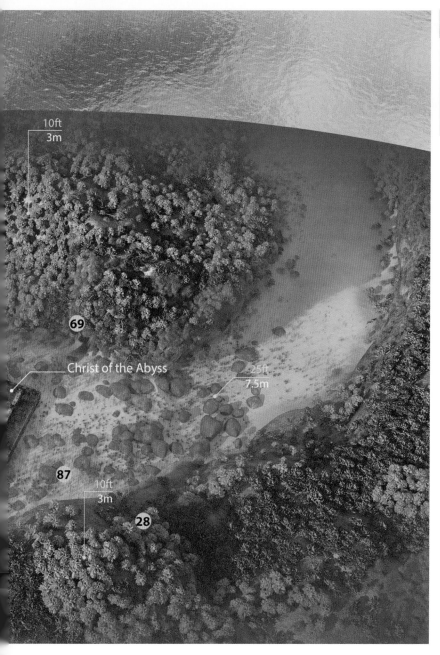

10ft
3m

69

Christ of the Abyss

25ft
7.5m

87

10ft
3m

28

urs means that divers and snorkelers may
xperience wave surge at times.

EMERALD LAGOON

Difficulty ● ○ ○
Current ● ○ ○
Depth ● ○ ○
Reef ★★☆
Fauna ★☆☆

Level Open Water

Location Key Largo
GPS   GPS 25° 07.996'N, 80° 23.946'W

Getting there

Jules' Undersea Lodge and the Emerald Lagoon are located just north of the John Pennekamp Coral Reef State Park. When traveling north on the Overseas Highway turn right onto Transylvania Avenue, which is just

0.5 miles (0.8 kilometers) past the entrance to the Pennekamp State Park. If traveling south on the Overseas Highway, turn left onto Transylvania Avenue just 0.31 miles (0.5 kilometers) after crossing over the Marvin Adams Waterway – the narrow canal that connects the bay side to the ocean side of Key Largo. There is no light at this turn, so be careful of oncoming traffic. Head east along Transylvania Avenue until it ends at Shoreline Drive after 0.42 miles (0.67 kilometers). The

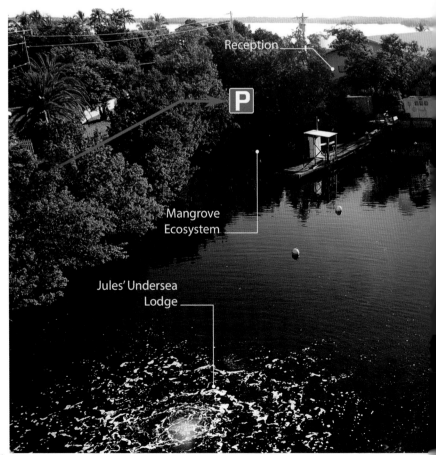

Reception

P

Mangrove
Ecosystem

Jules' Undersea
Lodge

entry to the property is on your right as you come to the end of Transylvania Avenue. The official address is 51 Shoreland Drive, Key Largo.

Access

The property surrounding the lagoon is private and there is an entry fee to access the water. Currently, the fee is $15 USD per person for snorkelers and $40 USD per person for divers (prices do not include a 7.5 percent sales tax). The site is open from 8am to 3pm most days except Monday, when it is closed all day, and Tuesday when it closes at 1pm. For more information, check out their website at **Jul.com.**

Description

This site is popular with divers and snorkelers who are looking to get wet when the ocean is too rough due to the weather. It has a maximum depth of 30 feet (9 meters) and offers shelter from the wind and waves, although it is still considered open water. This makes it ideal as an open water diver training location, particular for navigation tests. The site boasts training platforms as well as a marine archaeology exhibit and the MarineLab underwater research and education habitat. Perhaps most interesting to visitors is Jules' Undersea Lodge, which is the world's first underwater hotel. Guests literally scuba dive down to enter the lodge and stay in the underwater bedrooms and common area, complete with a viewing porthole.

Snorkelers and divers will see plenty of fish species in the lagoon, including rainbow parrotfish, barracuda, Atlantic spadefish and bluestriped grunts. Many snapper species frequent the lagoon as well, and there is a section of mangrove habitat in the northwestern corner that is interesting to explore.

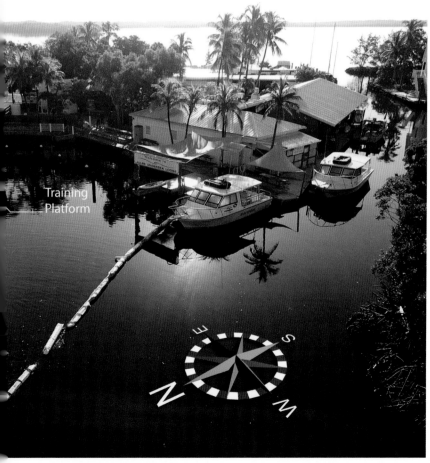

Training Platform

GRECIAN ROCKS

Difficulty ● ○ ○
Current ● ○ ○
Depth ● ○ ○
Reef ★★☆
Fauna ★★☆

Access 🛥 6.5mi (10.5km) from Key Largo

Level Open Water

Location Key Largo

GPS
GR1 25° 06.463'N, 80° 18.420'W
GR2 25° 06.535'N, 80° 18.366'W
GR3 25° 06.557'N, 80° 18.397'W
GR4 25° 06.599'N, 80° 18.404'W
GR5 25° 06.643'N, 80° 18.353'W
GR6 25° 06.658'N, 80° 18.337'W
GR7 25° 06.687'N, 80° 18.324'W
GR8 25° 06.711'N, 80° 18.312'W
GR9 25° 06.745'N, 80° 18.301'W
GR10 25° 06.766'N, 80° 18.285'W
GR11 25° 06.801'N, 80° 18.246'W
GR12 25° 06.591'N, 80° 18.212'W

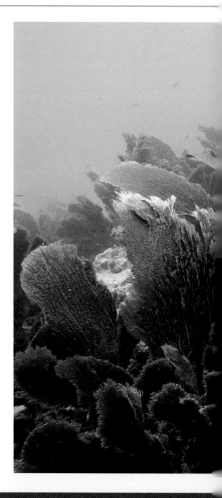

Getting there

Grecian Rocks is another large section of shallow reef located off the coast of Key Largo. The 0.4-mile (0.7-kilometer) reef sits on the inner reef line, often called the "mid-grounds" just to the south of the Key Largo Dry Rocks. The reef is just a 25-minute boat ride from Key Largo.

Access

Grecian Rocks is only accessible by boat given its distance from shore. The reef is suitable for divers and snorkelers of all levels and is largely sheltered from waves and currents. Most of the 12 mooring buoys are located on the shallower west side, however, which makes the reef generally more popular as a destination for snorkeling rather than diving. Even so, the diver-friendly buoy on the deeper eastern side, along with the buoy to the south, remain popular with divers.

DID YOU KNOW?

Sponge diving in the United States began in the early 19th century in Key West. Early boats were known as hook boats because they used poles with a series of hooks, similar to a garden rake, to remove sponges from the shallow reefs. Sponges were big business in the Florida Keys and by 1900 the industry boasted 350 vessels and employed close to 1,500 fishers. Around this time Greek sponge divers who used hard hat diving to collect sponges, started emigrating to the United States and established a sponge diving community in Tarpon Springs, Florida, which developed into the sponge capital of the world.

Description

Grecian Rocks reportedly gets its name from the Greek sponge divers who used to frequent the site to harvest sponges many decades ago. The reef is currently inside a Sanctuary Preservation Area (SPA), which means fishing or other harvesting of any kind is no longer permitted.

The shallow side buoys are anchored in the sand and rubble west of the reef at a depth of around 10 feet (3 meters) with the reef itself getting as shallow as 2 feet (0.5 meters). This shallow reef was once dominated by elkhorn and staghorn corals back in the 1970s, but it is now predominantly covered in sea fans and other soft corals and gorgonians. The shallow reef shelters plenty of fish species, however, including bluestriped and French grunts, blue tangs, stoplight parrotfish and smooth trunkfish. The presence of smaller fish also

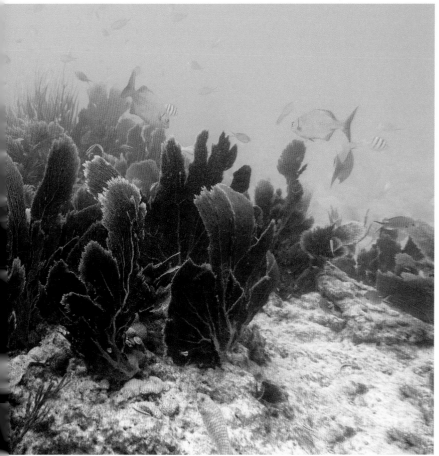

Sea fans dominate the shallow reefs off Key Largo.

means that predatory fish are commonly seen here, including barracuda and some larger grouper.

The lone buoy (GR12) on the eastern side of the reef is anchored at a depth of 30 feet (9 meters) next to a large, healthy patch reef. This site is often called Grecian Proper by local dive operators. Nurse sharks and southern stingrays are regularly seen on this side of the reef, with moray eels hiding in the crevices of the reef. This sheltered site is more dominated by brain and star corals on the patch reef and on the deeper sections of the reef ledge that runs northeast and southwest next to the sand.

The southernmost buoy on the reef (GR1) is called Banana Reef or Banana Patch, and it gets its name from the slope in the reef that matches the shape of a banana. Other named sites include Barracuda

GRECIAN ROCKS

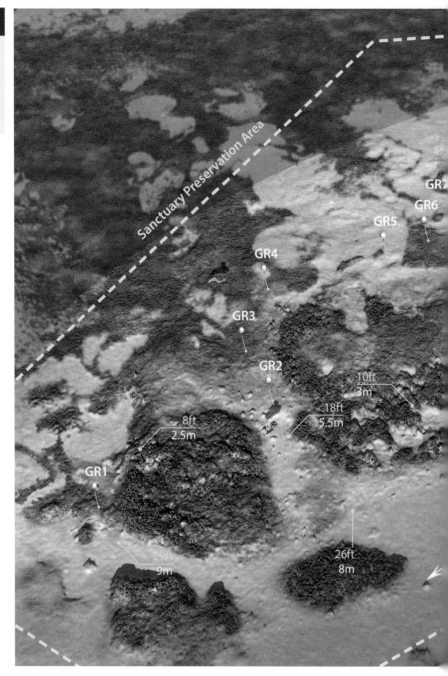

Alley (GR2) and Hamburger Corals, which is a shallow site just to the south of GR1 that gets its name from coral heads that resemble hamburgers.

Route

The best route for exploring the reef will depend on the starting point. For snorkelers, there is plenty to explore along the western edge of the reef. Durin calm weather, the shallow water above the reef ca provide excellent viewing of the ecosystem. Bu during higher wind and swell events, the top of th reef can become surgy and choppy, so snorkeler should steer clear of this area to avoid injury c damaging the fragile reef.

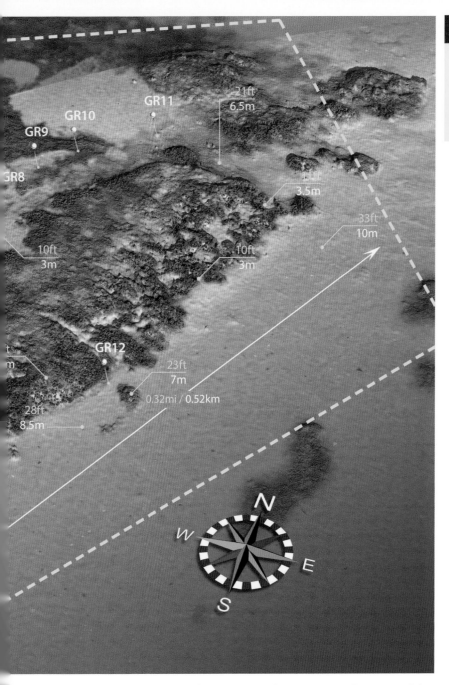

GR11

21ft
6.5m

GR10

GR9

GR8

3.5m

33ft
10m

10ft
3m

10ft
3m

GR12

23ft
7m

0.32mi / 0.52km

28ft
8.5m

he best route for Grecian Proper involves first xploring the patch reef next to the mooring uoy before moving on to explore the edge of the eef and the biodiverse reef-sand transition area. epending on the current, divers can choose to ead north or south along the reef ledge before ooping around to return along the shallower part of the reef. For Banana Patch, most snorkelers explore the southern face of this smaller section of reef, while divers can make their way north to explore the ledge along the larger reef.

JOHN PENNEKAMP CORAL REEF STATE PARK

Difficulty ● ○ ○
Current ● ○ ○
Depth ● ○ ○
Reef ★★☆
Fauna ★☆☆

Access 🚙 2 min from Key Largo
🏊 1 min from shore

Level n/a

Location Key Largo
GPS 25° 07.550'N, 80° 24.317'W

Getting there
This state park is in the middle of Key Largo, on the southeastern (or Atlantic Ocean) side. When heading north on the Overseas Highway, turn right into the park next to the large sign indicating the entrance. For those heading south, there is a dedicated turning lane but no traffic light, so use caution when turning across oncoming traffic. There is a fee station located 0.1 miles (0.16 kilometers) from the highway. Continue another 0.25 miles (0.4 kilometers) to a parking lot on the left. Cannon Beach is the main swimming and snorkeling beach in the park and one of two shore-accessible sites in the park. The official address for the state park is 102601 Overseas Highway, Key Largo (mile-marker 102.5).

Access
Pennekamp State Park has an $8 vehicle fee and $0.50 per person entry fee. The park is open 365 days a year, and provides ample parking, as well as bathroom and shower facilities. Covered picnic tables are also available in the beach area.

Description
John Pennekamp Coral Reef State Park covers 70 square nautical miles (240 square kilometers) and

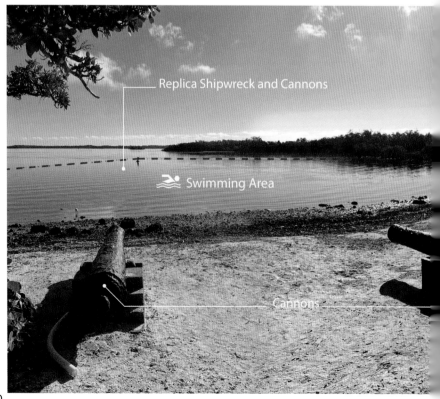

Replica Shipwreck and Cannons

Swimming Area

Cannons

JOHN PENNEKAMP CORAL REEF STATE PARK

extends nearly 3 miles (5 kilometers) offshore. Cannon Beach gets its name from the cannons currently located on the beach. They were discovered on a shipwreck near Carysfort Reef back in the 1930s. Through close examination of the raised designs on the cannons, they were traced back to the *HMS Winchester*. A buoy line marks the swimming area around the beach, which may prove a little shallow for most divers, but snorkelers will still find the water and reef life here interesting. For instance, snorkelers are likely to see gray snapper, French grunts, sergeant majors, bar jacks and hogfish. Given the proximity to the mangroves, these waters also support juveniles of many reef fishes, particularly grunts and snapper, while larger fish, such as barracuda and tarpon, are not uncommon. The second beach is found just beyond Cannon Beach. The aptly named Far Beach is another 0.25 miles (0.4 kilometers) past the parking lot at Cannon Beach. It too has a buoy line that marks the boundaries of the swimming area, and it features many of the same fish species found at Cannon Beach, despite being smaller in area.

The park also features hiking trails, a short boardwalk and miles of kayak and canoe paddling trails. There are a few dive and snorkel sites in Hawk Channel, including Turtle Reef and Three Sisters, which are featured in this book on pages 42 and 105, respectively. But the park's fleet of dive and snorkel boats provide additional access to all the popular dive sites listed for Key Largo, including nearby Dry Rocks, Grecian Rocks and the Spiegel Grove, to name just a few.

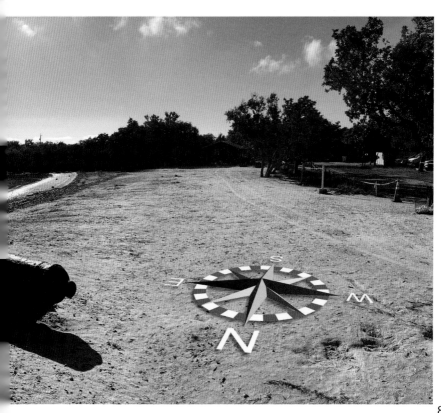

SPIEGEL GROVE

Difficulty ● ● ●
Current ● ● ○
Depth ● ● ●
Reef ★★☆
Fauna ★★★

Access 🚤 8mi (13km) from Key Largo

Level Advanced

Location Key Largo
GPS   25° 03.969'N, 80° 18.735'W

Getting there

Spiegel Grove rests in deep water, just 0.4 miles (0.7 kilometers) beyond the outer reef line and 8 miles (13 kilometers) off the coast of Key Largo. It is a relatively short 30- to 40-minute boat ride to reach the site for most of the local dive operators.

Access

Spiegel Grove is only accessible by boat given its distance from shore. The artificial reef is accessible to advanced divers only because of its depth. The seabed bottoms out at 134 feet (41 meters) while the highest point of the wreck is 72 feet (22 meters) deep. There are usually eight mooring buoys anchored to various parts of the wreck, which provide ample access even during busy dive days when multiple dive boats visit the site.

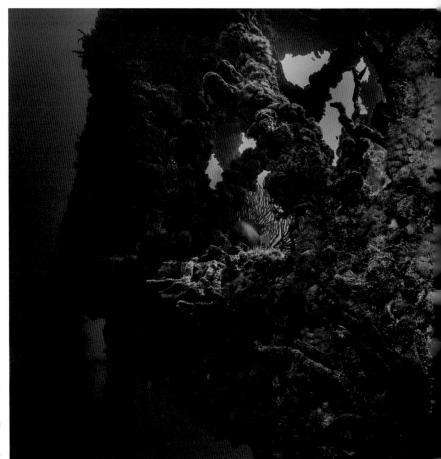

Corals and sponges (and the invasive orange cup corals) cover the crane arms of the *Spiegel Grove*.

RELAX & RECHARGE

The Fish House (102401 Overseas Highway) specializes in fresh seafood, all sourced locally from commercial Keys fishers and filleted on the premises so it is guaranteed to be fresh. Popular dishes include yellowtail snapper, mahi mahi, grouper, lobster and stone crab, served in a range of styles, including blackened, Jamaican Jerk or Matecumbe. The smoked fish is their specialty – smoking is done on the premises – and they can even arrange for smoked fish to be shipped direct to you in case you are still craving their food after you return home. The Fish House has received numerous People's Choice awards over the years, including Best Restaurant and Best Service in the Upper Keys. They have also been voted Best Key Lime Pie in Florida by Florida Living Magazine, so make sure to stay for dessert.
Visit: **Fishhouse.com**

Description

USS Spiegel Grove was originally the fifth of eight Thomaston-class landing ship docks built for the U.S. Navy. She was launched on November 10, 1955, out of Pascagoula, Mississippi, and began her career completing a circuit through the Caribbean before her first major tour in the Mediterranean. She conducted many training and joint operations over her decades of service, operating primarily along the eastern seaboard of the United States and in the Caribbean, but with a brief stint in the Arctic as well. She participated in multiple goodwill tours, including one along the coast of Africa in 1963 and another in the Caribbean in 1981. However, she made the biggest headlines for her role in helping evacuate 282 Americans and other foreign nationals from Beirut in 1976 during the civil war in Lebanon.

She was ultimately decommissioned in October 1989, and eventually transferred to the State of Florida Fish & Wildlife Conservation Commission in 2001 for deployment as an artificial reef off the coast of Key Largo. She was cleaned and prepared for sinking up in Norfolk, Virginia, before being towed down to the Keys. The deployment on May 17, 2002, did not go as planned, however. The vessel started sinking six hours ahead of schedule, forcing the rapid evacuation of her surprised deployment crew who were unable to complete the flooding procedure. As a result, she listed heavily to her starboard side as she sank, leaving her stern touching the bottom while her bow remained floating at the surface due to air trapped in some of her forward holds. She stayed there, floating upside down for a few weeks before crews were able to complete the sinking with the help of air pumps, air bladders and tugs. She finally settled onto the seafloor on her starboard side.

Her story was not over, however. In July 2005, Hurricane Dennis passed just south of the Florida Keys. Winds and currents from the major hurricane were felt throughout the Keys, including east of Key Largo, where they rolled the ship back onto her keel. She now sits upright in the exact position planned in the original deployment, largely parallel to the shoreline with the bow pointing roughly northeast. Her upper decks are accessible to advanced divers, while

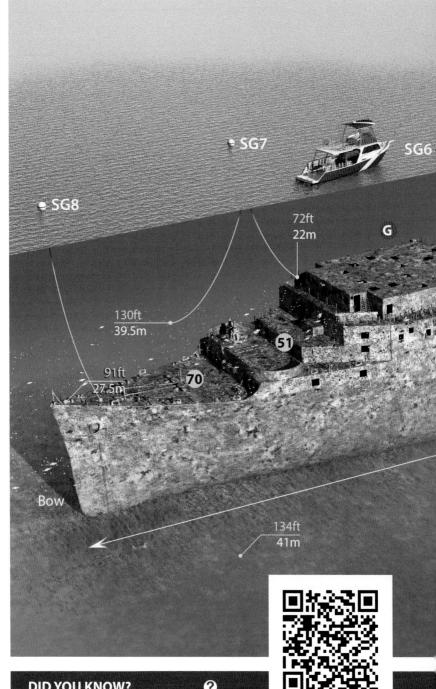

SG7

SG6

SG8

72ft
22m

G

130ft
39.5m

51

91ft
27.5m

70

Bow

134ft
41m

DID YOU KNOW?

Use your phone or tablet to scan this QR code and view a digital three dimensional (3D) model of the Spiegel Grove. You can also use your device to view this 3D model in augmented-reality.

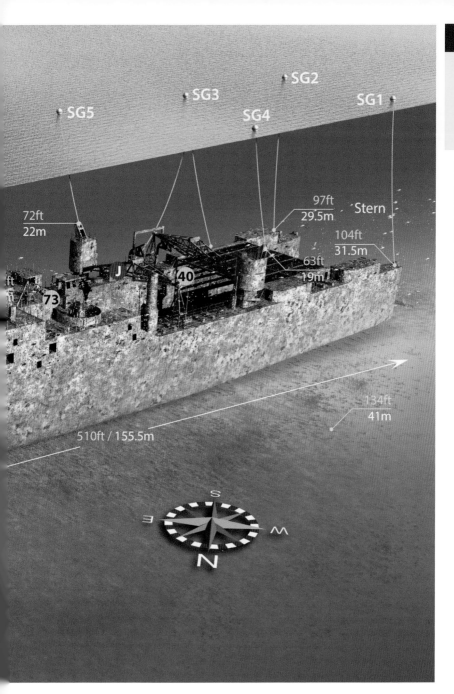

SG2

SG3

SG5

SG4

SG1

97ft
29.5m   Stern

72ft
22m

104ft
31.5m

63ft
19m

ft
n

73

J

40

134ft
41m

510ft / 155.5m

S

E

W

N

her interior and lower decks provide plenty of exploration potential for technical divers using mixed gases.

At the time of her deployment, *Spiegel Grove* was the biggest ship ever deployed as an artificial reef. She is 510 feet (155 meters) in length and offers more than 60 feet (18 meters) of relief off the sandy seafloor. With the many holes cut in her hull and superstructure prior to deployment, there are ample penetration opportunities for those with the necessary experience, including some swim-throughs in the wheelhouse.

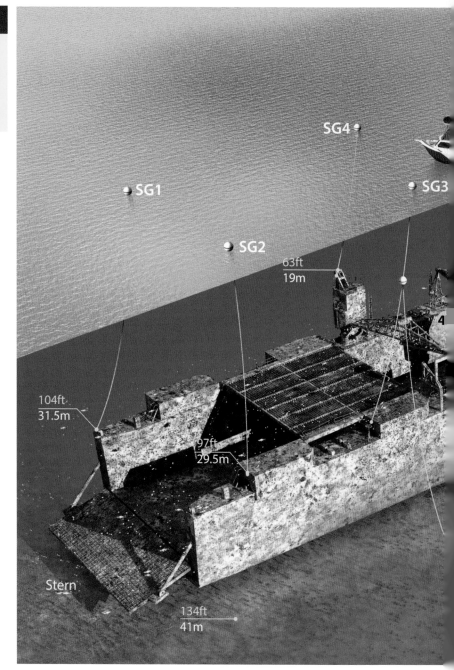

SG4

SG1

SG3

SG2

63ft
19m

104ft
31.5m

97ft
29.5m

Stern

134ft
41m

The massive landing bay will make any diver feel tiny – when in operation, the bay could hold up to nine LCM-8s (landing craft mechanized) or 50 AAVs (assault amphibious vehicles). The tall cranes that span the bay are heavily encrusted with corals and sponges, making them interesting for divers to explore up close. Marine life was quick to colonize the artificial reef, and most of the surfaces of the wreck are well covered. The diversity of the coral cover helps support a variety of reef fish including damselfish, blue tangs, surgeonfish

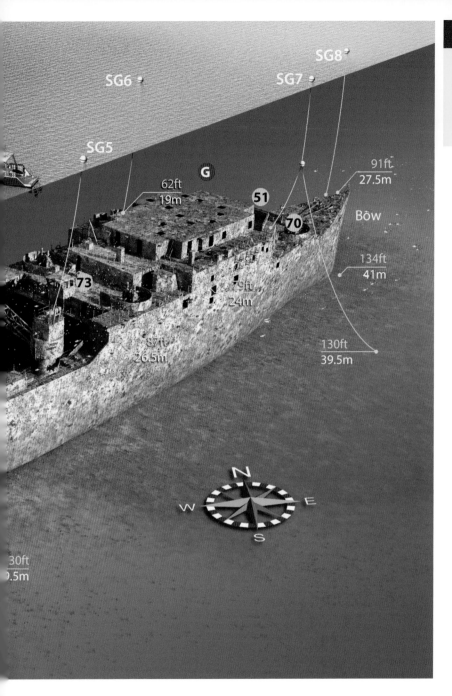

SG8

SG6

SG7

SG5

62ft
19m

G

51

70

91ft
27.5m

Bōw

134ft
41m

73

79ft
24m

87ft
26.5m

130ft
39.5m

N
W   E
S

30ft
9.5m

eef butterflyfish and the rare black-capped basslet. The assortment of smaller species, in turn, support the larger predators that requent the site, including barracuda, goliath grouper and reef sharks. Great hammerheads ave occasionally been spotted here as well.

Route

The best route to explore this site depends largely on the buoy used to access the wreck. It is next to impossible to adequately explore *Spiegel Grove* in a single dive, which is why many operators choose to complete back-to-

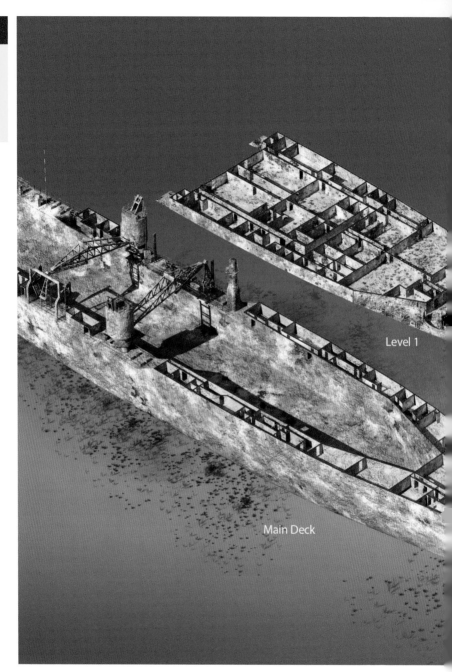

Level 1

Main Deck

back dives on the wreck, which allows for a better, more thorough, exploration of the site.

Tying up to the bow or forward buoys is typically best for dive planning as the current generally runs from the stern toward the bow. Divers can therefore begin their dive by heading into the current, allowing them to drift back and complete their dive by exploring the superstructure or the cranes. The current can be strong at this site, but the high amount of intact structure on the upper decks help provide shelter.

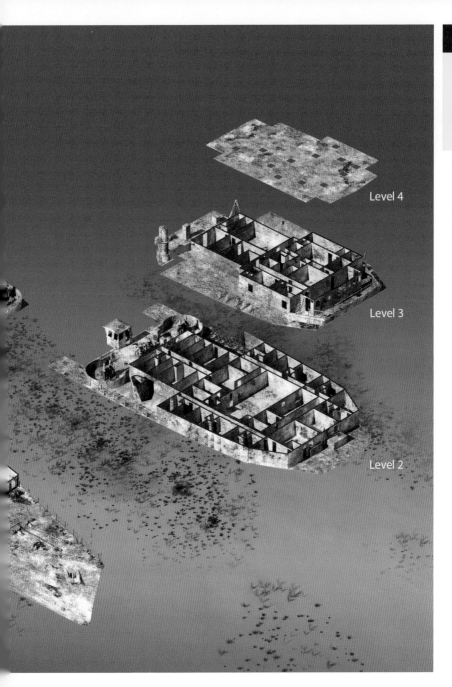

Level 4

Level 3

Level 2

SCIENTIFIC INSIGHT

Orange cup corals (*Tubastraea sp.*) are originally from the Indo-Pacific region. These non-reef building corals were first observed in Puerto Rico and Curacao in 1943. Scientists believe they arrived attached to the hulls of vessels traveling from the Pacific to the Atlantic. Today, these invasive corals have established themselves on many of the wrecks in the Keys, often outcompeting native corals and sponges.

SPIEGEL GROVE

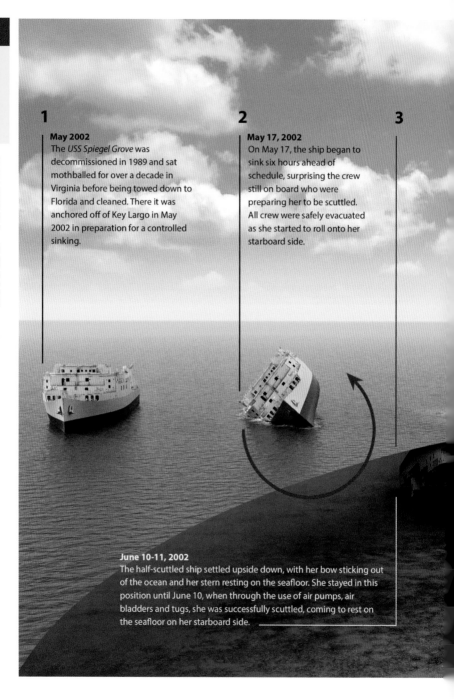

1

May 2002
The USS Spiegel Grove was decommissioned in 1989 and sat mothballed for over a decade in Virginia before being towed down to Florida and cleaned. There it was anchored off of Key Largo in May 2002 in preparation for a controlled sinking.

2

May 17, 2002
On May 17, the ship began to sink six hours ahead of schedule, surprising the crew still on board who were preparing her to be scuttled. All crew were safely evacuated as she started to roll onto her starboard side.

3

June 10-11, 2002
The half-scuttled ship settled upside down, with her bow sticking out of the ocean and her stern resting on the seafloor. She stayed in this position until June 10, when through the use of air pumps, air bladders and tugs, she was successfully scuttled, coming to rest on the seafloor on her starboard side.

4

June 26, 2002
The *Spiegel Grove* was opened to recreational divers on June 26. At the time, she was the biggest ship to be purposefully sunk in order to create an artificial reef. Divers and marine life took to her quickly, although her significant depth means that only advanced divers can share in the experience.

5

July 2005
Hurricane Dennis passed to the west of the Keys in early July. The hurricane caused minor damage to the Keys but in a stroke of luck, the currents generated by the hurricane shifted the wreck onto her keel and into the position originally intended when she was first scuttled.

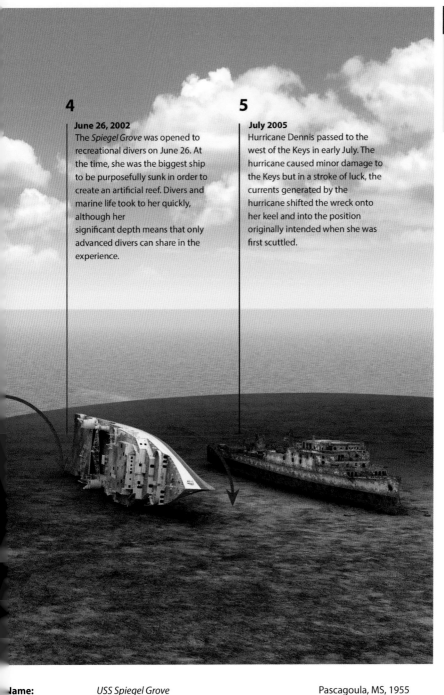

Name:	*USS Spiegel Grove*		Pascagoula, MS, 1955
Type:	Landing Ship	**Last owner:**	U.S. Navy
Previous names:	*LSD-32*	**Sunk:**	May 17, 2002
Length:	510ft (155m)		
Tonnage:	8,899t (11,300t fully loaded)		
Construction:	Ingalls Shipbuilding Corp,		

BENWOOD

Difficulty ● ○ ○
Current ● ○ ○
Depth ● ○ ○
Reef ★★★
Fauna ★★☆

Access 🚤 7.5mi (12km) from Key Largo

Level Open Water

Location Key Largo
GPS
BW1 25° 03.128'N, 80° 19.920'W
BW2 25° 03.141'N, 80° 19.936'W
BW3 25° 03.158'N, 80° 19.916'W
BW4 25° 03.166'N, 80° 19.950'W
BW5 25° 03.158'N, 80° 19.972'W
BW6 25° 03.139'N, 80° 20.026'W

Getting there

Benwood rests in shallow water right on the edge of the outer reef line, just 6.5 miles (10.5 kilometers) off the coast of Key Largo. Reaching the wreck site requires a boat ride of about 30 to 40 minutes via most of the local dive operators.

Access

Benwood is only accessible by boat given its distance from shore. The wreck is suitable for

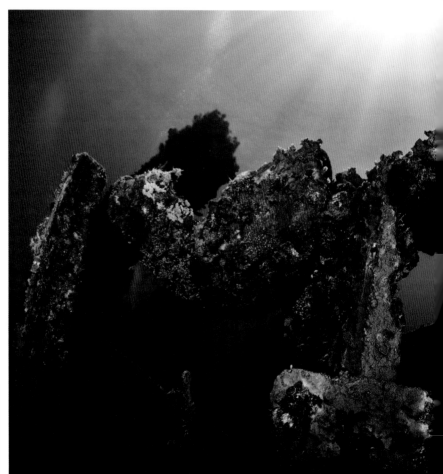

Sea fans and encrusting corals and algae coat the wreck of the *Benwood*.

SCIENTIFIC INSIGHT

Over the years, Florida has lost more than 90 percent of its total coral cover. A 2019 study conducted in the Florida Keys by the Harbor Branch Oceanographic Institute and University of South Florida concluded that nutrient pollution from coast development was a primary factor in coral loss in that area, but disease and overfishing can also play a significant role. Disease is the major cause in the loss of the beautiful branching elkhorn and staghorn corals, some of which can be found at *Benwood*. Great strides are being made to restore these species to Caribbean reefs by various coral restoration programs.

divers of all levels as its sits at a depth of just 5 feet (14 meters). However, the wreck offers just a few feet of relief from the bottom, so it is challenging for most snorkelers to explore. The site has six mooring buoys spaced around the edge of the site.

Description

S *Benwood* was originally a British-built

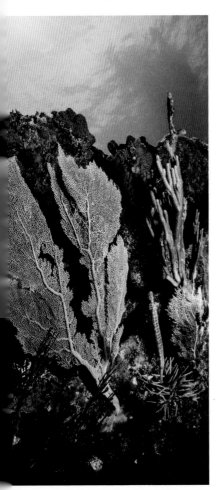

Norwegian merchant freighter. She was reportedly sailing north along the coast of Florida on the night of April 9, 1942, without the use of running lights, which was common during the Second World War to avoid the attention of prowling German U-boats. Unfortunately, the much larger *Robert C Tuttle* was traveling southbound along the coast, also without lights. According to the reports of the time, both captains saw a dark object ahead and signaled that they were turning. The *Tuttle* allegedly turned to starboard, and the *Benwood* turned to port, which placed them on a collision course. At the last minute, the captain of the *Benwood* ordered a full reverse of the engines, but it was too late: the *Benwood* hit the *Tuttle* on the latter ship's port side.

Benwood's bow crumpled, and she started taking on water quickly. Her captain attempted to steer the ship toward shore in order to ground her, but she only made it as far as the reef line before foundering. Her crew abandoned ship with all hands accounted for, and the ship sank to the bottom with her stern pointing toward shore at a depth of 25 feet (7.5 meters) and her large upright bow section pointing out to sea at a depth of 45 feet (14 meters).

The wreck of the *Benwood* is located just north of French reef. The debris field includes many identifiable elements, including hull plates, bracket frames, an engine mount a crank and an internal buklhead. The bow section remains upright and is the tallest part of wreck, rising up nearly 20 feet (6 meters) off the seabed and reaching a depth of 28 feet (8.5 meters). Her bow anchor was partially uncovered by currents from Hurricane Irma in 2017.

The site has become well colonized with corals, mostly encrusting corals and gorgonians. Divers will see plenty of sergeant majors on the site, along with porkfish, yellowtail snapper, blue tangs, bicolor damselfish and brown chromis. Atlantic trumpetfish can be seen hanging vertically in the water column as they hunt next to the soft corals, while spotted moray eels and

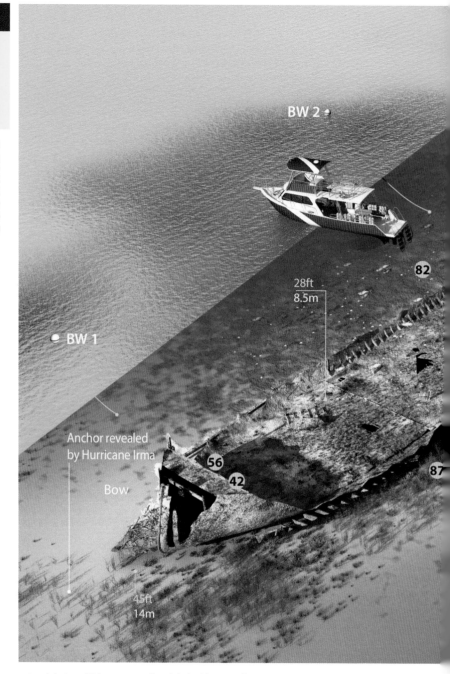

BW 2

82

28ft
8.5m

BW 1

Anchor revealed
by Hurricane Irma

56

Bow

42

87

45ft
14m

spiny lobsters hide among the debris. Nurse sharks are frequently seen resting against the hull plates scattered around the site, while a stand of elkhorn coral can be found near the stern. *Benwood* is also popular with divers as she is one of nine wrecks on the Florida Keys National Marine Sanctuary Shipwreck Trail.

Route

While debris covers a large area of the site, shallow nature means there is plenty of botto time to explore every nook and cranny. Mc divers make their way around the site in a circu pattern, with their starting point chosen based c

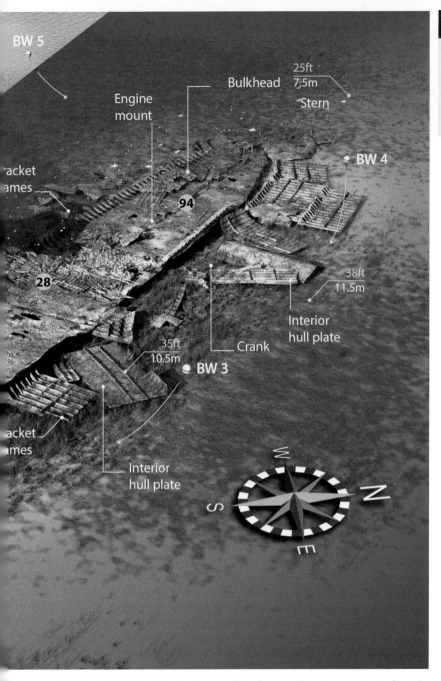

BW 5

Engine mount

Bulkhead

25ft
7.5m

Stern

BW 4

acket
ames

94

28

38ft
11.5m

Interior
hull plate

35ft
10.5m

Crank

BW 3

acket
ames

Interior
hull plate

hatever mooring buoy their dive boat has tied to. ter exploring the wreck, some divers choose to sit the ledges located just shoreward of the stern. ᵼother option is to explore the steep slope known Benwood Wall, which is located about 330 feet 00 meters) seaward of the ship's bow. However, s feature is a significant swim from the wreck

and is often considered a separate site from the *Benwood* itself.

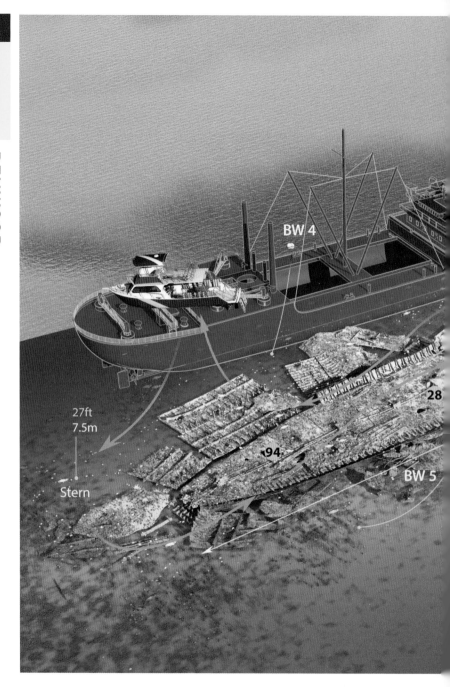

BW 4

27ft
7.5m

Stern

94

28

BW 5

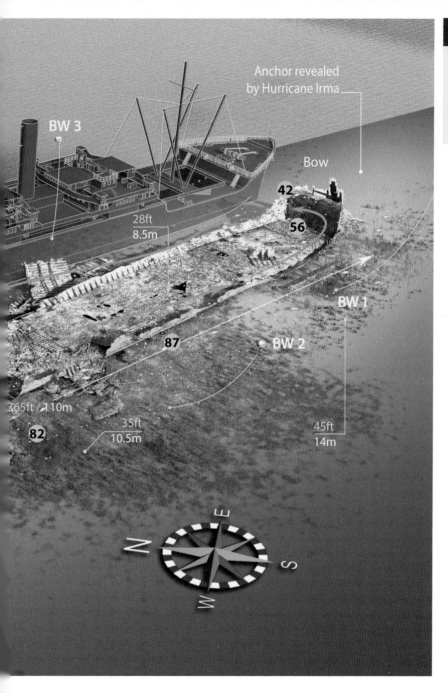

Anchor revealed by Hurricane Irma

BW 3

Bow

42

56

28ft
8.5m

BW 1

87

BW 2

365ft / 110m

82

35ft
10.5m

45ft
14m

ame:	SS Benwood		Stockton-on-Tees, UK, 1910
pe:	Cargo ship	Last owner:	Skejelbred, O.A.T. Rederi
evious names:	n/a		A/S Kristiansand
ngth:	365ft (109m)	Sunk:	April 9, 1942
nnage:	3,931 grt		
nstruction:	Craig, Taylor & Co.,		

97

FRENCH REEF

Difficulty ● ○ ○
Current ● ○ ○
Depth ● ○ ○
Reef ★★☆
Fauna ★★☆

Access 🚤 7.5mi (12km) from Key Largo

Level Open Water

Location Key Largo
GPS   FR1 25° 01.980'N, 80° 20.981'W
       FR2 25° 02.007'N, 80° 20.964'W
       FR3 25° 02.020'N, 80° 20.939'W
       FR4 25° 02.049'N, 80° 20.913'W
       FR5 25° 02.057'N, 80° 20.893'W
       FR6 25° 02.069'N, 80° 20.877'W
       FR7 25° 02.113'N, 80° 20.873'W
       FR8 25° 02.147'N, 80° 20.855'W
       FR9 25° 02.173'N, 80° 20.839'W
       FR10 25° 02.162'N, 80° 20.760'W
       FR11 25° 02.044'N, 80° 20.824'W
       FR12 25° 02.006'N, 80° 20.867'W
       FR13 25° 02.025'N, 80° 20.908'W
       FR14 25° 02.092'N, 80° 20.916'W
       FR15 25° 02.059'N, 80° 20.953'W
       FR16 25° 02.034'N, 80° 20.980'W
       FR17 25° 02.014'N, 80° 21.007'W
       FR18 25° 01.987'N, 80° 20.945'W
       FR19 25° 02.323'N, 80° 20.691'W
       FR20 25° 02.232'N, 80° 20.606'W

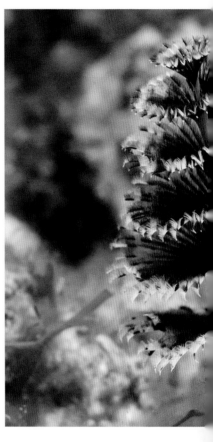

Getting there

French Reef is a large section of relatively shallow reef located 6 miles (9.5 kilometers) off the coast of Key Largo. The entire reef system stretches nearly a mile (0.8 kilometers) along the outer reef line, just north of the popular Molasses Reef. The reef is located about a 30- to 40-minute boat ride from Key Largo.

Access

French Reef is only accessible by boat given its distance from shore. The reef is suitable for divers and snorkelers of all levels although currents can sometimes prove challenging as the reef is located on the edge of the shelf that runs parallel to the coast. As many as 25 mooring buoys are concentrated along a 0.3-mile (0.5-kilometer) stretch of spur and groove habitat located in the middle of the reef.

Description

French Reef sits inside a Sanctuary Preservation Area (SPA), which means fishing and harvesting of any kind is not permitted. The remains of

Totten Beacon "G," once an important navigation beacon for ships, can be found in shallow wate just seaward of the shoal. These remains are rare explored, however, as they are located too far fro the well-developed spur and groove area of th reef where divers and snorkelers typically spen most of their time.

The grooves on French Reef are particular interesting for divers as the sand has been washe away in many sections, allowing divers to swi beneath the spurs and into large, open "cave Many of the sites at French Reef are named aft the caves found nearby, such as Sand Botto

Cave (FR5), Hourglass Cave (FR1) and Christmas Tree Cave (FR3). The latter is depicted on page 102 of this guidebook. While not true caves, these formations are more like swim-throughs so only those experienced with overhead environments and good buoyancy should enter them.

The reef itself is dominated by soft corals, including sea fans and other gorgonians. Small heads of hard corals such as brain and star corals are scattered around the complex structures of the spurs, providing shelter to a variety of reef fish species. Divers and snorkelers may see blue, stoplight and Queen parrotfishes, alongside various species of surgeonfish and damselfish. Sergeant majors dance above the reef while glassy sweepers are often spotted schooling in the shadows of the reef's many swim-throughs. Nurse sharks are also commonly seen here, as they are along many of the reefs in the Florida Keys and lucky visitors

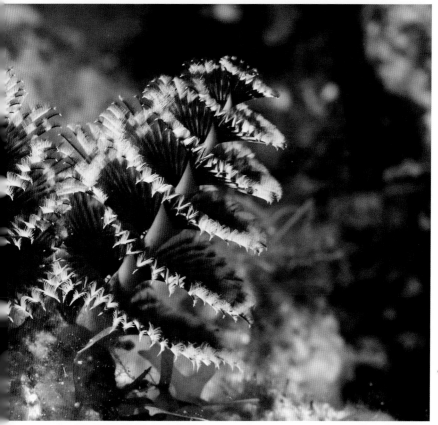

Christmas tree worms are common on French Reef and even lend their name to a popular cave.

SCIENTIFIC INSIGHT

Parrotfish are a common sight on many shallow reefs throughout the Caribbean, including those found in the Florida Keys. They feed by literally breaking off pieces of reef with their powerful beak-like teeth and crushing them into sand to access the algae. Scientists have determined that parrotfish teeth consist of hundreds of tiny fibers woven together into a single fused structure that represents one of the toughest biominerals on the planet. The sand that parrotfish produce through their feeding is excreted onto the reef and ultimately becomes the beaches that we love to relax on during our vacations in tropical countries. Research has shown that each parrotfish can produce a huge amount of sand per year: depending on the species, between 200 and 1,000 pounds (91 and 454 kilograms) of coral sand per year, per fish.

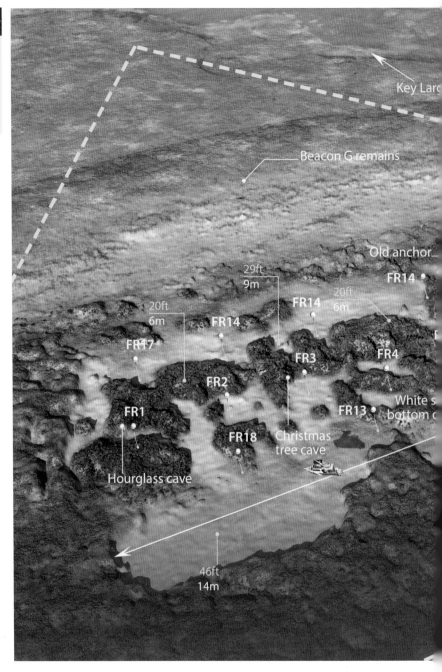

Key Largo

Beacon G remains

Old anchor

29ft
9m

20ft
6m

FR14

20ft
6m

FR14

FR17

FR14

FR3

FR4

FR2

White s
bottom c

FR1

FR13

FR18

Christmas
tree cave

Hourglass cave

46ft
14m

may also spot eagle rays and loggerhead turtles cruising through the site.

The tops of the reef spurs generally reach a depth of around 20 feet (6 meters), but some sections extend as shallow as 16 feet (5 meters) or less, such as the section of spur above the Christmas

Tree Cave. The rubble bottom that covers most the reef averages between 30 and 35 feet (9 a 10.5 meters) which makes French Reef deep than some of the mid-ground reefs farther to t north. However, it is still within easy viewing of t surface by snorkelers.

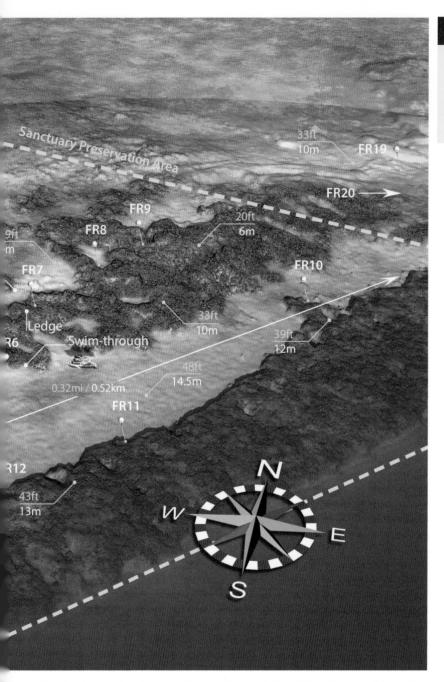

Sanctuary Preservation Area

33ft
10m   FR19

FR20 →

FR9

20ft
6m

FR8

9ft
m

FR10

FR7

Ledge

33ft
10m

39ft
12m

R6   Swim-through

48ft
14.5m

0.32mi / 0.52km

FR11

R12

43ft
13m

N
W   E
S

ristmas Tree Cave is a popular swim-through on
nch Reef. The formation is located just 50 feet
meters) west of the anchor point for mooring
by FR3. The spur here runs roughly north to
th, getting thinner as it tapers to a point in the
ble groove that bounds it on both sides. The
ry point to the swim-through is marked by a

tall mound of coral that rises toward the surface
of the water, while the spur itself remains heavily
undercut where it meets the sand. The swim
through is short – only around 15 to 20 feet (4.5 to 6
meters) in length. It is tight enough that divers can
only pass through in single file. Light from the exit
is visible as divers enter the swim-through, which

CHRISTMAS TREE CAVE

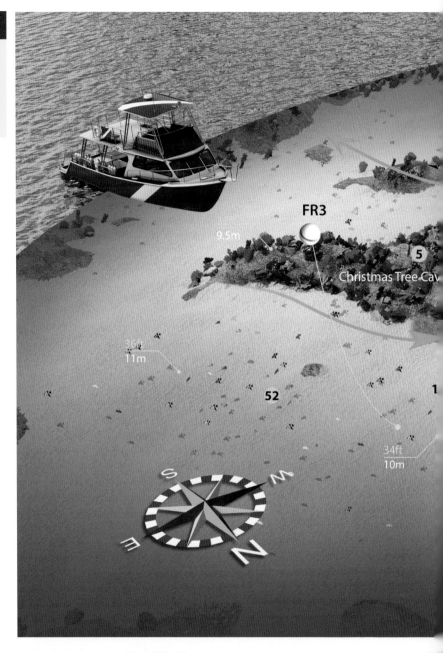

FR3

9.5m

5

Christmas Tree Cave

36ft
11m

52

1

34ft
10m

DID YOU KNOW?

The name of this site comes from the many Christmas Tree worms that cover the surrounding spurs. These marine worms feed with hair-like appendages that protrude from its body. When deployed, these appendages have a striking similarity to colorful little Christmas trees. However, when startled they retract their appendages and are often hard to differentiate from other small holes in the reef.

CHRISTMAS TREE CAVE

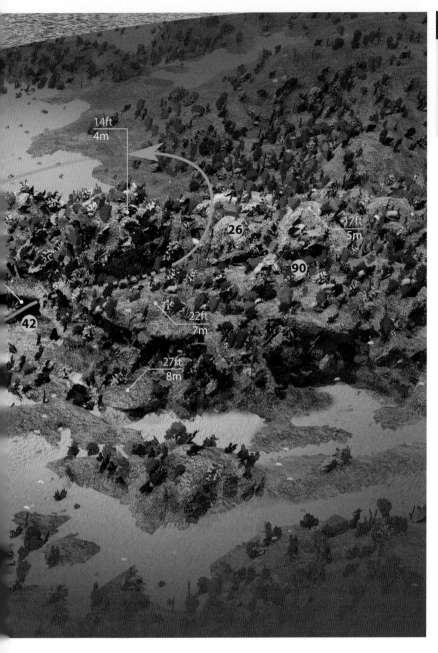

14ft
4m

26

17ft
5m

90

42

22ft
7m

27ft
8m

plifies navigation. However, neutral buoyancy essential to traverse the swim-through without maging the reef.

ute

ers can explore wherever they wish at French f. It does not matter what buoy is used, as most relatively close to one another, allowing divers d snorkelers to explore two or three buoys in

either direction. When exploring Christmas Tree Cave, it is easier to explore the swim-through by first entering from the open space adjacent to the mooring buoy anchor. The reverse direction requires more buoyancy control and care to not damage the fragile corals surrounding the exit points, as it involves swimming downward then taking a relatively sharp turn to exit onto the flat rubble groove by the mooring buoy.

WHITE BANKS

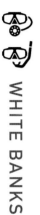

Difficulty	● ○ ○
Current	● ○ ○
Depth	● ○ ○
Reef	★★☆
Fauna	★★☆

Access

7.5mi (12km) from Key Largo

Level Open water

Location Key Largo
GPS   WB1 25° 02.332'N, 80° 22.400'W
       WB2 25° 02.405'N, 80° 22.359'W
       WB3 25° 02.431'N, 80° 22.330'W
       WB4 25° 02.584'N, 80° 22.158'W
       WB5 25° 02.633'N, 80° 22.191'W
       WB6 25° 02.674'N, 80° 22.204'W
       WB7 25° 02.314'N, 80° 22.275'W
       WB8 25° 02.703'N, 80° 22.176'W

Getting there
White Banks is a series of shallow patch reefs that sit nearly 5 miles (8 kilometers) east of Rodriguez Key. Getting there involves a 30- to 40-minute boat ride from Key Largo.

Access
These patch reefs are suitable for divers and snorkelers of all levels. Visibility is sometimes poor but currents are usually mild. White Banks is only accessible by boat due to the distance from shore. There are eight mooring buoys at White banks, which means boats will not need to anchor.

Description
White Banks is more popular as a snorkel site than a dive site, although divers often use it for training and for refresher dives. The tops of the reefs reach as shallow as just 3 feet (1 meter) in some places, while the sand channel between the two main sets of patch reefs drops as deep as 21 feet (6.5 meters). The coral cover is dense with plenty of sea fans and other gorgonians. A scattering of smaller hard corals can also be seen at this site. Because these patch reefs are surrounded by so much sand, they act as small islands of biodiversity. The reefs are home to plenty of surgeonfish, sergeant majors, yellowtail snapper and barracuda, among other species.

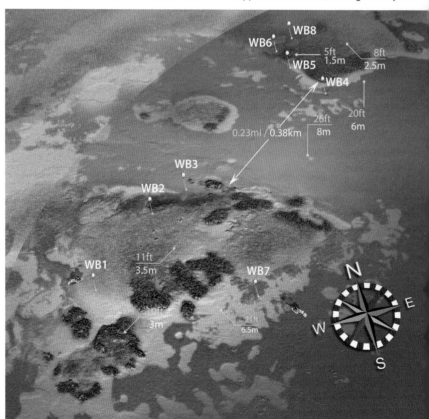

THREE SISTERS

Difficulty	● ○ ○
Current	● ○ ○
Depth	● ○ ○
Reef	★★★
Fauna	★☆☆

Access 🚤
7.5mi (12km) from Key Largo

Level Open water

Location Key Largo
GPS   TS1 25° 01.776'N, 80° 23.884'W

Getting there

Three Sisters is a small collection of patch reefs located inside the boundary of the John Pennekamp Coral Reef State Park. The site is nearly 5 miles (8 kilometers) east southeast of Rodriguez Key. Getting there involves a 35- to 40-minute boat ride from Key Largo.

Access

These patch reefs are suitable for divers and snorkelers of all levels. Visibility is sometimes poor, but currents are usually mild. Three Sisters is only accessible by boat due to its distance from shore. There is a single mooring buoy located at this site. There is no lobstering within the boundaries of the Pennekamp Park,

Description

An often-overlooked site, the reef at Three Sisters is shallow at about 14 feet (4 meters) deep, while the surrounding sand gets as deep as 20 feet (6 meters). The resulting relief makes this site a great place to see a variety of reef fish species, including gray and French angelfish, hogfish, highhats, bar jacks and Bermuda chub. Bluestriped grunts are also a common sight here, as are numerous wrasse species. Green morays and barracuda are also spotted here on a regular basis.

Seagrass beds surround the patch reefs, set back from the reef by a stretch of sand. This habitat supports a host of other marine creatures, including sea turtles, goatfish and stingrays. Divers can focus their time on the reefs or the seagrass, depending on their preference.

THREE SISTERS

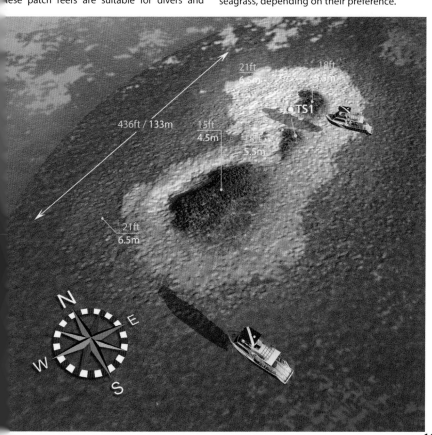

WOLFE REEF

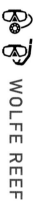

Difficulty ● ○ ○
Current ● ○ ○
Depth ● ○ ○
Reef ★☆☆ Access 🚤
Fauna ★☆☆ 8.5mi (13.5km) from Key Largo

Level Open water

Location Key Largo
GPS   WR1 25° 01.300'N, 80° 23.782'W

Getting there

Wolfe Reef is a collection of small coral mounds located on a hard-bottomed area just outside the boundary of the John Pennekamp Coral Reef State Park. The site is nearly 5 miles (8 kilometers) east southeast of Rodriguez Key. Getting there involves a 35- to 40-minute boat ride from Key Largo.

Access

The site is suitable for divers and snorkelers of a levels. Visibility is sometimes poor, but currents ar usually mild. Wolfe Reef is only accessible by boa due to its distance from shore. There is a singl mooring buoy located at this site.

Description

Wolfe (sometimes spelled Wolf) Reef is a shallo bottomed site at a depth of just 18 feet (5. meters) The handful of coral mounds that ar located here rise about 5 feet (1.5 meters) off th hard seabed. The limited structure is enough t attract a broad range of fish species, however.

Divers and snorkelers to this site will regularl see Bermuda chub, surgeonfish, sergea majors, and various wrasse and grunt specie The biodiversity helps attract predatory fis including black grouper, red grouper, bar jac and barracuda. Nurse sharks are also often see resting near the mounds.

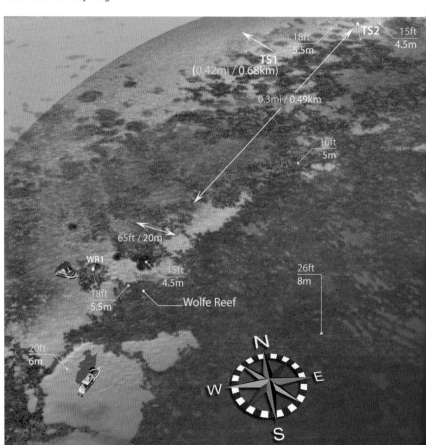

SAND ISLAND

Difficulty	● ○ ○	
Current	● ○ ○	
Depth	● ○ ○	
Reef	★★★☆	Access
Fauna	★☆☆	8.5mi (13.5km) from Key Largo

Level Open water

Location Key Largo

GPS
SI1 25° 01.081'N, 80° 22.089'W
SI2 25° 01.109'N, 80° 22.044'W
SI3 25° 01.146'N, 80° 22.004'W
SI4 25° 01.104'N, 80° 22.007'W

Getting there

Sand Island is located just 0.5 miles (0.8 kilometers) north of Molasses Reef, along the outer reef line near Key Largo. Getting there involves a 40- to 45-minute boat ride from Key Largo.

Access

Sand Island is suitable for divers and snorkelers of all levels. Currents are generally mild, and the visibility is usually good. The site is only accessible by boat due to its distance from shore. There are four mooring buoys located at this site.

Description

Sand Island gets its name from the fact that there was reportedly an island with a long palm tree on it that once existed here. As the story goes, a hurricane in 1960 washed it away. While the topside ecosystem is long gone, the fragmented coral spurs that are just seaward of the reef still support plenty of life. Large patches of healthy elkhorn coral thrive at this shallow site which has a maximum depth of about 26 feet (8 meters). The tops of the corals reach up to a depth of 13 feet (4 meters), making this reef a great place to snorkel. Visitors will see yellowtail snapper, wrasses, grunts and bicolor damselfish, and a variety of butterflyfish, including banded and foureye. Barracuda are common here as well, and some operators report seeing a particularly large and curious individual that is often present to greet boats when they tie up to the mooring buoy.

SAND ISLAND

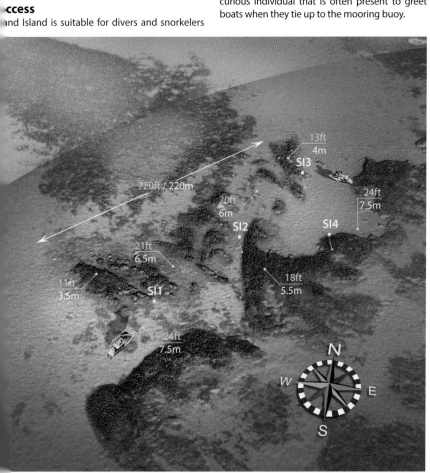

MOLASSES REEF

Difficulty ● ○ ○
Current ● ○ ○
Depth ● ○ ○
Reef ★★★
Fauna ★★★

Access 9mi (14.5km) from Key Largo

Level Open Water

Location Key Largo
GPS
MR1 25° 00.483'N, 80° 22.661'W
MR2 25° 00.494'N, 80° 22.634'W
MR3 25° 00.505'N, 80° 22.607'W
MR4 25° 00.516'N, 80° 22.582'W
MR5 25° 00.539'N, 80° 22.542'W
MR6 25° 00.551'N, 80° 22.500'W
MR7 25° 00.547'N, 80° 22.471'W
MR8 25° 00.579'N, 80° 22.471'W
MR9 25° 00.551'N, 80° 22.436'W
MR10 25° 00.582'N, 80° 22.438'W
MR11 25° 00.599'N, 80° 22.411'W
MR12 25° 00.612'N, 80° 22.395'W
MR13 25° 00.624'N, 80° 22.432'W
MR14 25° 00.611'N, 80° 22.460'W
MR15 25° 00.594'N, 80° 22.507'W
MR16 25° 00.571'N, 80° 22.541'W
MR17 25° 00.553'N, 80° 22.569'W
MR18 25° 00.543'N, 80° 22.602'W
MR19 25° 00.445'N, 80° 22.672'W
MR20 25° 00.470'N, 80° 22.637'W
MR21 25° 00.485'N, 80° 22.602'W
MR22 25° 00.492'N, 80° 22.584'W
MR23 25° 00.497'N, 80° 22.549'W
MR24 25° 00.515'N, 80° 22.519'W
MR25 25° 00.530'N, 80° 22.448'W
MR26 25° 00.434'N, 80° 22.525'W
MR27 25° 00.439'N, 80° 22.468'W
MR28 25° 00.455'N, 80° 22.405'W
MR29 25° 00.628'N, 80° 22.342'W
MR30 25° 00.645'N, 80° 22.388'W
MR31 25° 00.637'N, 80° 22.403'W
MR32 25° 00.608'N, 80° 22.330'W

Getting there

Molasses Reef is located just over 5 miles (8 kilometers) southeast of Rodriguez Key near Key Largo. The reef sits on a bend in the outer reef line, leaving it projecting out into the open water. Getting there involves a 50-minute boat ride from Key Largo.

Access

Molasses Reef is suitable for divers and snorkelers of all levels. It is by far the most popular reef in Key Largo and accessibility is facilitated by the 29 mooring buoys spaced evenly across the defined spur and groove formations and the three mooring buoys located on the deeper reef slope. Currents can be brisk given the reef's exposure to the prevailing currents from the south, but that also means visibility is usually good. The site is only accessible by boat due to its distance from shore.

Description

Molasses Reef is the most visited reef in the entire

DID YOU KNOW? ❓

On August 4, 1984, a 400-foot (122-meter) freighter named *MV Wellwood* ran aground on Molasses Reef. The ship spent 12 days lodged on the reef causing untold damage to the ecosystem. Wave action further ground the vessel's hull against the reef, and additional damage was caused by prop wash and cable scrapes from the efforts to free her. She was finally released from the reef, but the area of greatest impact is now termed the "parking lot" because of the limited reef structure that remained after the vessel was freed. In total, the grounding destroyed more than 1.4 acres (5,805 square meters) of living coral and damaged a further 18.5 acres (75,000 square meters) of reef habitat. It took nearly two and half years to reach a financial settlement with the shipping company that owned the vessel. The $6.75 million settlement was paid out as an annuity over 15 years. Extensive restoration of the coral reef in the damaged area began in 2002. The site is marked by an underwater brass monument (GPS coordinates: 25° 00.633'N, 80° 22.366'W). The marker is used to help with survey efforts during ongoing monitoring of the reef. A spar buoy usually marks the monument's location.

Florida Keys. With 32 mooring buoys stretching across a reef system that measures over 0.5 miles (0.8 kilometers) in length, this reef offers something for everyone. The area is a veritable maze of defined coral spurs that rise to depths of as little as 10 feet (3 meters), interspersed with sand and rubble-bottom grooves with maximum depths between 33 and 40 feet (10 and 12 meters). The tops of the corals are covered in dense stands of sea fans and soft corals, interspersed with large boulder corals, barrel sponges and yellow tube sponges. The entire Molasses Reef area falls within a Sanctuary Preservation Area (SPA) which prohibits the removal, harvest or possession of any marine life.

Visitors to Molasses have the choice of many different named sites to explore on this massive

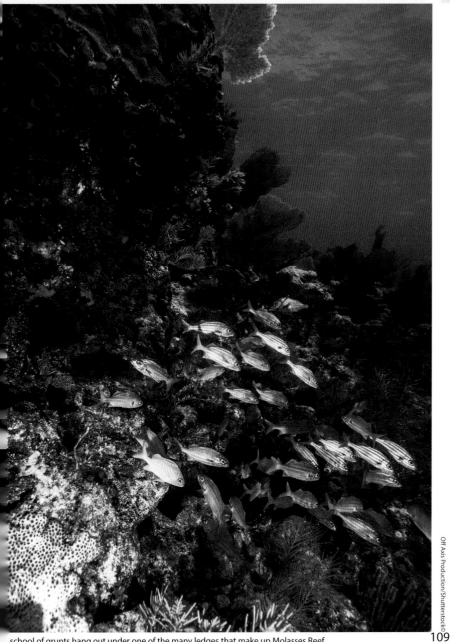

Off Axis Production/Shutterstock©

school of grunts hang out under one of the many ledges that make up Molasses Reef.

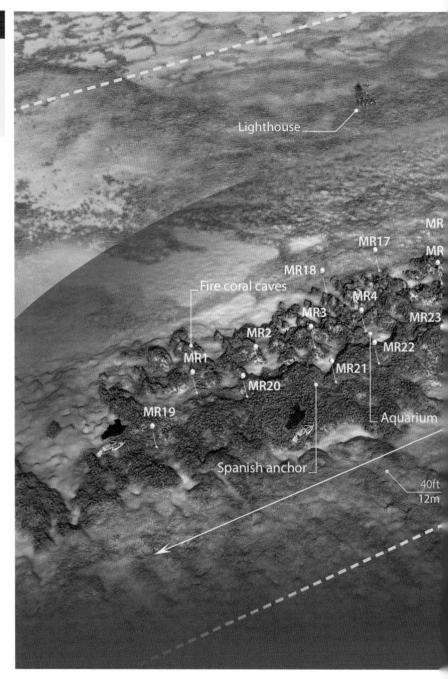

Lighthouse

MR

MR17

MR18

MR

Fire coral caves

MR4

MR3

MR23

MR2

MR1

MR22

MR21

MR20

Aquarium

MR19

Spanish anchor

40ft
12m

reef. From Spanish Anchor located near MR21 to Winch Hole near MR7 and MR8 - each location has its own story and provides its own experience. For instance, the 10-foot (3-meter) winch in Winch Hole is part of what remains of the windlass that was originally part of the sailing bark *Slobodna*. The vessel ran aground on Molasses Reef in

1887 and was hammered the following year b a massive hurricane that spread parts of the sh across a wide area.

Other named sites include North Star near MR1 which is on the barrier edge of the reef and hold debris from the many ships that have wrecked o

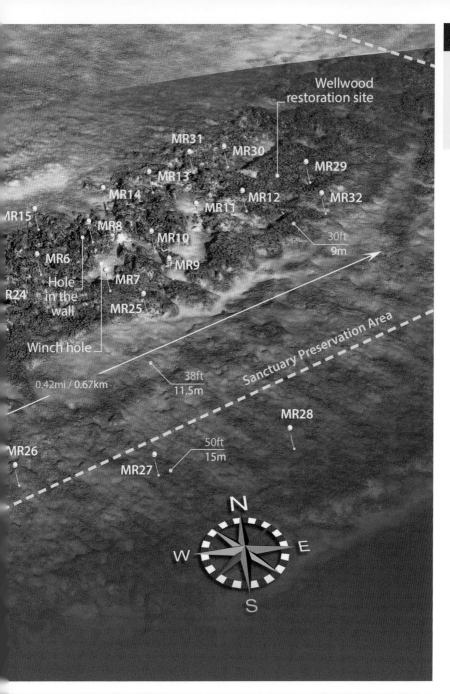

Wellwood restoration site

MR31
MR30
MR29
MR13
MR14
MR12
MR32
MR15
MR11
MR8
30ft
9m
MR10
MR6
MR9
Hole in the wall
MR7
R24
MR25
Winch hole
0.42mi / 0.67km
38ft
11,5m
Sanctuary Preservation Area
MR28
MR26
50ft
15m
MR27

N
W   E
S

ECO TIP

The presence of sharks on a coral reef poses little threat to divers and snorkelers but is a very good indicator of reef health. You can learn about sharks and ecosystem health in **Beneath the Blue Planet** – a guide to the coral reef ecosystem for divers and snorkelers – published by **Reef Smart Guides**.

MOLASSES REEF

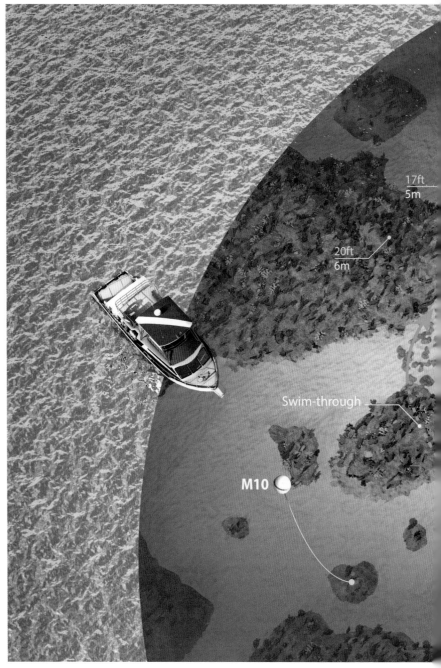

17ft
5m

20ft
6m

Swim-through

M10

the reef. Aquarium is located near MR4 and gets its name from the schools of fish that frequent the big open space bracketed on all sides by tall spurs, almost like fish in an aquarium bowl. The self-explanatory Coral Canyons is near buoy MR7, while another popular site, Hole in The Wall, is located just west of MR8. The main feature of

that site is a large square-shaped swim-throug located in a sand channel running north fror Winch Hole. The northern buoys on the reef mar the Wellwood Preservation area.

Molasses Reef slopes downward at the seawar edge of the spur and groove zone. The ha

MOLASSES REEF

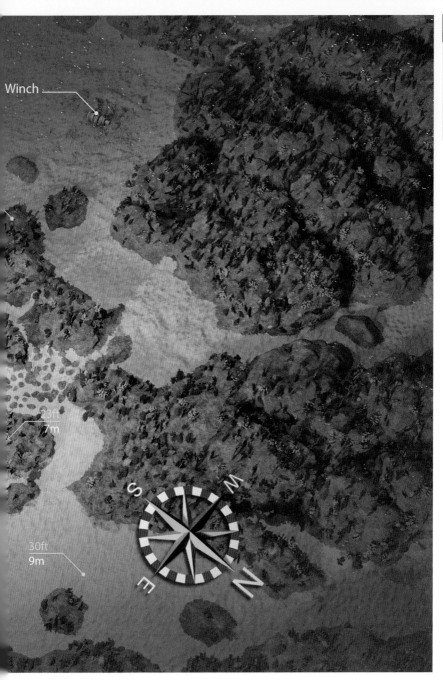

Winch

23ft
7m

30ft
9m

ottomed reef slope is cut through with narrow
and chutes and is covered in a scattering of hard
nd soft corals and medium-sized barrel sponges.
he top of this slope is at a depth of 39 to 46 feet
2 to 14 meters) and descends to between 70 and
00 feet (21.5 and 30.5 meters).

There is an incredible array of marine life present at
Molasses Reef. Schools of French and bluestriped
grunts are common, along with yellowtail,
schoolmaster and mahogany snapper. Divers
and snorkelers often find green sea turtles on the
reef, while southern stingrays shelter in the sand-
bottomed grooves. Nurse sharks are also commonly

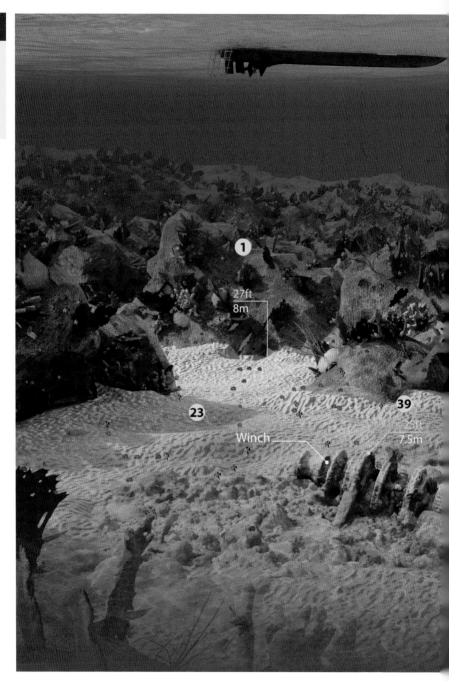

27ft
8m

① 1

② 23

39

25ft
7.5m

Winch

seen resting against the sides of coral spurs, while reports of higher numbers of Caribbean reef sharks suggest that the Molasses ecosystem is recovering to a healthy level.

Route

The route taken to explore Molasses Reef will depend on the buoy used as a starting poin Pretty much any buoy a dive boat ties into wi have a named site (or two) associated with it. is impossible to explore the whole reef in eve an entire week of diving, which is why diver and snorkelers keep returning to Molasses Re time and again.

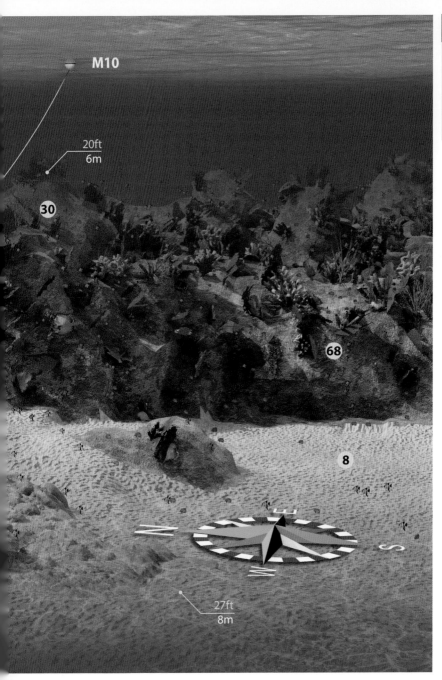

M10

20ft
6m

30

68

8

N E W S

27ft
8m

he reef is shallow enough that dives will
ost likely be limited by air and not bottom
me. As divers and snorkelers explore the
eef, it is important to be mindful of their
tarting point. The twisting and turning spurs
nd grooves can be disorienting to many,
nd it is easy to end up returning to the
wrong mooring buoy. Receiving a proper dive
briefing at the start of the dive can help divers
and snorkelers keep their bearings as they
explore this incredible reef.

BIBB

Difficulty ● ● ●
Current ● ● ●
Depth ● ● ●
Reef ★★★
Fauna ★★★

Access 🚤 10mi (16km) from Key Largo

Level Advanced

Location Key Largo
GPS   24° 59.710′N, 80° 22.770′W

Getting there

Bibb is located nearly 7.5 miles (12 kilometers) off the coast of Key Largo, just under a mile (1.5 kilometers) off the outer reef line. Getting there involves a boat ride of around 50 minutes from Key Largo.

Access

Bibb is only suitable for advanced divers because of the wreck's depth – her shallowest point is just 95 feet (29 meters) deep while the maximum depth of the seabed is 135 feet (41 meters). There is a single mooring buoy on the *Bibb* that allows boats to access the site without having to anchor or tie into the wreck itself. Due to its exposed position beyond the reef line, the site can experience strong currents. This site is only accessible by boat due to its distance from shore.

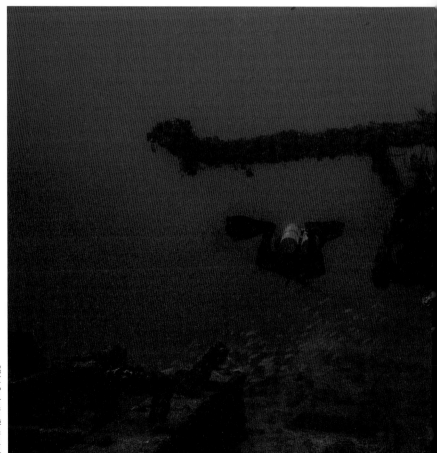

The *Bibb* settled on its side when it sank, but it still created great habitat for marine organisms

RELAX & RECHARGE

Sharkey's Sharkbite Grill (522 Caribbean Drive, Key Largo) is a waterfront restaurant located just across the canal from the Sundiver boat dock and Rainbow Reef Dive Center. On the ground floor, Sharkey's Pub and Taphouse is a popular sports bar with big screen TVs and a menu that has something for everyone. There are 32 beer taps serving a range of popular beers as well as the latest micro brews from across Florida. The dining experience is a little quieter on the 2nd floor. Sharkey's is known for its Baja-style jumbo fish tacos, but they also serve a range of other options, including sandwiches and salads. Do not miss "Fish Fryday" – all you can eat Mahi Mahi experience every Friday night. There is a lot of outdoor space to unwind in as you watch the boats arrive and depart the busy marina and sip on a nice, cold drink. It is a relaxing way to end the day.
Visit: **Sharkeysgalley.com**.

Description

USCG Bibb was a steel-hulled cutter built for the U.S. Coast Guard in Charleston, South Carolina in March 1937. She was one of the Treasury or Secretary class of cutters – they were all named for former secretaries of the Treasury. In the *Bibb's* case, she was named after George M. Bibb, a U.S. senator from Kentucky who was appointed Secretary of the Treasury in 1844 by President Tyler.

Bibb served as a patrol ship in the North Atlantic to help protect shipping at the start of the Second World War. Her duties changed in 1940, and she was assigned to provide weather information during 21-day tours patrolling a 100-square mile (260-square kilometer) area in the mid-Atlantic. Weather data was no longer being collected by the merchant fleet because of the war, and the Coast Guard's cutters were tasked with hosting meteorologists who took readings with weather balloons. In 1941, she was fitted with anti-submarine weaponry and transferred to the Navy where she received the designation WPG-31. She conducted multiple patrols along the northeast coast of the United States and was also tasked with protecting trans-Atlantic convoys. She engaged submarines on multiple occasions and participated in the rescue of sailors from boats that had been torpedoed, including one instance in 1943 when she disobeyed orders to return to a torpedoed boat to rescue a total of 202 survivors from the frigid waters of the North Atlantic.

Later in the war she helped protect convoys bound for North Africa, and even spent some time in the Pacific, where she was stripped of her heavy armament and refitted with anti-aircraft guns. A large radio room was also added, and she was converted to a command-and-control vessel for amphibious landings. Her designation was also officially changed to WAGC-31.

At the end of the war, *Bibb* was transferred back to the Coast Guard and converted back to her original configuration as a cutter. Once refitted, she returned to service conducting weather patrols, operating out of Boston. While on patrol, she participated in multiple rescues, including a particularly challenging one involving the passengers and crew of the *Bermuda Sky Queen* in October 1947. The "flying boat" had made an

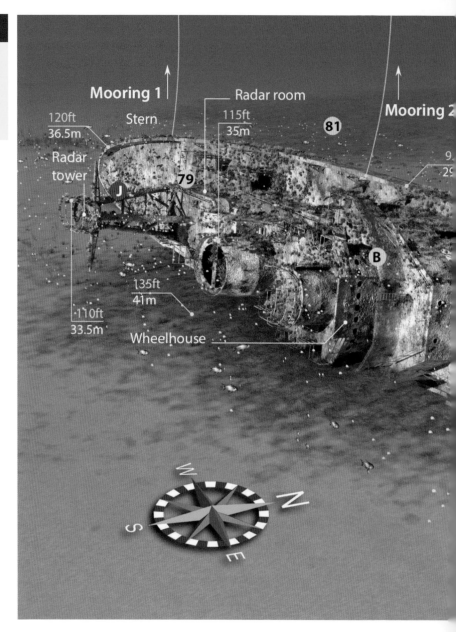

Mooring 1

Stern

120ft
36.5m

Radar
tower

J

79

Radar room

115ft
35m

81

Mooring 2

9.
29

B

135ft
41m

110ft
33.5m

Wheelhouse

emergency landing in 30-foot (9-meter) seas on its way from Ireland to Newfoundland, Canada, after burning too much fuel battling stronger-than-expected headwinds.

In 1967, she once again assumed wartime duties in support of the Navy, this time in Vietnamese waters. She engaged the enemy multiple times but is perhaps best known for transporting Senator John Kerry after he was shot on his

Swift boat. She was finally decommissioned in September 1984 and was then stripped and deployed as an artificial reef in 1987 alongside her sister ship, *USCG Duane* (see page 122).

During the deployment, she settled on her starboard side, placing most of her superstructure and the main body of the wreck below a depth of 100 feet (30.5 meters). She represents one of the deepest wrecks in the Florida Keys because

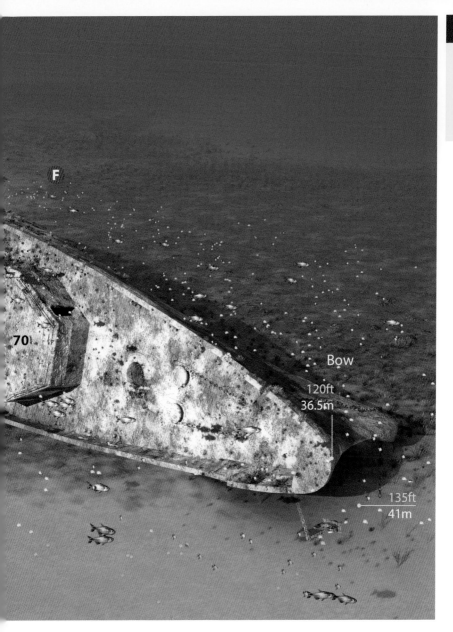

of this positioning. The wreck offers plenty of penetration opportunities for divers with the necessary training.

Her depth and position out in the waters of the Gulf Stream make *Bibb* a great site to experience large marine life, such as great hammerhead sharks and even the occasional whale shark. Barracks, barracuda and cobia are commonly seen in the waters around the wreck, while French and Queen angelfish and tomtate schools are common closer to the superstructure and inside the holds. Goliath grouper have also been known to frequent the wreck.

Route

Due to her depth, divers will need to carefully plan their route through the wreck. The wheelhouse offers limited penetration and the orientation, while challenging to navigate, can provide an interesting

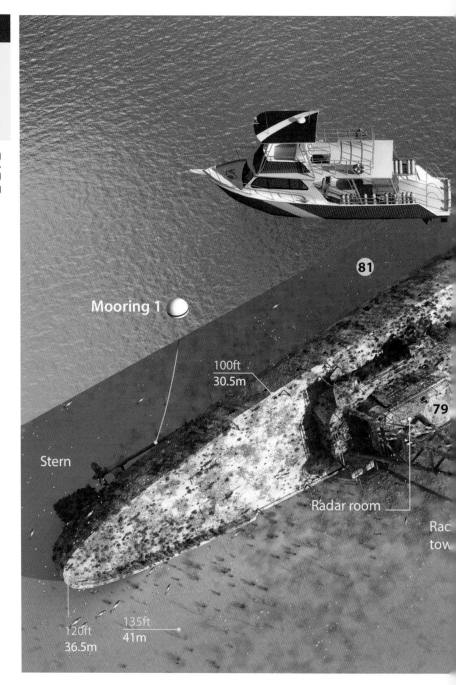

81

Mooring 1

100ft
30.5m

79

Stern

Radar room

Rac
tow

120ft
36.5m

135ft
41m

perspective on the vessel's interior. With limited
bottom time, most divers focus their attention on
the wheelhouse, the funnel region of the wreck and
the open radar tower.

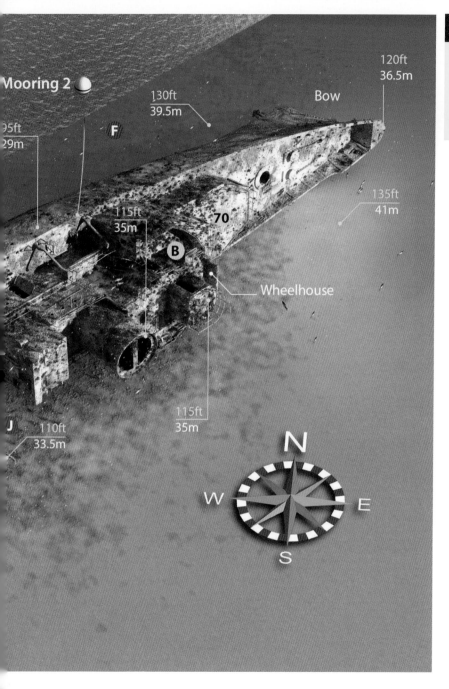

Mooring 2

95ft
29m

F

130ft
39.5m

Bow

120ft
36.5m

115ft
35m

70

B

135ft
41m

Wheelhouse

115ft
35m

J   110ft
33.5m

N

W   E

S

Name:	USCG Bibb		Charleston, SC, 1937
Type:	Coast Guard Cutter	**Last owner:**	U.S. Coast Guard
Previous names:	WPG-31, WAGC-31, WHEC-31	**Sunk:**	Nov. 27, 1987
Length:	327ft (100m)		
Tonnage:	2,350grt		
Construction:	Charleston Shipbuilding,		

DUANE

Difficulty	● ● ●
Current	● ● ○
Depth	● ● ○
Reef	★★★
Fauna	★★★

Access 🚤 10.5mi (17km) from Key Largo

Level Advanced

Location Key Largo
GPS   24° 59.384'N, 80° 22.888'W

Getting there

Duane is located nearly 7.5 miles (12 kilometers) off the coast of Key Largo. The wreck rests just under a mile (1.5 kilometers) off the outer reef line. Getting there involves a boat ride of about 50 minutes from Key Largo.

Access

Duane is suitable for divers with advanced experience because of the wreck's depth. Although her highest point reaches a depth of 60 feet (18 meters) at her radar tower, the bulk of the wreck sits at 90 feet (27.5 meters) and below. There are three mooring buoys attached to the wreck (although the third one is often missing), which provide access to the site without having to anchor or tie-in to the wreck itself. Due to its exposed position beyond the reef line, the site can experience strong currents, although the upright nature of the wreck creates some sheltered areas when the current is strong. The site is only accessible by boat due to its distance from shore.

Description

USCG Duane was a steel-hulled cutter built for the Coast Guard in Philadelphia, Pennsylvania in June 1936. She was one of the Treasury or Secretary class of cutters – they were all named for former secretaries of the U.S. Treasury. She was named after Irish-born William J. Duane who served as Secretary of the Treasury for just four months under President Jackson in 1833.

This period in U.S. history was marked by the "Bank War," during which time President Jackson wanted to withdraw government deposits from the Second Bank of the United States. His first Secretary of the Treasury refused to approve the withdrawal, so Jackson replaced him with Duane who was opposed to the Bank on principle. In the end however, Duane also refused to approve the withdrawal, believing it would cause financial

chaos and panic, and so Jackson fired him as well. *USCG Duane* served a much longer term of duty than her namesake. Her first responsibilities were in the Pacific, helping provide supplies and machinery to the colonists on the Line Islands south of Hawaii and then patrolling the Bering Sea. She was transferred to Boston in 1939 to help patrol the Grand Banks in the North Atlantic. When those patrols stopped in 1940, her duties changed to providing weather information via 21-day tours spent patrolling a 100-square mile (260-square kilometer) area in the mid-Atlantic. Weather data was no longer being collected by the merchant fleet because of the war, and the Coast Guard's cutters were tasked to host meteorologists who took readings with weather balloons.

In 1941, she was fitted out with anti-submarine weaponry and transferred to the Navy where she received the designation WPG-33. She continued to conduct weather patrols, however, until she was transferred over to convoy escort duty in 1942. Shortly after rearmament, she ran aground near the Cape Cod canal and required dry dock repairs. She then joined the *USCG Bibb* (see page 116) on anti-submarine exercises in April 1942 ahead of escorting convoys through the North Atlantic. She engaged numerous submarines and rounded up straggling merchant ships many times over the following year. She even participated in the sinking of the German submarine *U-175* on April 2, 1943, while on a convoy bound from Argentina to Londonderry, Ireland.

In the summer of 1944, *Duane* participated in the maritime landing invasion of southern France. The complex operation involved coordinating aerial bombardment and naval bombardment of the shore-based defenses, in conjunction with waves of landing craft that deposited men and machinery on the beaches.

At the end of the war, *Duane* was transferred back to the Coast Guard and converted back to her original configuration as a cutter. Once refitted, she returned to service conducting weather patrols in the north and mid-Atlantic. The weather information collected by *Duane* and her sister ships was essential for the successful expansion of international air travel between Europe and North America.

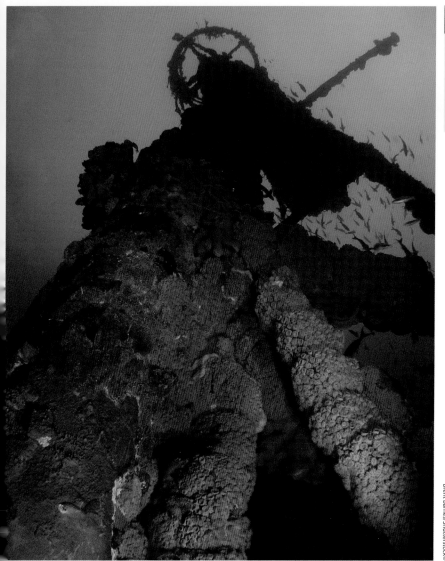

The *Duane* is heavily encrusted with colorful corals, algae and sponges, including invasive orange cup corals..

In 1967, she once again assumed wartime duties in support of the Navy in Vietnamese waters. She engaged the enemy multiple times including the destruction of an observation post and associated bunkers, tunnels and fortifications on her first day of patrol. Following the war, she returned to her duties on weather patrol until those responsibilities were shut down in 1973 in favor of electronic shore-based weather monitoring. *Duane* served out her remaining years on patrol in the waters around Portland, Maine. Her planned decommissioning in the late 1970s was delayed by Congressional fears that the Coast Guard lacked the capacity to successfully engage in its new mandate to intercept drug smugglers.

She was finally decommissioned in August 1985 after 49 years in services – at the time, she was the oldest U.S. warship on active duty.

Duane was donated to the Keys Association of Dive Operators in 1987, and she was prepared for sinking as an artificial reef before being towed out and deployed just south of Molasses Reef. She sank alongside her sister ship, *USCG Bibb* in November 1987. She settled upright on a sandy bottom at a depth of 125 feet (38 meters). *Duane* is a popular site to visit as part of the Florida Keys National Marine Sanctuary Shipwreck Trail.

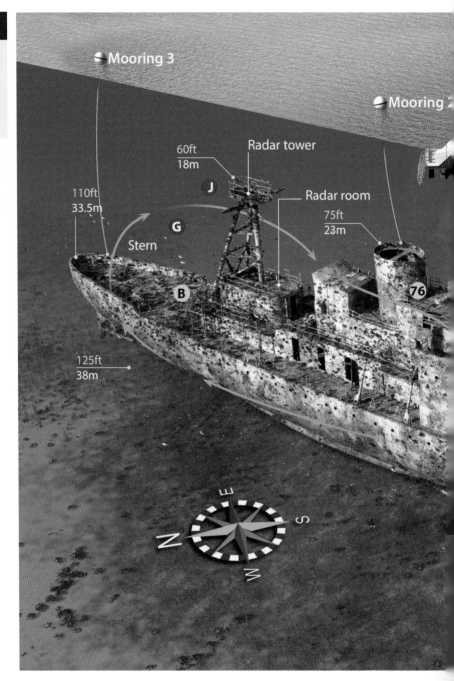

Mooring 3

Mooring 2

60ft
18m

Radar tower

110ft
33.5m

J

Radar room

75ft
23m

G

Stern

B

76

125ft
38m

Her depth and position out in the waters of the Gulf Stream make *Duane* a great site to experience larger marine life, such as great hammerhead sharks, bull sharks, and even the occasional giant manta ray. Bar jacks, barracuda and cobia are commonly seen in the waters above the wreck, while French, Queen and gray angelfish patrol the decks. Bluestriped grunt, porkfish and tomtates are all frequently seen schooling on the wreck, often inside the holds. Goliath grouper have been known to frequent the wreck as well.

Route

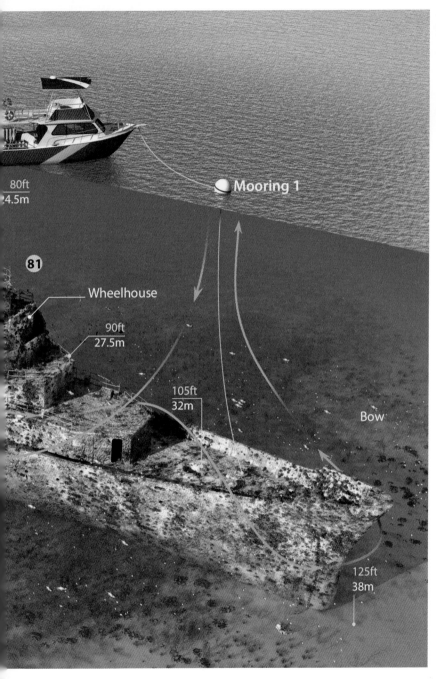

80ft
24.5m

Mooring 1

81

Wheelhouse

90ft
27.5m

105ft
32m

Bow

125ft
38m

ue to her depth, divers will need to carefully
an how they explore the wreck. The
heelhouse offers limited penetration while full
enetration is possible through the four levels of
ecks, including the main deck, superstructure,
heelhouse and radar room. The most common
ute involves descending to the main deck at a

depth of 105 feet (32 meters) before exploring
the superstructure and wheelhouse. Divers can
finish off their dive in the radar room located on
top of the superstructure or around the radar
tower located just aft of midship, depending on
which mooring buoy line they descended.

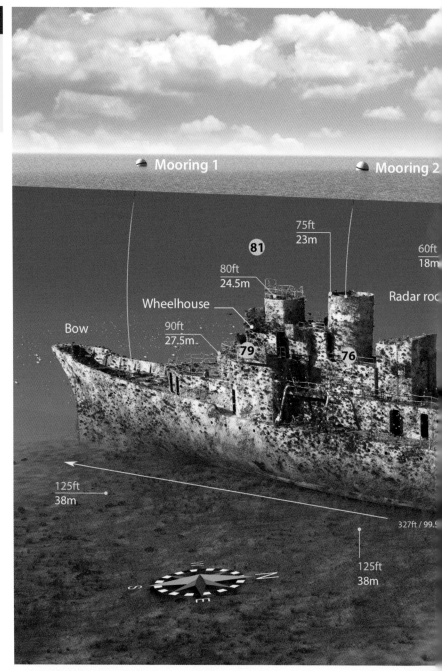

Mooring 1

Mooring 2

75ft
23m

81

60ft
18m

80ft
24.5m

Radar roc

Wheelhouse

Bow

90ft
27.5m

79

76

125ft
38m

327ft / 99.

125ft
38m

SCIENTIFIC INSIGHT

Invasive species such as orange cup corals (*Tubastraea sp.*) and the lionfish (*Pterois volitans*) pose a threat to reef ecosystems because they have the potential to cause the extinction of native organisms. They compete for scarce resources, such as hard surfaces on which to settle in the case of orange cup corals. Without room to settle and grow, native corals and sponges may decline in abundance, causing knock on effects throughout the

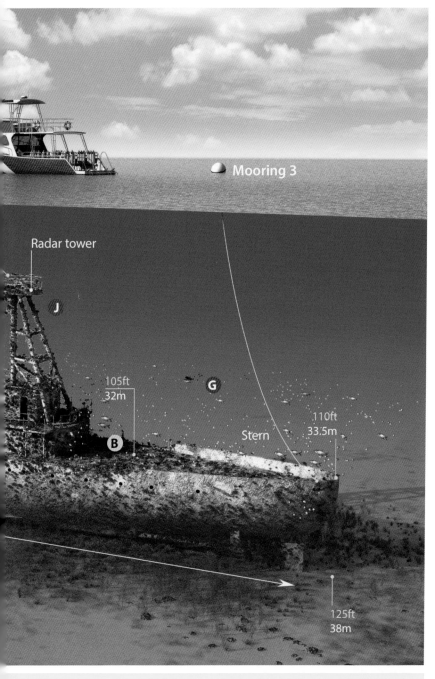

Mooring 3

Radar tower

J

105ft
32m

G

B

110ft
33.5m

Stern

125ft
38m

rest of the system. Invasives typically have a competitive advantage over similar native species as they are unfamiliar to predators and potentially less susceptible to local diseases and parasites. As a result, they face fewer pressures than do local populations, allowing them to thrive at the expensive of the locals. Not every non-native species is considered invasive, however. The label invasive is reserved for organisms that actually hinder or prevent the survival of other organisms within the ecosystem.

DUANE AND BIBB DECK PLAN

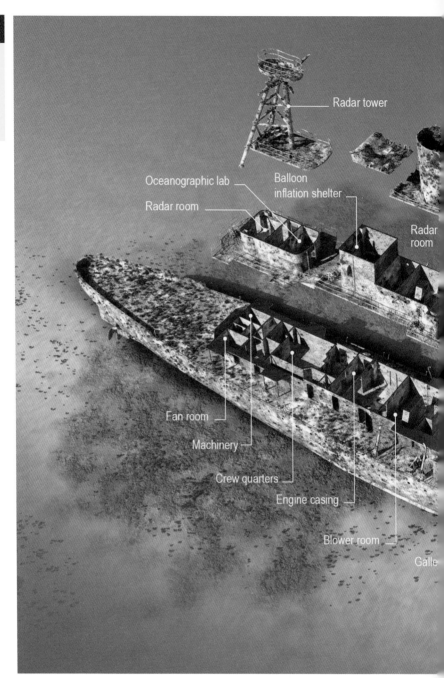

Radar tower

Oceanographic lab

Balloon inflation shelter

Radar room

Radar room

Fan room

Machinery

Crew quarters

Engine casing

Blower room

Galle

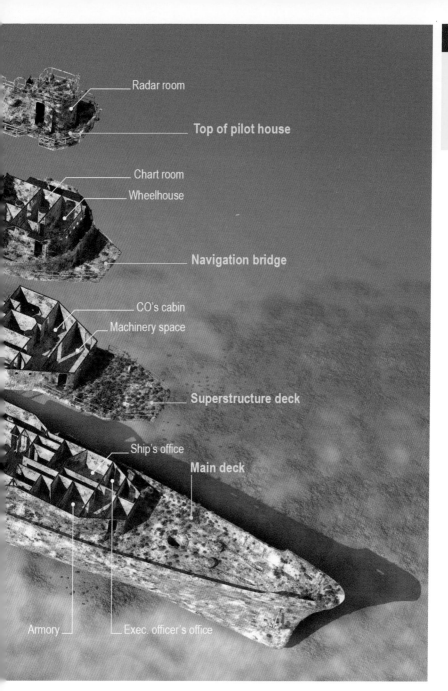

Radar room

Top of pilot house

Chart room

Wheelhouse

Navigation bridge

CO's cabin

Machinery space

Superstructure deck

Ship's office

Main deck

Armory

Exec. officer's office

ame:	*USCG Duane*	Philadelphia, PA, 1936
ype:	Coast Guard Cutter	**Last owner:** U.S. Coast Guard
evious names:	*WPG-33, WAGC-33, WHEC-33*	**Sunk:** Nov. 27, 1987
ength:	327ft (100m)	
•nnage:	2,589grt	
•nstruction:	Philadelphia Naval Shipyard,	

PICKLES REEF

Difficulty ● ○ ○
Current ● ○ ○
Depth ● ○ ○
Reef ★★★☆
Fauna ★★★☆

Access 🚤 12mi (19.5km) from Key Largo

Level Open Water

Location Key Largo
GPS   PR1 24° 59.085′N, 80° 24.965′W
      PR2 24° 59.148′N, 80° 24.903′W
      PR3 24° 59.229′N, 80° 24.864′W
      PR4 24° 59.497′N, 80° 24.540′W
      PR5 24° 59.541′N, 80° 24.524′W

Getting there

Pickles Reef is located 6.2 miles (10 kilometers) off the coast of Tavernier. The large reef is nearly 2.5 miles (4 kilometers) southwest of Molasses Reef, and slightly closer to shore than its more popular neighbor. Getting there involves a boat ride of around 50 minutes to an hour from Key Largo.

Access

Pickles Reef is only accessible by boat given its distance from shore. The reef is suitable for divers and snorkelers of all levels. It generally has good visibility due to its position on the outer reef line, but currents are rarely strong here. The site has five mooring buoys – three on the main southern section of reef and two in the smaller northern portion – so there is no need for boats to anchor at this site.

Description

Pickles Reef is a shallow reef with a large area of sand and rubble flanked on its seaward edge by well-defined spurs and grooves. The origin of its name remains unclear – although some attribute it to a story about the historic wreck located on the reef and cement-filled pickle barrels.

While there is indeed a wreck on the reef, it has little to do with pickle barrels. The wreck is an iron-hulled sailing vessel that remains unidentified, which is believed to have foundered sometime before the 1900s. Later, in 1914, a steamship by the name of the *Times* also ran aground at the same spot on the reef as the historic wreck.

To lighten their load and free their vessel from the reef, the crew rolled overboard barrels of the cement mix they were carrying as cargo. The water mixed with the cement and then set,

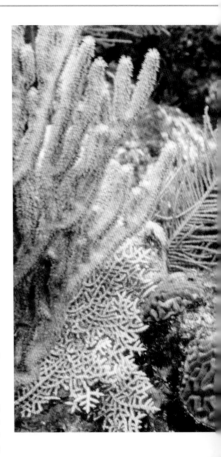

leaving replicas of the barrels' interiors on th wreck once the wood rotted away. The wrec became known locally as the Pickles Reef Barr Wreck, but very little remains of the origin shipwreck. except the "concrete barrels," whic are now largely incorporated into the reef nez buoy PR3 on the northern edge of the ma section of reef.

Pickles Reef was an important navigational poi in the early days of sailing along the coast, as marked the entrance to safe anchorages ne Rodriguez Key and Tavernier. In fact, Pickl Reef hosted one of the historic Totten Beacor Beacon "F." The remains of this beacon are fou

RELAX & RECHARGE

What The Fish Rolls & More (80775 Old Highway, Tavernier) is a great place to pick up lunch or dinner after a day on the water. This quality seafood shack, located right next door to Captain Slate's Scuba Adventures, specializes in fresh fish rolls. They also serve shrimp, chicken and pork options, as well as a range of delicious salads. The crab cakes, lobster roll and spicy calamari roll are particularly popular. If your day of diving is complete, an ice-cold beer makes the perfect accompaniment. There's plenty of parking, an outdoor seating area and free WiFi. Visit: **Whatthefishrolls.com**

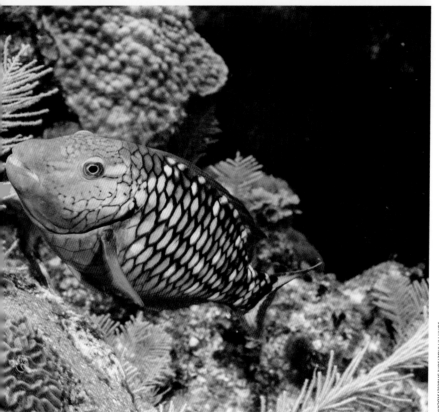

John A. Anderson/Shutterstock©

stoplight parrotfish swims by some hard corals and gorgonians like the ones found on Pickles Reef.

around 8 feet (2.5 meters) of water between e spur and groove section and the large sand d rubble berm that dominates this site. In tal, there are three posts that remain visible, anding at an angle, which represent successive enerations of Totten Beacons as they failed the elements and were replaced with newer rsions. Debris from the beacons is visible on e seafloor just seaward of the posts. Due to eir distance from the main mooring buoys, e posts are not easily explored by divers and orkelers. Boaters should avoid anchoring here ue to the risk of disturbing the debris from the storic beacons.

The spurs along the main section of reef reach a depth of around 11 feet (3.5 meters), while the grooves extend to a depth of about 26 feet (8 meters). Seaward of the spur and groove zone is a hard-bottomed slope that contains numerous shallow sand channels. The slope descends to a depth of nearly 70 feet (21.5 meters) where it meets sand.

The spurs of Pickles Reef are covered in a variety of corals, including mustard hill coral, smooth starlet coral, finger coral and fire corals. Sea fans and other soft corals are plentiful on this shallow reef, as are a variety of sponges, including red rope sponge and encrusting orange sponge.

131

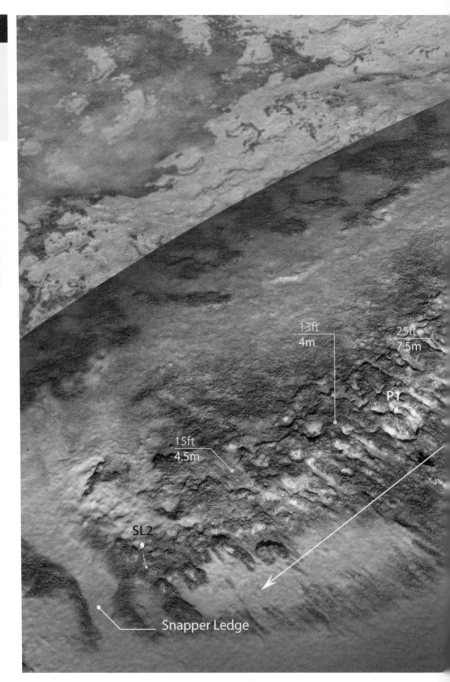

13ft
4m

25ft
7.5m

P1

15ft
4.5m

SL2

Snapper Ledge

The complex structures provide plenty of shelter for a variety of damselfish species, including bicolors, yellowtails, cocoas and sergeant majors. Striped, stoplight, and princess parrotfish are also plentiful on the reef as they graze on the macroalgae covering the surface of the coral spurs and the rubble-bottomed grooves. French and bluestriped grunts school on the reef, wh ocean surgeonfish and blue tangs pick their w. across the tops of spurs seeking their own alg to graze on.

A large collection of pillar corals can be fou between the two northern buoys, PR4 and PF

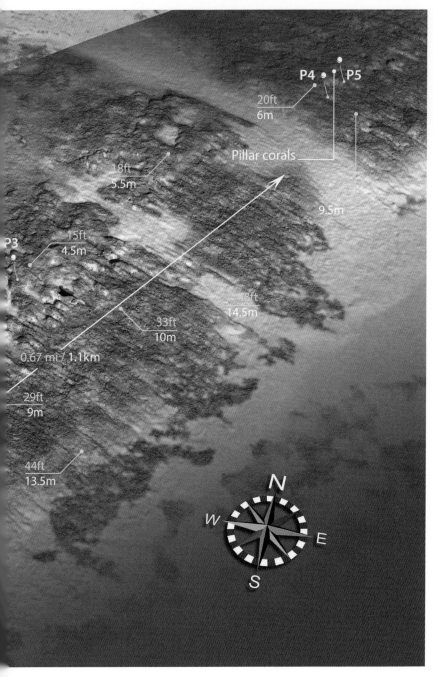

P4 • P5

20ft
6m

Pillar corals

18ft
5.5m

9.5m

P3

15ft
4.5m

48ft
14.5m

33ft
10m

0.67 mi / 1.1km

29ft
9m

44ft
13.5m

N
W E
S

ese pillar corals can be difficult to locate and y require a little searching. The two northern oys and their associated pillar corals are located arly 0.5 miles (0.8 kilometers) northeast of the in buoys and so would need to be visited on eparate dive. Most divers spend their time in shallower part of the reef, exploring the many

spurs and grooves found here. A second dive can be done on the northern section of reef, looking for the pillar corals anchored to a hard bottom at a depth of 16 feet (5 meters).

SNAPPER LEDGE

Difficulty	●	○	○	
Current	●	●	○	
Depth	●	○	○	
Reef	★	★	☆	
Fauna	★	★	☆	

Access 🛥 12mi (19.5km) from Key Largo

Level Open Water

Location Key Largo
GPS   SL1 24° 58.901′N, 80° 25.310′W
            SL2 24° 58.963′N, 80° 25.149′W

Getting there

Snapper Ledge is located 6.2 miles (10 kilometers) off the coast of Tavernier, directly off the southern terminus of Pickles Reef. Getting there involves a boat ride of around 50 minutes to an hour from Key Largo.

Access

Snapper Ledge is only accessible by boat give its distance from shore. The reef is suitable fe divers and snorkelers of all levels. This site ha good visibility due to its position on the oute reef line, although currents can sometime be strong which can make snorkeling mor challenging at times. The site is accessible via tw mooring buoys – one on either side of the wid sand channel. The southern buoy is the main t in to access the ledge features that give this si its name.

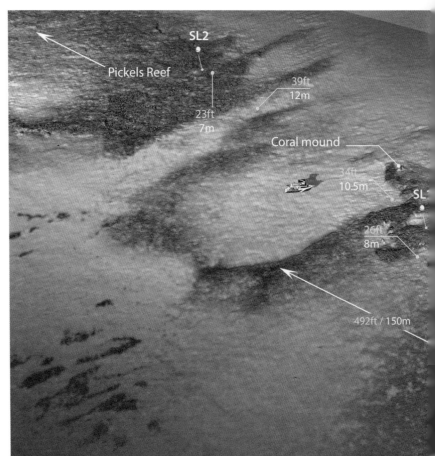

Description

Snapper Ledge actually consists of two main ledges, rather than one. The first runs roughly parallel to shore with its shallowest point at around 20 feet (6 meters) and its deepest point at 26 feet (8 meters). The second ledge starts perpendicular to the first on its northeastern end and turns at a right angle halfway along. This second ledge is deeper, with its shallowest point at roughly 30 feet (9 meters) and its deepest point at around 35 feet (10.5 meters). A tall pinnacle of coral rises over 10 feet (3.5 meters) from the top of the reef just to the east of the second ledge. A collapsed swim-through midway along the first ledge leads through to an open depression in the top of the ledge known as the "fishbowl."

This section of reef gets its name from the large schools of snapper and grunts that frequent the site. Yellowtail snapper dominate the group, but schoolmaster, gray and mahogany snapper are also common. Among the grunts, bluestriped, french, Spanish and white grunts are the most common, along with porkfish. Blue parrotfish are also a regular sight here as they forage on algae along the top of the ledge. Nurse sharks are often spotted resting around the base of the ledge while reef sharks frequently patrol the deeper waters. The ledge is dominated by soft corals, although there are numerous brain corals dotted across the reef.

Route

Most divers focus their attention along the two main ledges located adjacent to the southwestern mooring buoy. They typically spend equal parts of their time along the interesting sand-reef interface at the base of the ledges, as well as exploring along the top of the ledge. The fishbowl, located close to the western edge of the site, and the tall pillar of coral at the eastern end offer useful landmarks for turning around while on the dive.

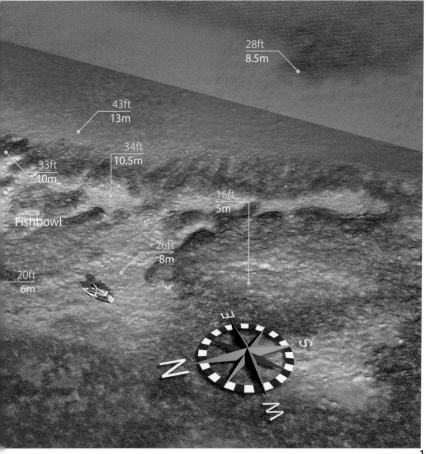

135

FLORIDA KEYS

CONCH REEF, CONCH WALL & LITTLE CONCH REEF

Difficulty ● ● ○
Current ● ○ ○
Depth ● ● ○
Reef ★★★
Fauna ★★☆

Access 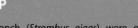 11mi (17km) from Islamorada

Level Open Water

Location Islamorada
GPS   CR1 24° 57.115'N, 80° 27.564'W
          CR2 24° 57.307'N, 80° 27.462'W
          CR3 24° 57.369'N, 80° 27.432'W

          CRW1 24° 56.784'N, 80° 27.394'W
          CRW2 24° 56.798'N, 80° 27.369'W
          CRW3 24° 56.830'N, 80° 27.326'W

Getting there

Conch Reef and the adjacent sites of Conch Wall and Little Conch Reef are located just over 5 miles (8 kilometers) southeast of Plantation Key. Getting there involves a boat ride of around 45 minutes from Islamorada.

Access

The three sites are only accessible by boat given their distance from shore. Conch Reef and Little Conch Reef are suitable for divers and snorkelers of all levels as they are the shallowest of the three sites with a seabed that reaches 25 feet (7.5 meters). Conch Wall is a steep slope, which bottoms out at a depth of 95 to 110 feet (29 to 33.5 meters). Conch Reef and Conch Wall are accessible via three mooring buoys per reef. Little Conch does not have any mooring buoys. Both Conch Wall and Little Conch Reef are often explored via drift dives. Conch Reef is protected by a Sanctuary Preservation Area (SPA) and thus no harvesting of marine life is allowed except for catch-and-release trolling, which is permitted here.

Description

Conch Reef gets its name from the presence of

Queen conchs at this site. Although no longer present in the number they once were, the are still commonly seen thanks to the extensiv seagrass beds in the area, which are the conch preferred habitat. It is illegal to harvest or remov a conch or its shell in Florida waters.

Conch Reef offers divers a chance to explore nearly 10-foot (2.5-meter) ledge that stretche approximately half a mile (0.8 kilometers) alon the seabed. The top of the ledge reaches 16 fee (5 meters) in some places, whereas the bottom of the ledge reaches an average depth of 2 feet (7.5 meters). Divers have an opportuni to see stands of rare pillar coral along the to of the ledge, while sea fans and barrel sponge are also plentiful. The reef supports plenty reef fishes, including bicolor and yellowt damselfish, along with brightly colored Spanis hogfish and wrasses. Nurse sharks are frequent spotted resting at the base of the ledge, whi hammerhead and reef sharks are sometim seen in the deeper parts of the slope along th seaward edge of the reef. Conch can be found the shallower sandy edge of the ledge, often patches of seagrass.

The deeper Conch Wall site is one of the be wall or slope dives in the Florida Keys. It star at a depth of 50 feet (15 meters) in the bro sand channel the separates the wall from t shallower section of reef at Conch Reef to t northwest. The slope is dominated by lar barrel sponges and small hard corals. Black cor are also present on the lower half of the slo here. The deeper waters support larger anima including spotted eagle rays, bull sharks a both green and loggerhead sea turtles. The us complement of reef fishes are also found here

CONCH REEF, CONCH WALL & LITTLE CONCH

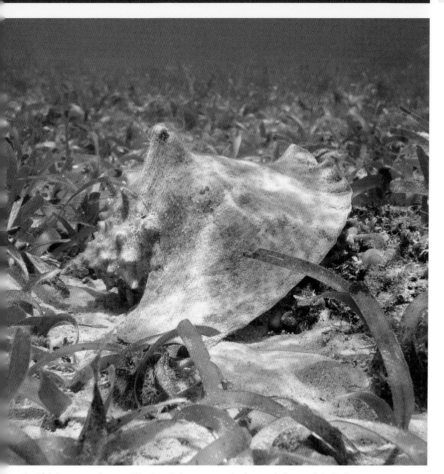

ce plentiful, Queen conchs can still be found along seagrass beds near shallow reefs in the Keys.

ge numbers, including creole wrasses, Atlantic mpetfish and large hogfish. There is often re current along this deeper section of reef as s farther out into the Gulf Stream. As a result, ers often explore this site as a drift dive.

le Conch Reef sits to the southwest of the er two sites. It has a ledge that sits at a similar oth to Conch Reef and offers divers and rkelers a chance to explore similar habitat. e historic wreck of the Spanish galleon,

El Infante, rests just seaward of the ledge, around half a mile (0.8 kilometers) beyond the northern terminus of Little Conch Reef (see page 12 for more on the Spanish Fleet of 1733). The wreckage is well incorporated into the surrounding coral rubble at a depth of just 20 feet (6 meters). Timbers and ballast stones are still visible from the armed galleon that was one of the largest vessels in the historic 1733 fleet that wrecked along the coast of the Florida Keys.

CONCH REEF, CONCH WALL & LITTLE CONCH

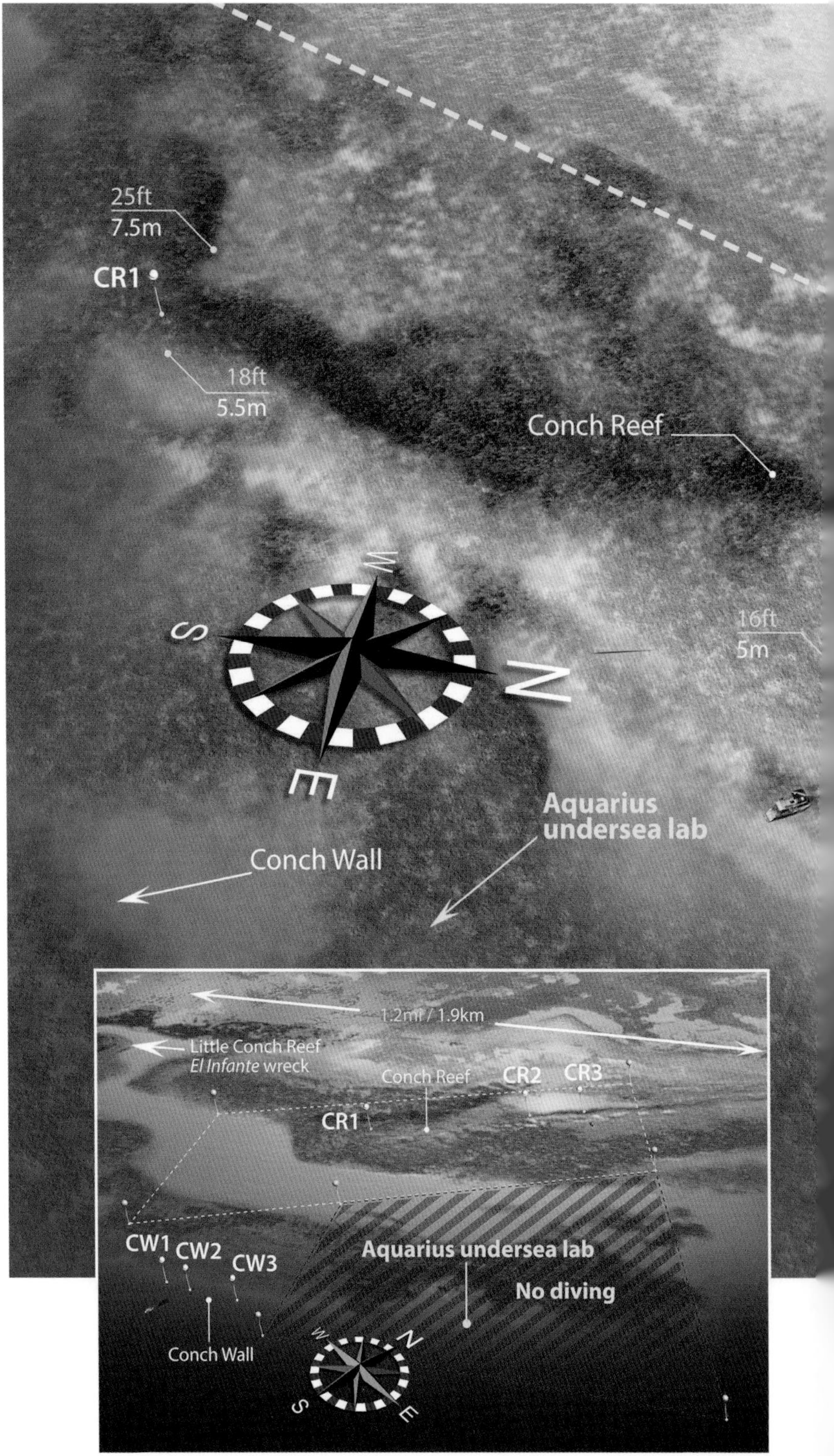

25ft
7.5m

CR1

18ft
5.5m

Conch Reef

16ft
5m

Conch Wall

Aquarius
undersea lab

1.2mi / 1.9km

Little Conch Reef
El Infante wreck

Conch Reef

CR2   CR3

CR1

CW1   CW2   CW3

Conch Wall

Aquarius undersea lab

No diving

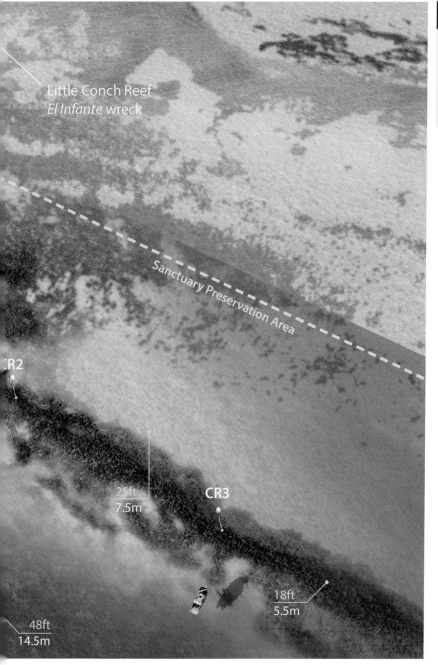

Little Conch Reef
El Infante wreck

Sanctuary Preservation Area

R2

25ft
7.5m

CR3

18ft
5.5m

48ft
14.5m

DAVIS REEF

Difficulty ● ○ ○
Current ● ● ○
Depth ● ● ○
Reef ★★☆
Fauna ★★☆

Access 🚤 8mi (13km) from Islamorada

Level Open Water

Location Islamorada

GPS   DR1 24° 55.302'N, 80° 30.357'W
DR2 24° 55.340'N, 80° 30.330'W
DR3 24° 55 363'N, 80° 30.206'W
DR4 24° 55.404'N, 80° 30.283'W
DR5 24° 55.080'N, 80° 30.372'W
DR6 24° 55.501'N, 80° 29.933'W

Getting there

Davis Reef is located just over 4 miles (7

kilometers) southeast of Plantation Key. Gettin
there involves a boat ride of around 30 minute
from Islamorada.

Access

This site is only accessible by boat given i
distance from shore. Davis Reef is suitable fc
divers and snorkelers of all levels along the set c
four mooring buoys anchored near the shallo
ledge. The two deeper buoys are only accessib
to divers. The four shallow buoys are within th
Davis Reef Sanctuary Preservation Area (SP/

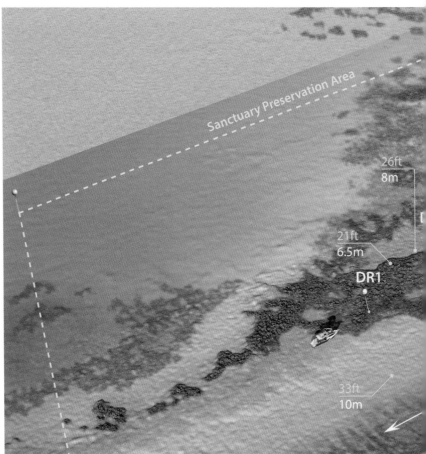

which was designated to protect the many well-developed gorgonians found at this site, including sea fans, sea rods, sea whips and sea plumes. No harvesting of any kind is permitted in the SPA.

Description

The shallow section of Davis Reef focuses on a 7- to 10-foot-tall (2- to 3-meter) ledge that runs parallel to the shoreline. The ledge is shallow enough for snorkelers and divers to enjoy the forests of well-established gorgonians located at this site. Hard corals are also found here, intermixed with the soft corals, including a particularly large brain coral located near the south end of the site between buoys DR1 and DR2. Out in the sand, around 25 feet (7.5 meters) toward shore from the large brain coral, sits a small statue of a Buddha. The origin of this statue has largely been lost to time, but it was replaced in 2001 after being removed (possibly as a prank) in the summer of 2000. The new Buddha rests on concrete blocks at a depth of 20 feet (6 meters).

The ledge area is home to nurse sharks, moray eels and lobsters given the many overhangs and crevices. Divers and snorkelers are also likely to see plenty of sergeant majors, stoplight parrotfish, rock beauties, yellowtail snapper and gray snapper. Both spotted and yellow goatfish are often seen in the sand patches around the reef, along with brown garden eels, which can be found sticking their heads out of the sand and rubble-covered areas.

The two deeper buoys (DR5 and DR6) are positioned outside of the SPA boundaries to the east and the south of the main ledge. These buoys are popular with commercial and recreational fishers, but also with divers, as the reef slope here is largely hard bottomed reef with shallow sand channels cutting through it. The area is covered in a scattering of hard and soft corals, which provide cover to a range of marine species, from hogfish to green sea turtles.

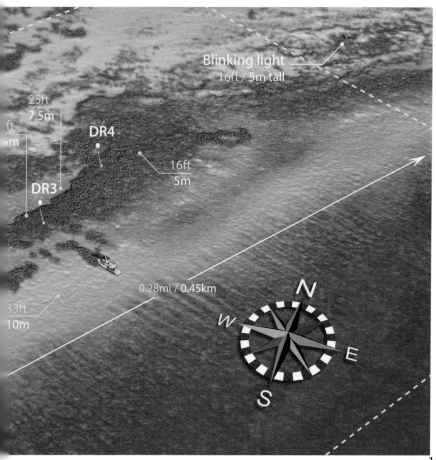

FLORIDA KEYS

DAVEY CROCKER & CROCKER REEF

Difficulty ● ○ ○
Current ● ○ ○
Depth ● ● ○
Reef ★★★☆
Fauna ★★★

Access 🚤 6mi (10km) from Islamorada

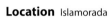

🤿 **Level** Open Water

🤿 **Location** Islamorada
GPS CR1 24° 54.151'N, 80° 31.843'W
CR2 24° 54.241'N, 80° 31.574'W
CR3 24° 54.496'N, 80° 31.176'W
CR5 (Davey Crocker)
24° 54.836'N, 80° 30.914'W

Getting there

Davey Crocker and Crocker Reef are located on the outer reef line just 4 miles (6.5 kilometers) southeast of Plantation Key. Getting to these adjacent sites involves a boat ride of around 15 to 20 minutes from Islamorada.

Access

These sites are only accessible by boat given their distance from shore. Davey Crocker is a shallow

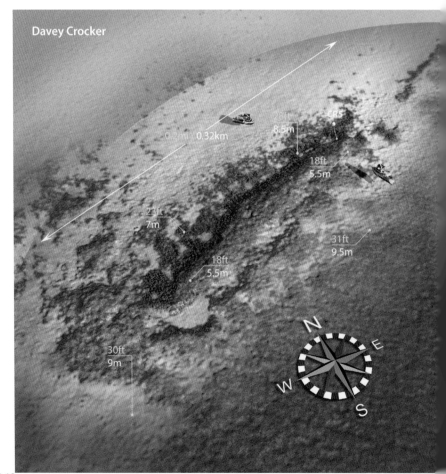

Davey Crocker

RELAX & RECHARGE

As you might expect, the **M.E.A.T. Eatery and Taproom** (88005 Overseas Highway, Islamorada) is famous for its burgers and beer, but this is certainly not your average burger joint. All the meats are smoked on site, and they even create their own condiments from scratch. There are a range of incredible burger options, as well as fish, chicken and pulled-pork sandwiches. All burger and sandwiches come with French fries, smoked potato salad or coleslaw, but you can upgrade to onion rings, zucchini fries, salads or their bistro fries, which are made with truffle oil and parmesan cheese. On the liquid side of life there are a dozen craft beers on tap, as well as organic wines, floats, and "adult milkshakes," like the mind-boggling Guinness and Nutella banana bread ale and vanilla bean shake! It's no wonder M.E.A.T., which also has a Boca Raton location, has won multiple awards over the years. Visit: **Meateatery.com**

ledge that is suitable for divers and snorkelers of all skill levels via a single mooring buoy. Crocker Reef is accessible via three mooring buoys anchored at depths ranging between 50 and 60 feet (16 and 18 meters). The reef slope here descends to depths of 100 to 110 feet (30.5 to 33.5 meter). The deeper buoys of Crocker Reef are only accessible to divers, although snorkelers may enjoy the shallow ledge adjacent to these deeper buoys. Accessing this southern ledge would require anchoring in the sand near the ledge as it is over 0.25 miles (400 meters) from the nearest buoy.

Description

Davey Crocker is technically part of the larger Crocker Reef site. It gets its name from its position midway between Davis Reef and Crocker Reef. Davey Crocker is a shallow ledge that supports an incredible array of fish species. The ledge stretches around 0.2 miles (320 meters) in length from southwest to northeast and tops out at a depth of 18 feet (5.5 meters). It reaches a depth of between 23 and 28 feet (7 and 8.5 meters) along the bottom of the ledge, where divers are likely to see nurse sharks and moray eels. The ledge site is popular with French and bluestriped grunts, as well as schoolmaster, gray and yellowtail snapper. Divers also regularly spot turtles along the ledge.

Crocker Reef is a hard bottom reef slope marked with shallow ravines and small grooves that provide plenty of complex structure to support the marine life found here. The deeper waters at this site make it more likely to see megafauna, including reef sharks and spotted eagle rays. The usual complement of grunts and snapper are also found here in high numbers, along with French, gray, Queen and blue angelfish. Scamp, red grouper, coney and black grouper can also be seen waiting in ambush among the soft corals and large barrel sponges that pepper the reef slope.

The mooring buoy anchored to the south of this site is the shallowest of the three buoys, sometimes called Crocker 35 or Crocker Orbit. The northern buoy of these three deep mooring buoys is also called Dropoff or Crocker Wall, and it is the deeper of the three buoys. This site rarely experiences much current, but usually has good visibility given its location out on the outer reef line. When there is current, it is popular to explore the site as a drift dive.

DID YOU KNOW?

The size and shape of a fish's teeth and mouth can help determine what it eats. It can be a useful tool for divers and snorkelers looking to identify the fish swimming around them on the reef. Most dive sites in the Florida Keys support enough biodiversity to allow divers to compare and contrast a variety of mouth and teeth sizes and shapes. Fishes with a large gape (the size of the mouth when opened wide) such as members of the predatory grouper family, are designed to accommodate a wide variety of prey. Diminutive mouths with comb-like teeth, such as those seen in butterflyfishes, are perfectly designed for grasping tiny food such as coral polyps and marine worms. Meanwhile, the crescent-shaped mouth of angelfishes are perfect for taking bites out of sponges – just like the ones that cover Davey Crocker and Crocker Reef. Wherever you are exploring, take the time to look around and pay attention to the story unfolding nearby.

CROCKER REEF

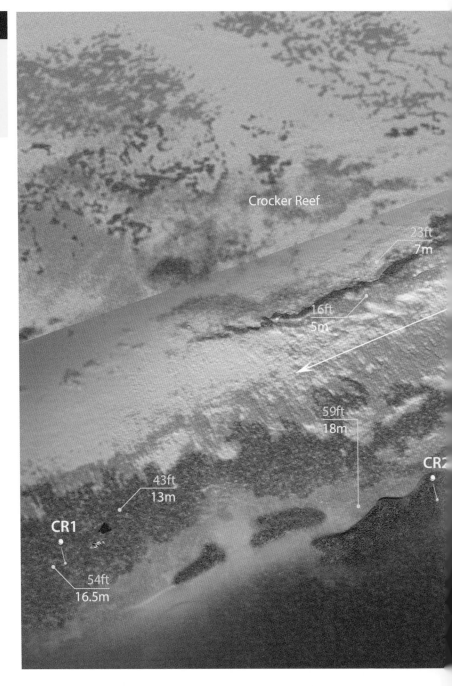

Crocker Reef

23ft
7m

16ft
5m

59ft
18m

43ft
13m

CR1

54ft
16.5m

CR2

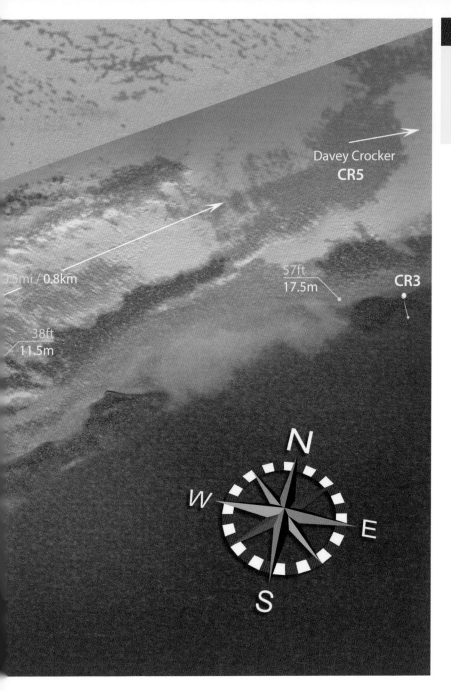

Davey Crocker
CR5

1.5mi / 0.8km

57ft
17.5m

CR3

38ft
11.5m

N

W

E

S

HEN & CHICKENS

HC8 24° 56.220'N, 80° 32.862'W
HC9 24° 56.253'N, 80° 32.839'W
HC10 24° 56.012'N, 80° 33.050'W

Difficulty	● ○ ○		
Current	● ○ ○		
Depth	● ○ ○		
Reef	★★☆	Access	⛵
Fauna	★★☆	4mi (6.5km) from Islamorada	

Level Open Water

Location Islamorada
GPS
HC1 24° 56.033'N, 80° 33.029'W
HC2 24° 56.039'N, 80° 32.988'W
HC3 24° 56.025'N, 80° 32.958'W
HC4 24° 56.039'N, 80° 32.934'W
HC5 24° 56.085'N, 80° 32.924'W
HC6 24° 56.105'N, 80° 32.873'W
HC7 24° 56.143'N, 80° 32.912'W

Getting there

Hen & Chickens Reef is a group of patch reefs located in shallow water less than 2 miles (3 kilometers) offshore of Plantation Key. Visiting this site involves a boat ride of around 10 to 15 minutes from Islamorada.

Access

Despite being closer to shore than most dive sites in the Florida Keys, Hen & Chickens is still only accessible by boat. The site features four large sections of reef patches located in just 23 feet (7 meters) of water that are suitable for snorkelers and divers alike. Dive boats can access the reef via one of the 10 mooring buoys anchored throughout the site. Currents are rarely strong here in Hawk Channel, but that also means

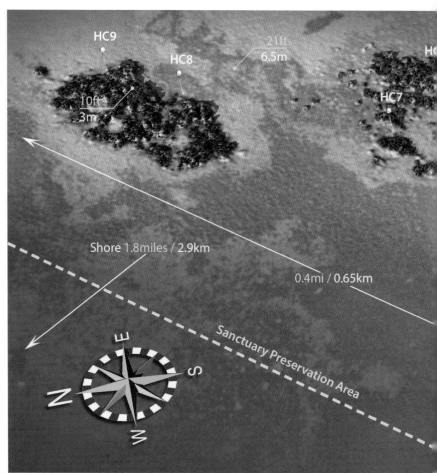

HC9
HC8
21ft
6.5m
HC
HC7
10ft
3m
Shore 1.8miles / 2.9km
0.4mi / 0.65km
Sanctuary Preservation Area

visibility can be poor if the wind and waves have stirred up sediment. These patch reefs are located within the boundaries of a Sanctuary Preservation Area (SPA) and so fishing of any kind or anchoring when a mooring buoy is available is not permitted.

Description

Hen & Chickens Reef (also sometimes called Hens & Chickens Reef) is very popular with divers and snorkelers as it provides complex structure despite its relatively shallow depth. The reef gets its name from its resemblance, when viewed from above, to a hen and her chicks. The site is easy to locate as it is marked by a large, lighted channel tower.

The site is very shallow, with the tops of corals reaching up to just 10 feet (3 meters) or less below the surface of the water. These large coral mounds of brain and star coral help create a labyrinthine feel to the site. The reef itself is covered in a forest of purple sea fans and other gorgonians, helping provide habitat for enough colorful reef fish to keep even the most experienced divers engaged for a full dive.

Along with the usual complement of bluestriped grunts, porkfish and French grunts, divers and snorkelers may also see Queen and gray angelfish, stoplight parrotfish, hogfish and both spotfin and foureye butterflyfish. The high density of reef fish supports larger predators, including barracuda, black grouper and a variety of snapper species, including yellowtail, lane and schoolmaster snapper. Divers and snorkelers have reported seeing nurse sharks resting in the sand next to small reef ledges and overhangs, while sea turtles are also seen cruising through the area, including green, hawksbill and loggerheads. Some locals report a friendly green moray eel is also located at this site.

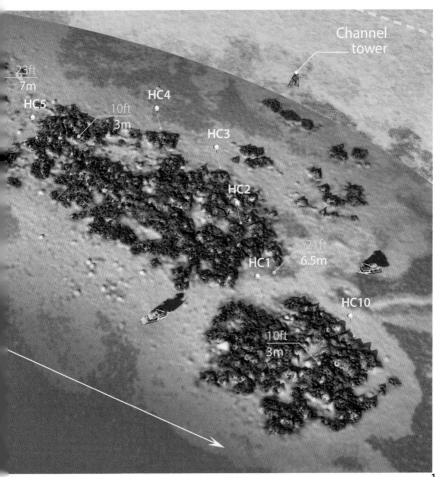

VICTORY REEF

Difficulty	● ○ ○
Current	● ● ○
Depth	● ● ○
Reef	★★☆ Access
Fauna	★☆☆ 5mi (8km) from Islamorada

Level Open water

Location Islamorada
GPS   24° 53.298'N, 80° 32.957'W

Getting there
Victory Reef is a site along the outer reef that sits just 5 miles (8 kilometers) offshore from Islamorada. Visiting this site involves a boat ride of around 10 to 15 minutes from Islamorada.

Access
Victory Reef is only accessible by boat. At its shallowest point, the reef is around 37 feet (11.5 meters) deep, making it better suited to divers than snorkelers. There are no mooring buoys at this site, so boats should aim to anchor in the large V-shaped sand patch that gives this site its name. Currents can be strong along this stretch of outer reef line, but the visibility is generally good.

Description
Victory Reef features a large area of sand bounded on both sides by low reef spurs and a hard substrate bottom. The area of sand measures 330 feet (100 meters) across and slopes from 37 feet (11.5 meters) down to 54 feet (16.5 meters) where it gives way to the hard-bottomed reef slope common along this section of the Keys. It can take about 10 minutes to swim out to the ledge, which contains spur and groove formations that drop down to sand at about 90 feet (27.5 meters). The reef supports a variety of fish species, including reef sharks and barracuda.

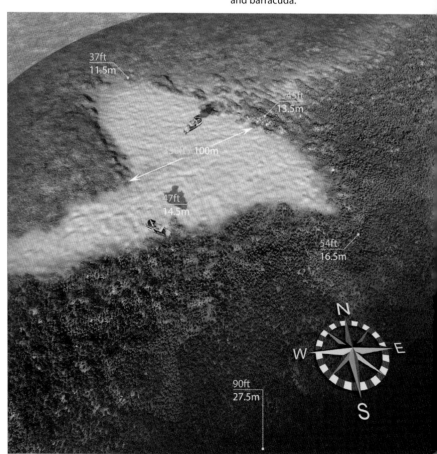

ISLAMORADA FINGERS

Difficulty ● ○ ○
Current   ● ● ○
Depth   ● ● ○
Reef   ★★☆   Access 🚤
Fauna   ★★☆   5.5mi (9km) from Islamorada

Level Open water

Location Islamorada
GPS   24° 52.927'N, 80° 33.528'W

Getting there

Islamorada Fingers is a site along the outer reef that sits just 5 miles (8 kilometers) offshore from Islamorada. Visiting this site involves a boat ride of around 10 to 15 minutes from Islamorada.

Access

Islamorada Fingers (sometimes just called Fingers) is only accessible by boat. The site ranges in depth from 35 to 75 feet (10.5 to 23 meters), making it more suitable for divers than snorkelers. There are no mooring buoys at this site, so boats should aim to anchor in the main sand channel immediately adjacent to the GPS coordinates provided above. Currents can be strong along this stretch of the outer reef line, but the visibility is generally good.

Description

The site gets its name from the resemblance of the reef to a hand with spurs of coral (the "fingers") pointing out toward sea, interspersed with grooves of sand and rubble. There is a ledge at 70 feet (21.5 meters) where the fingers meet the sand, bottoming out at a depth of 85 feet (26 meters). The main sand channel running out to sea has 3-foot (1-meter) ledges on either side and represents a starting point for most dives. Divers have a chance to see a range of creatures, from hogfish and rock beauties to eagle rays and dolphins, while yellowhead jawfish are common in the sand and rubble areas of the reef.

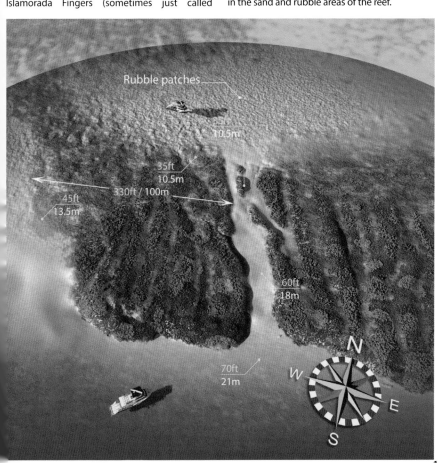

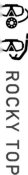

ROCKY TOP

Difficulty ● ○ ○
Current   ● ○ ○
Depth   ● ○ ○
Reef   ★★★☆   Access 🛥
Fauna   ★★★   3.5mi (6km) from Islamorada

Level Open water

Location Islamorada
GPS   RT1 24° 53.715'N, 80° 34.339'W

Getting there
Rocky Top is a small patch reef located just inside of the outer reef line, about 3.5 miles (6 kilometers) offshore from Islamorada. Visiting this site involves a boat ride of around 10 minutes from Islamorada.

Access
Rocky Top is only accessible by boat. The reef bottoms out in sand at a depth of just 25 feet (7.5 meters) making it suitable for divers and snorkelers of all experience levels. There is a single mooring buoy at this site, so boats should aim to tie into it to avoid anchoring near the reef and damaging the corals. Currents are generally mild here, but visibility can be poor when wind and waves stir up the sediments.

Description
Rocky Top is a popular oasis of reef life in the otherwise sandy region inland of the outer reef line. The sea fan-covered reefs support a variety of fish species including large schools of bluestriped and French grunts. Yellowtail and gray snapper are also common here, along with hogfish and goatfish. Nurse sharks can be spotted hanging out under reef ledges while southern stingrays are commonly seen out in the sand and rubble areas that surround the reef.

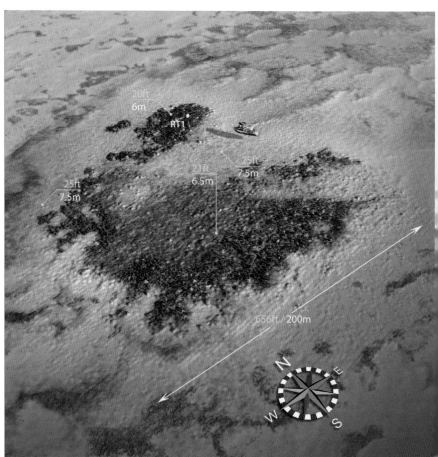

MORADA

Difficulty	● ○ ○	
Current	● ○ ○	
Depth	● ○ ○	
Reef	★★★	Access 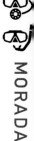
Fauna	★☆☆	3.5mi (6km) from Islamorada

Level Open water

Location Islamorada
GPS   24° 53.614'N, 80° 34.664'W

Getting there

Morada is a small patch reef located in the sandy area that sits just 3.5 miles (6 kilometers) offshore from Islamorada and just inside of the outer reef line. Visiting this site involves a boat ride of around 10 minutes from Islamorada.

Access

Morada is only accessible by boat. The reef bottoms out in sand at a depth of just 20 feet (6 meters) making it suitable for divers and snorkelers of all experience levels. There are no mooring buoys at this site, so boats should aim to anchor in the sand well clear of any corals. Currents are generally mild at this site, but visibility can be poor when wind and waves stir up the sediments.

Description

Morada means purple in Spanish and this small set of patch reefs gets its name from its dense covering of purple sea fans and purple sponges. This site is popular with divers looking for a colorful reef to explore in shallow water. The patch reef shelters yellowtail snapper, ocean surgeonfish and bicolor damselfish among other species. Nurse sharks and stingrays are often seen in the sand and rubble areas that surround the coral patches, while bonnethead sharks (the smallest members of the hammerhead family) frequent these reefs for much of the year.

MORADA

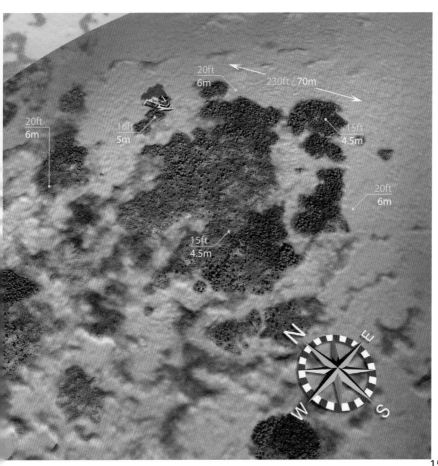

EAGLE

Difficulty ● ● ○
Current ● ○ ○
Depth ● ● ○
Reef ★★★☆
Fauna ★★☆☆

Access 6.5mi (10.5km) from Islamorada

Level Advanced

Location Islamorada
GPS   24° 52.199'N, 80° 34.230'W

Getting there
Eagle is an artificial reef located just 5 miles (8 kilometers) offshore from Islamorada, just beyond the outer reef line that runs parallel to the coast. Visiting this site involves a boat ride of around 25 to 30 minutes from Islamorada.

Access
This site is only accessible by boat due to its distance from shore. The highest point of the wreck sits at 70 feet (21.5 meters) making it better suited to advanced divers with experience at depth. The seabed is 110 feet (33.5 meters) deep, which is slightly shallower than many of the other wrecks along the coast. There are two surface mooring buoys at this site and one submerged mooring buoy. Currents are generally mild here.

Description
Eagle was originally a cargo freighter built in Holland in 1962. She launched under the name *Raila Dan* to begin what, by all accounts, was a short and troubled career. She operated as *Raila Dan* for the first seven years of her existence under a Danish flag. She experienced a serious fire during this period and was sold and renamed *Barok* in 1969. She changed names and owners

once again seven years later, now operating under the name *Carmela*. Successive name changes followed, including *Ytai* in 1976 and *Etai* in 1977. It was in 1977 that she experienced yet another serious fire. In 1981 she changed hands again and was renamed *Carigulf Pioneer*, before ultimately being sold to a Caymanian company, the Jonaz Corporation, in 1984 and renamed *Arron K*.

On October 6, 1985, she caught fire, once again, while en route from Miami to Venezuela with a shipment of scrap paper. Two U.S. Coast Guard cutters intervened and helped rescue the crew, but the fire caused massive damage to the ship's superstructure, and she was declared a total loss. She was towed back to Miami and remained docked in the Miami River until the Florida Keys Artificial Reef Association purchased her with financial support from a collection of divers and businesses, including Joe Teitelbaum, owner of the North River Terminals and the Eagle Tire Co. In all, the ship cost $30,000 to purchase and clean before she was rechristened the *Eagle Tire Co.* and towed out for deployment.

She was moored next to the *Alexander Barge* in preparation for deployment, just past the outer reef line offshore of Islamorada. She was scuttled on December 19, 1985, with the help of explosives from the Miami-Dade County Bomb Squad, and she sank within just a few minutes, coming to rest on her starboard side. She is

---

DID YOU KNOW? ❓

Explosives have been a popular method of scuttling vessels and creating artificial reefs for decades. The practice was effective at getting the ship to the bottom as quickly as possible and often made for a good show. The famous *Oriskany* just offshore Pensacola, Florida, required 500 pounds of C-4 to successfully scuttle her. Today, most deployments rely on controlled flooding, where during the clean and prep phase of deployment, holes are cut in the hull just above the waterline. When it is time to sink

the ship, water is pumped into the hull until the boat sinks enough for the cut holes to drop below the waterline, and then physics takes over. Not only does it do less damage to the wreck, but this strategy also causes less damage to the environment. It was not uncommon for the concussive blast from a large explosion used during a deployment to stun and possibly kill large schools of fish in the vicinity of a vessel as it went down. While controlled flooding takes longer than blasting, it is better for everyone when a wreck is scuttled this way rather than through a spectacular explosion.

one of nine wrecks included in the Florida Keys National Marine Sanctuary Shipwreck Trail.

In 1998, Hurricane Georges swept through the Keys and the resulting currents generated by the storm caused the wreck to break in two, just in front of the superstructure. Over the years, the underwater environment has taken its toll, causing the main holds to collapse in on themselves. But the bow and superstructure remain largely intact, along with the two kingposts or mast-like towers that are used to support a ship's cargo booms. The forward kingpost remains attached to the bow and lies parallel to the sandy seabed, while the midships kingpost has collapsed onto the sand along with much of the midships hull.

The wreck offers plenty of swim-throughs, as well as some deeper penetration opportunities

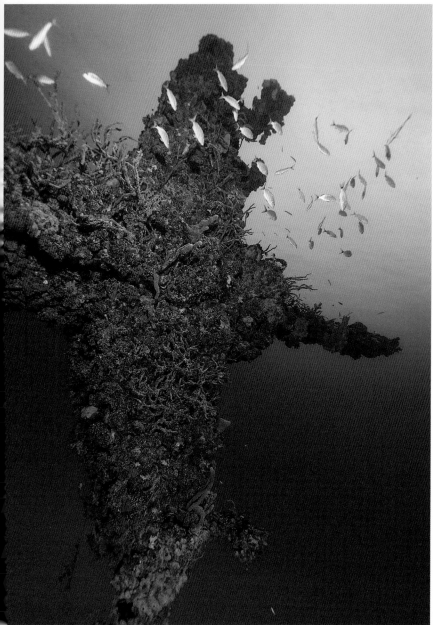

Kurt Tidd ©

The kingmast on the wreck of the *Eagle* is heavily encrusted with corals and sponges.

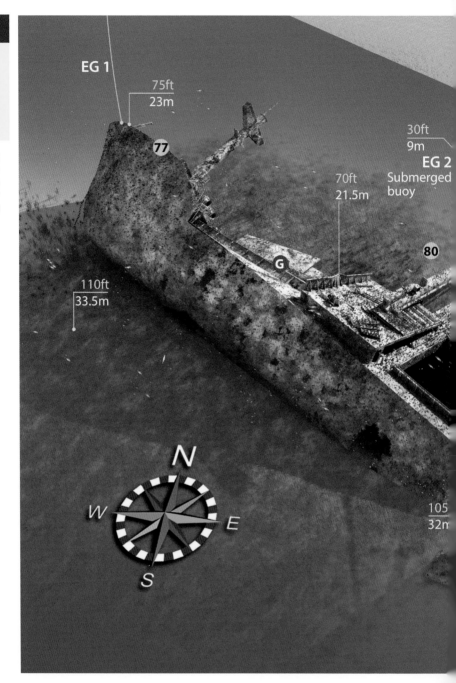

EG 1

75ft
23m

77

30ft
9m

EG 2
Submerged
buoy

70ft
21.5m

80

G

110ft
33.5m

105
32m

for those divers with experience. Large holes in the wreck's hull allow divers to see into the lower holds, while the bridge and wheelhouse are also accessible.

Corals, sponges and all manner of marine life have colonized the wreck over the years. The depth and position of the wreck mean it support large fish, including goliath grouper, eagle ray and bull sharks. Large tarpon and barracuda are also commonly seen here, along with a variet of smaller reef fish, including bar jacks, ree butterflyfish, graysbies, Queen angelfish and sharpnose puffers.

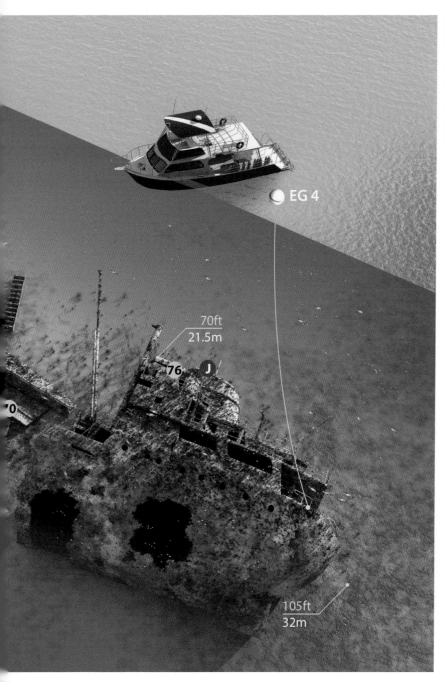

EG 4

70ft
21.5m

76

J

0

105ft
32m

Route

Divers often start their route exploring the stern area of the wreck with its relatively intact superstructure and exposed propeller. The wheelhouse provides an interesting swim-through, while the rest of the superstructure allows for some penetration. The central cargo hold has collapsed around midship, but there are still opportunities to explore the structure created by the debris, including overhanging hull plates and the heavily encrusted kingposts. The bow remains relatively intact with access points along the stern edge. Given the average depth of the site, bottom time can be somewhat limited. The superstructure

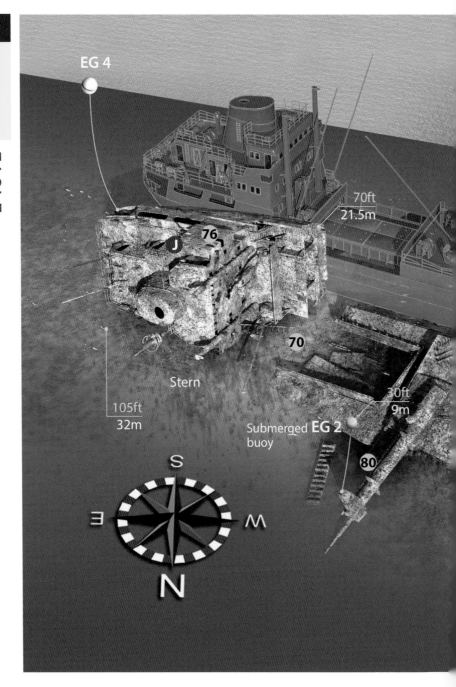

EG 4

70ft
21.5m

76

J

70

Stern

30ft
9m

105ft
32m

Submerged EG 2
buoy

80

S

E

W

N

therefore presents the most interesting area to
explore and is also the shallowest, allowing divers
to potentially extend their bottom time.

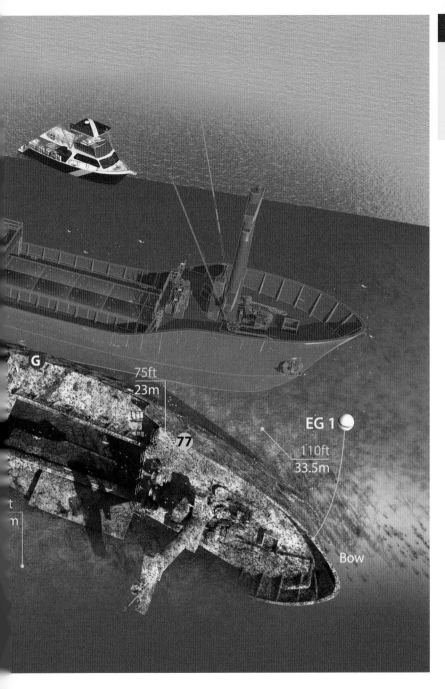

75ft
23m

EG 1

110ft
33.5m

Bow

Name:	*MV Eagle Tire Co.*	**Construction:**	Bijkers Aannemingsbedrijf,
Type:	Cargo freighter		Werf Gorinchem, Holland,
Previous names:	*Raila Dan, Barok, Carmela, Ytai,*		December 1962
	Etai, Carigulf Pioneer, Arron K	**Last owner:**	Florida Department of
Length:	287ft (81.5m)		Natural Resources
Tonnage:	1,768grt	**Sunk:**	Dec. 19, 1985

ALEXANDER BARGE

Difficulty ● ● ○
Current ● ○ ○
Depth ● ● ○
Reef ★★☆
Fauna ★★☆

Access 🚤 6.5mi (10.5km) from Islamorada

Level Advanced

Location Islamorada
GPS   24° 52.154'N, 80° 34.323'W

Getting there

Alexander Barge is an artificial reef located just 5 miles (8 kilometers) offshore from Islamorada, just beyond the outer reef line that runs parallel to the coast. Visiting this site involves a boat ride of around 25 to 30 minutes from Islamorada.

Access

This site is only accessible by boat due to its distance from shore. The wreck has just 15 feet (4.5 meters) of relief from a sandy seafloor that reaches a depth of approximately 100 feet (30.5 meters). As such, this site is more suited to advanced divers. There are no mooring buoys at this site, so boats need to either tie into the wreck or hot-drop and explore the site as a drift dive.

Description

Alexander Barge was a 120-foot (36.5-meter) long, 40-foot (12-meter) wide push barge that was deployed as an artificial reef in 1984. Bridge rubble, either from the Snake Creek Bridge or the Whale Harbor bridge (accounts vary), was dropped at this location just one year later. The two deployments combine to add an incredible level of complexity to an otherwise flat and featureless sandy seabed. The site is just 600 feet (183 meters) southwest of the *Eagle*, making this pair of artificial reefs popular as a two-tank dive.

Divers exploring the site are likely to find plenty of lobster hidden in the crevices and overhangs created by the piles of rubble and the barge, which remains largely intact. Plenty of large grouper, amberjack and hogfish have been reported at the site, along with the usual complement of bluestriped grunts and yellowtail snapper that are found schooling around the wreck. Careful penetration is possible through large holes in the side of the barge, but only for those with experience in overhead environments. The hull of the overturned barge is well encrusted with soft corals and sponges, offering shelter to a host of damselfish species including bicolor and cocoa damselfish, as well as reef butterflyfish and highhats.

DID YOU KNOW?

Artificial reefs are human-made structures that have been placed underwater to achieve a range of different goals from coastal protection to the augmentation of local fisheries. Perhaps the earliest documented use of artificial reefs was by the ancient Persians dating back to around 250 BCE, when they sunk ships to block pirates from accessing the Tigris River. For millennia, fishers have known that fish are attracted to underwater structures, particularly in areas with flat and featureless seabeds. This principle is why fish traps work – the fish choose to enter the trap because they are attracted to the structure, believing it to be a safe place to shelter. In the 1800s, large artificial reef structures were created from logs and placed in the marine ecosystem off the coast of Southern Carolina and other U.S. states. During the 20th century through today, various countries have created artificial reefs from a range of novel structures, including ships, cars, trains, planes, military vehicles, bridges and even oil rigs, to dispose of waste while also providing habitat for marine life and an attraction for divers and snorkelers. More recently, artists have started creating fascinating underwater sculptures from marine cement, which have become tourist attractions.

ALEXANDER BARGE

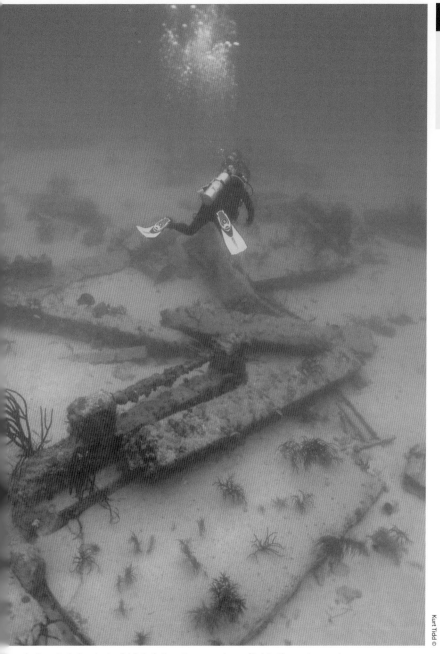

Kurt Tidd ©

xander Barge includes plenty of debris that creates a complex reef habitat for marine species.

me:	*Alexander Barge*	**Last owner:**	n/a
)e:	Push barge	**Sunk:**	1984
vious names:	n/a		
gth:	120ft (36.5m)		
nnage:	n/a		
nstruction:	n/a		

CHEECA ROCKS (AKA THE ROCKS)

Difficulty	● ○ ○	
Current	● ○ ○	
Depth	● ○ ○	
Reef	★★★	Access 🚤
Fauna	★★☆	3.5mi (5.6km) from Islamorada

Level Open Water

Location Islamorada

GPS
CR1 24° 54.216'N, 80° 36.952'W
CR2 24° 54.296'N, 80° 36.920'W
CR3 24° 54.245'N, 80° 36.885'W
CR4 24° 54.255'N, 80° 36.994'W
CR5 24° 54.230'N, 80° 36.978'W
CR6 24° 54.252'N, 80° 37.066'W
CR7 24° 54.042'N, 80° 37.068'W
CR8 24° 54.262'N, 80° 36.618'W
CR9 24° 54.260'N, 80° 36.551'W

Getting there

Cheeca Rocks is a small set of patch reefs located in Hawk Channel just over 1 mile (2 kilometers) offshore from Upper Matecumbe Key. Visiting this site involves a boat ride of around 10 minutes from Islamorada.

Access

Cheeca Rocks is only accessible by boat despite its proximity to shore. The shallowness of the site makes it suitable for divers and snorkelers of all experience levels. There are nine mooring buoys distributed across three of the four patch reef sections, making access relatively easy at this site. Currents are generally mild in Hawk Channel, but visibility can be poor when wind and waves stir up the sediments. The site is one of the smallest Sanctuary Protected Areas (SPAs). Harvesting of any marine creatures or anchoring when a buoy is available is not permitted.

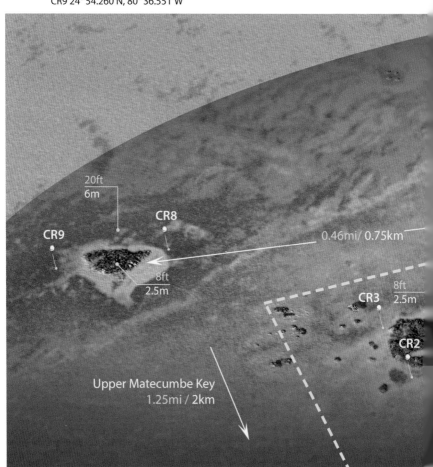

20ft
6m

CR8

CR9

0.46mi/ 0.75km

8ft
2.5m

8ft
CR3   2.5m

CR2

Upper Matecumbe Key
1.25mi / 2km

Description

Cheeca Rocks is an inshore patch reef that supports a variety of marine life in relatively shallow waters. The reef top is as shallow as just 8 feet (2.5 meters) in some places, while the sandy seabed bottoms out at a depth between 16 and 20 feet (5 and 6 meters). The reef supports a healthy coral covering, including mustard hill coral, star corals and brain corals. Sea fans and other gorgonians are also found at the site in relatively high numbers.

The high complexity of the site supports plenty of marine fishes, including bluestriped and white grunts, gray angelfish, blue tangs and various parrotfish, including both stoplight and striped parrotfish. Yellowtail and schoolmaster snapper are also commonly seen here, as are large barracuda. Nurse sharks are often spotted resting along the edges of the patch reefs.

SCIENTIFIC INSIGHT

Cheeca Rocks is one of seven sites across the Florida Keys National Marine Sanctuary that is part of a multi-million partnership between the National Marine Sanctuaries Foundation, Mote Marine Lab and the Coral Restoration Foundation, all under the project title of **Mission: Iconic Reefs**. The effort aims to restore nearly three million square feet (280,000 square meters) of coral in the Florida Keys. The hope is to counter the nearly 90 percent decline in live coral cover over the past 40 years. To learn more about the project, visit: **Marinesanctuary.org/mission-iconic-reefs/**

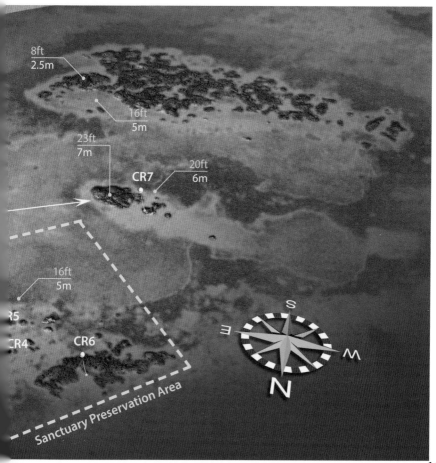

ALLIGATOR REEF & ALLIGATOR DEEP

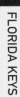

FLORIDA KEYS

Difficulty ● ○ ○
Current ● ● ○
Depth ● ○ ○
Reef ★★☆
Fauna ★★★

Access 🚤 8.5mi (13.5km) from Islamorada

Level Open Water/ Advanced

Location Islamorada
GPS   Alligator Wreck
     GPS 24° 51.065'N, 80° 37.083'W

     Alligator Reef
     AR0 24° 50.716'N, 80° 37.444'W
     AR1 24° 50.740'N, 80° 37.421'W
     AR2 24° 50.775'N, 80° 37.380'W
     AR3 24° 50.785'N, 80° 37.338'W
     AR4 24° 50.813'N, 80° 37.307'W

     Alligator Deep
     AR5 24° 50.465'N, 80° 37.355'W
     AR6 24° 50.523'N, 80° 37.174'W

Getting there

Alligator Reef is located just 4 miles (6.5 kilometers) off the southern tip of Upper Matecumbe Key. Getting there involves a boat trip of around 20 to 30 minutes, depending on the starting point. The reef is easy to locate based on the famous lighthouse that towers 136 feet (41.5 meters) over its northern end.

Access

Access to Alligator Reef is only possible by boat due to its distance from shore. The shallow reef is suitable for divers and snorkelers of all levels, but Alligator Deep is more accessible to advanced divers who might wish to explore the reef-sand interface that reaches depth

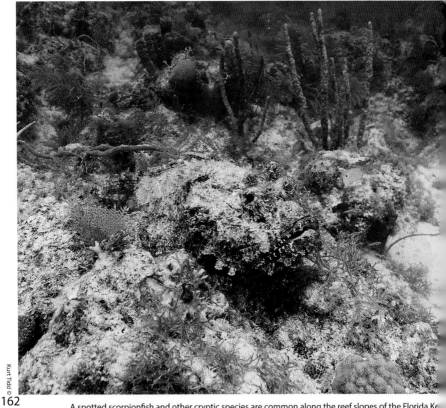

Kurt Tidd ©

A spotted scorpionfish and other cryptic species are common along the reef slopes of the Florida Ke

DID YOU KNOW?

USS Alligator was built to combat piracy in the Florida area, but also to enforce the Act Prohibiting Importation of Slaves, which was enacted by the U.S. government in 1807. The British government enacted a similar law, known as the Slave Trade Act, in the same year. Essentially, these two laws made it illegal to transport slaves across the Atlantic for the purposes of trade, while not abolishing the practice of owning slaves,

which continued in Britain until 1833 and until 1865 in the United States. *Alligator's* early missions took her across the Atlantic in 1821, where she captured several slave ships, including the schooners *Mathilde*, *L'Eliza* and *Daphne*, and captured the Portuguese pirate ship *Marianna Flora*. That same year, she conducted reconnaissance for land along the West African coast suitable for the repatriation of freed slaves. This work led to the establishment of a colony that would later become the Republic of Liberia.

of more than 90 feet (27 meters). Access is possible through five mooring buoys located along the shallow spurs and groove section of the reef, and two additional buoys anchored on the deeper seaward reef slope. There is a single mooring buoy near the wreck of the Alligator in the shallow waters at the foot of the lighthouse.

Description

Like many of the reefs to the north, Alligator Reef gets its name from its most famous shipwreck. *USS Alligator* was an armed schooner in the U.S. Navy. She was constructed in the Charlestown Navy Yard in Boston, Massachusetts, in 1820. She was built specifically to suppress piracy and the slave trade. She featured a new armament called the high pivot gun, which was a precursor to turret guns that allowed firing in multiple directions. Unfortunately, *Alligator's* career was brief.

On November 18, 1822, while escorting a convoy of seven merchant ships through the newly acquired territory of Florida – a region that had become rampant with piracy – *Alligator* ran aground on the reef that now bears her name. The crew attempted to refloat

the grounded vessel but was unable to budge her from the shallow reef. They salvaged what equipment they could and transferred it to the *Ann Maria* (a ship the *Alligator* had only recently liberated from pirates off the coast of Cuba). The sailors then set *Alligator* ablaze to avoid her being salvaged by pirates.

Officials have not been able to definitively show that the wreck of the *Alligator* is the same wreck that sits at the northern end of Alligator Reef. In fact, there are reasons to suspect it may not be the *Alligator*, since the two piles of ballast at the wreck site consist of stones and not the iron ballast the schooner supposedly carried. Even so, the wreck sits in just 3 to 12 feet (1 to 3.5 meters) of water, offering plenty of interest for snorkelers while divers may find the site a little too shallow for a comfortable dive.

The reef around the wreck is also worthy of exploration. The ledge that runs along the shallow portion of Alligator Reef is between 6 and 12 feet (2 and 3.5 meters) tall in some places. The ledge shelters an interesting assortment of marine life, including lobsters, moray eels and nurse sharks. Bonnethead sharks are also commonly spotted along this biodiverse reef. In fact, reef surveys have identified a total of 189

DID YOU KNOW?

It can be challenging to properly identify a historical wreck. Many wrecks are first located by identifying magnetic anomalies in the reef. Even wood-hulled sailing ships include iron components that will trigger a magnetic reading. Once located, these possible contacts are investigated with great care to remove the overlying sediment without disturbing living coral or the surrounding habitat. Divers work to identify the wreck by determining its size based on the pieces they uncover.

Archaeologists can compare the elements of the wreck they find, including sections of hull plating, construction styles and even the weight and makeup of the ship's ballast, to historical records from shipyards, manifests and even deduction based on the nature of the vessel and its occupation. Sometimes a survey team is lucky enough to uncover a bell or cannon or other component that is clearly marked with a ship's name or insignia. Despite the technology and tools available today, however, a positive identification is not always possible and the true identity of a historic wreck is lost to time.

ALLIGATOR REEF & ALLIGATOR WRECK

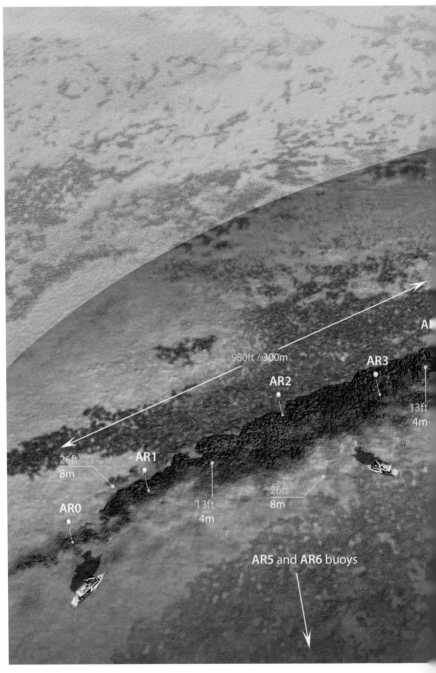

980ft / 300m

AR2

AR3

AR1

26ft
8m

AR0

13ft
4m

13ft
4m

26ft
8m

AR5 and **AR6** buoys

species on Alligator Reef, making it one of the most biodiverse in the area.

Alligator Deep sits just offshore of the shallower reef and represents two sections of deeper reef slope that are separated from the main reef by a wide sand channel. This rare double reef system

is dominated by shallow grooves that run out sea. The area is covered by a scattering of br and star corals as well as large barrel spong Forests of soft corals and sea fans provide shel for a variety of reef fishes, including Frer angelfish and large hogfish. A medium-si ledge and patch reefs mark the deep bound

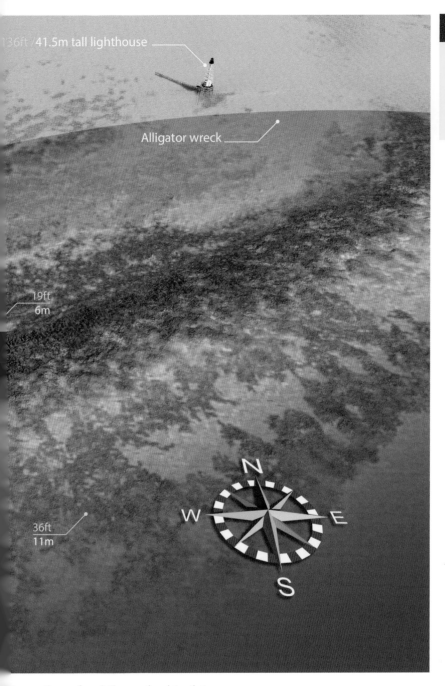

136ft / 41.5m tall lighthouse

Alligator wreck

19ft
6m

36ft
11m

N
W — E
S

tween the reef and the sandy plain that
tends seaward from the reef. Bull sharks and
at hammerhead sharks are commonly seen
trolling these deeper waters.

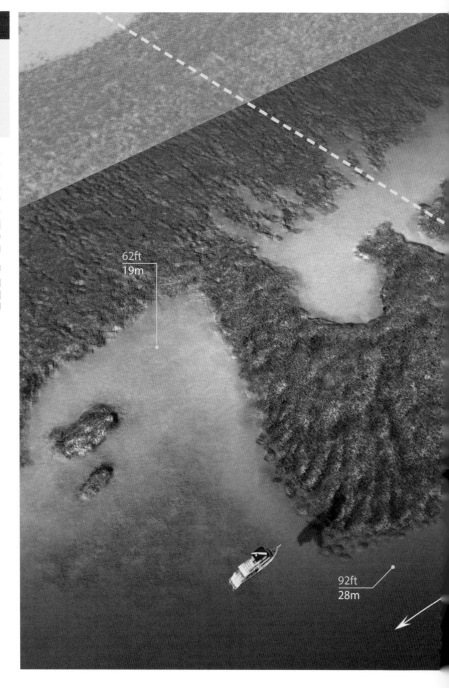

62ft
19m

92ft
28m

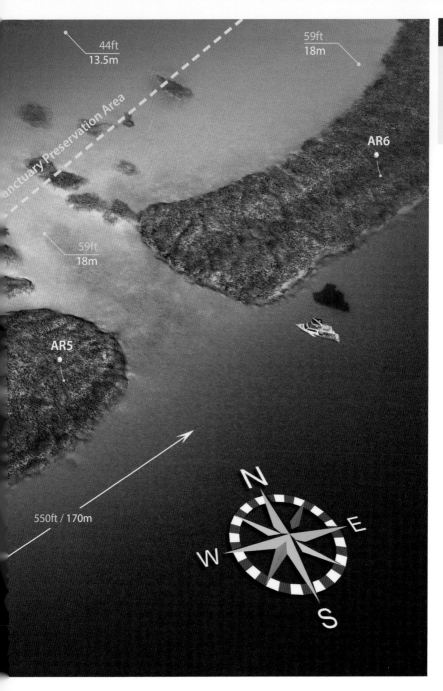

44ft
13.5m

59ft
18m

Sanctuary Preservation Area

AR6

59ft
18m

AR5

550ft / 170m

N
E
W
S

CANNABIS CRUISER

Difficulty ● ● ○
Current ● ● ○
Depth ● ○ ○
Reef ★★★
Fauna ★★☆

Access 🚤 11mi (18km) from Islamorada

Level Advanced

Location Islamorada
GPS   24° 49.506'N, 80° 38.573'W

Getting there
Cannabis Cruiser is located just 4.5 miles (7.5 kilometers) off the northern tip of Lower Matecumbe Key. The wreck lies about 1.6 miles (2.5 kilometers) southwest of Alligator Reef. Getting there involves a boat trip of around 30 to 45 minutes from Islamorada.

Access
Access to *Cannabis Wreck* is only possible by boat due to its distance from shore. Because of its depth and relatively low profile, the wreck is only suitable for advanced divers with experience at depth. There are no mooring buoys at this site, so boats will need to tie into the wreck itself, as the surrounding hard rubble seabed makes anchoring difficult.

Description
The history of *Cannabis Cruiser* (also called *Pot Wreck* and even *Ol' Yeller* by some locals) is wrapped in a fair amount of intrigue and mystery. Some sources suggest the 70-foot (21.5-meter) trawler was regularly used to smuggle marijuana into the United States during the 1970s. The crew apparently panicked during one smuggling run and scuttled the vessel with its full load of contraband to avoid getting caught by the Coast Guard. Years later, two divers discovered the wreck – and its full load of contraband – in the waters southwest of Alligator Reef. The story holds that all her navigational equipment was still in place at the time, although over the intervening decades the entire superstructure of the boat has torn off and been pushed well out of sight of the wreckage.

Today, the hull rests on her port side at a depth of 109 feet (33 meters). Her starboard side is the shallowest point on the wreck at 100 feet (30.5 meters), offering very little relief from the rubble seabed. It is enough to attract marine life, however, with schools of bluestriped grunts and tomtates using the wreck for shelter, while pairs of French angelfish also patrol the structure. Divers have

a good chance of spotting a nurse shark resting in the sandy depression around the stern of the wreck, while lane snapper and Spanish hogfish are often seen up around the bow.

The hull of the wreck is empty, and divers can peer inside via the forward hatch in the intact main deck. Penetration is not recommended due to the confined space. A shopping cart currently

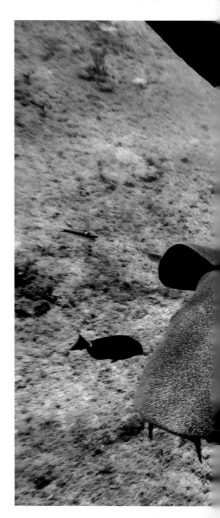

DID YOU KNOW?

Drug smuggling was a great source of artificial reefs in the 1980s and 90s. Coastal freighters were routinely seized during the war on drugs in an attempt to stem the flow of narcotics arriving in the United States from South and Central America. These seized ships were often either donated or purchased at auction by artificial reef associations, counties and even private citizens for redeployment as artificial reefs.

These vessels were often in disrepair and not suitable for continued use as ocean-going transport ships, so they ended up moored in local harbors awaiting interest from salvagers or for time and the elements to take their toll. Thankfully, the science of artificial reefs was showing the potential benefits of repurposing these vessels as underwater habitat that could help support the dive and fishing industries as well as take pressure off existing natural reefs.

ests near the forward hatch – likely an attempt y local divers to provide additional relief to the te – but it is unlikely to stay put for long given e exposed nature of the site and the thin metal f the cart.

Route

Due to her small size, it is easy to fully explore the *Cannabis Wreck* in a single dive. No particular route is required as visibility is generally good enough to see the entire length of the wreck

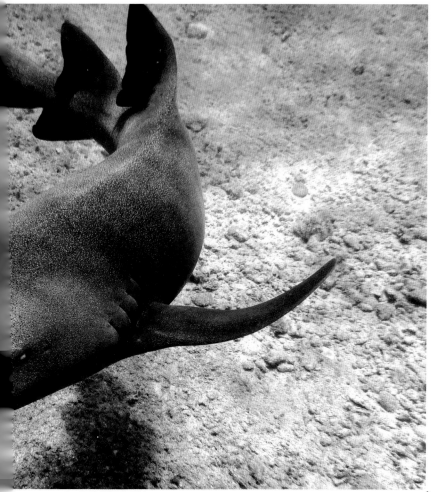

arturo baeza/Shutterstock©

se sharks are often seen resting or swimming slowly along the bottom of reefs and near wrecks in the Florida Keys.

CANNABIS CRUISER

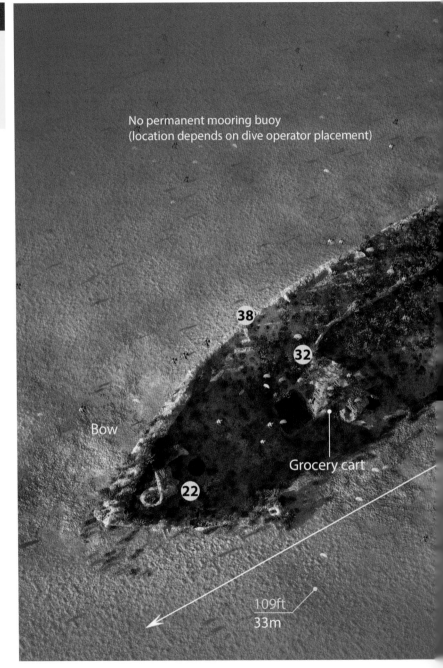

No permanent mooring buoy
(location depends on dive operator placement)

38

32

Bow

Grocery cart

22

109ft
33m

at a single glance. Divers can choose either a clockwise or counterclockwise route to tour the wreck, before spreading out and looking for cryptic marine life in the surrounding seafloor.

CANNABIS CRUISER

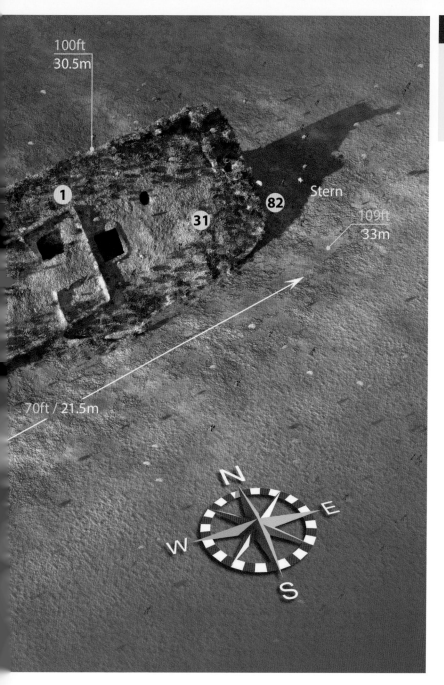

100ft
30.5m

①

82 Stern

31

109ft
33m

70ft / 21.5m

me:	*Cannabis Cruiser*	**Last owner:**	Unknown
e:	Trawler	**Sunk:**	1970s
vious names:	n/a		
gth:	70ft (21.5m)		
nage:	n/a		
struction:	n/a		

INDIAN KEY HISTORIC STATE PARK

Difficulty ● ○ ○
Current ● ○ ○
Depth ● ○ ○
Reef ★★☆
Fauna ★☆☆

Access 🚤 0.75mi (1.25km) Lower Matecumbe Ke

Level n/a

Location Islamorada
GPS   24° 52.688′N, 80° 40.603′W

Getting there
Indian Key sits just 0.5 miles (0.8 kilometers) away from the bridge connecting Islamorada to Lower Matecumbe Key. The site involves a boat ride of just a few minutes from Lower or Upper Matecumbe Key.

Access
Despite its proximity to shore, Indian Histori State Park is only accessible by boat, canoe c kayak. A few local operators on the mainland rer canoes and kayaks so that visitor can paddle ou to the island. There is an entry fee of $2.50 pe person payable at a self-pay kiosk located on th island. The island has no restrooms, water or foo facilities, and visitors must carry out their trash.

Description
Indian Key has an interesting and rich histor

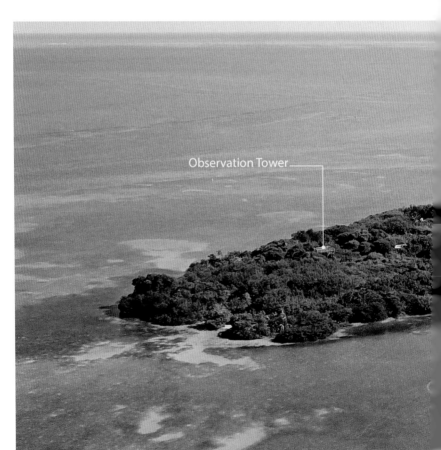

Observation Tower

At only 11 acres (4.5 hectares), it is relatively small compared to the surrounding keys. It was purchased in 1831 by Jacob Housman with the goal of building a wreck-salvage business that aimed to break the near monopoly enjoyed by similar businesses operating in Key West.

Housman built a community of "wreckers" on the island, which also included a hotel, warehouses, cisterns and wharves, remnants of which remain visible today. Just five years after buying the island, he had the Legislative Council name the island as the first county seat for Dade County in a bid to become independent from Key West. In 1840, the wrecking community came to an end when the island was attacked by Native Americans as part of the Second Seminole War. The attackers succeeded in burning most of the buildings to the ground. Thirteen residents were killed in the attack, which become known as the Indian Key Massacre, although Housman was able to escape. In later years the U.S. Navy occupied the island, establishing a squadron and building a hospital.

Today, visitors to the island can explore a recreation of Houseman's community, complete with a rebuilt dock, observation tower, shelter and trails. There are mooring buoys on the southwest corner of the island adjacent to the dock so boats should avoid anchoring in the delicate seagrass beds that surround the island. The waters are very shallow, and boats should approach from the southwest where depths are more easy to navigate. Paddlers can explore the seagrass beds from their kayaks and canoes while snorkelers can easily access the shallow rocky reefs that surround the island from a convenient access point located on the southeast corner of the island.

A shallow rocky reef encircles the island, providing visitors with the chance to see a range of marine creatures, from nurse sharks and barracuda to cocoa damselfish and sergeant majors. Snorkelers may also see Bermuda chub, scrawled filefish and highhats along the east side of the island. Meanwhile, bar jacks, banded butterflyfish and porkfish are common near the pier in the southwest corner.

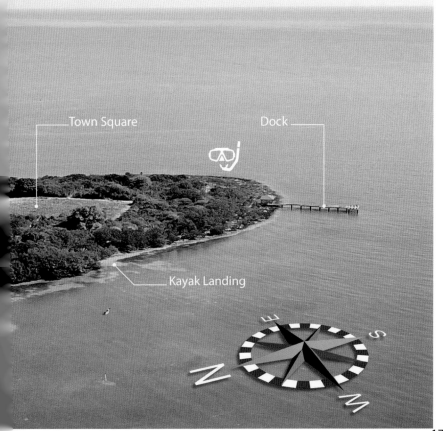

Town Square

Dock

Kayak Landing

SAN PEDRO

Difficulty ● ○ ○
Current ● ○ ○
Depth ● ○ ○
Reef ★★★
Fauna ★★★

Access 🚤
1.4mi (2.3km) from Lower Matecumbe Key

Level Open Water

Location Islamorada
GPS   SP1 24° 51.779'N, 80° 40.781'W
           SP2 24° 51.794'N, 80° 40.796'W
           SP3 24° 51.816'N, 80° 40.779'W
           SP5 24° 51.806'N, 80° 40.801'W

Getting there

The wreck of the *San Pedro* is located just over a mile (2 kilometers) off the northern tip of Lower Matecumbe Key. Getting there involves a boat trip of just a few minutes from shore.

Access

Despite its proximity to shore, the wreck of the *San Pedro* is only accessible by boat. The seabed has a depth of just 18 feet (5.5 meters) here, making it suitable for snorkelers and novice divers, although experienced divers with an interest in history might find this site worthwhile exploring. There are between four and six mooring buoys surrounding the site, so boats do not need to anchor near the historic area or the surrounding seagrass beds.

Description

San Pedro was part of a 22-vessel fleet of Spanish galleons that was caught in a hurricane as it sailed from Havana, Cuba, bound for Spain. A sudden wind change was all the warning the fleet received of the coming storm. The vessels scattered in an attempted to avoid the storm –

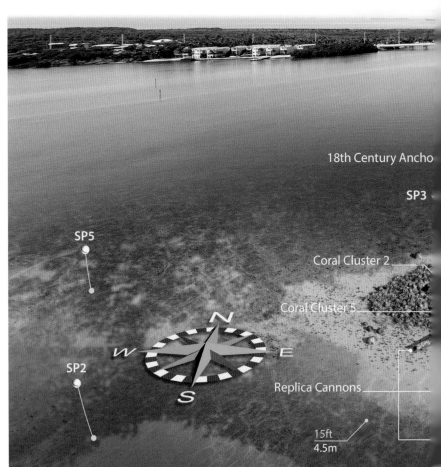

18th Century Ancho

SP3

SP5

Coral Cluster 2

Coral Cluster 5

SP2

Replica Cannons

15ft
4.5m

four where able to return to the safety of Cuba, one safely crossed Atlantic to Spain and 17 ended up running aground in the Keys. (See page 12 for more on the Spanish Fleet of 1733.)

San Pedro managed to cross the outer reef line before she sank in Hawk Channel, just off Lower Matecumbe Key. Her load of 16,000 pesos in Mexican silver, crates of Chinese porcelain, precious dyes such as cochineal and indigo, and other general cargo were successfully salvaged to a salvage camp established on nearby Indian Key.

The site is popular with snorkelers as it is designated an Underwater Archaeological Preserve and is part of the Florida Keys National Marine Sanctuary Shipwreck Trail. The vessel's original ballast stones are in a sandy hollow surrounded by seagrass beds at a depth of just 18 feet (5.5 meters). Replica cannons and a period-specific anchor have been added to the site to recreate what it originally looked like when first discovered. A small dedication plaque sits at the southeast end of the site. While exploring the area, snorkelers and interested divers may see black grouper, hogfish, bar jacks, barracuda and even a green moray eel, along with the usual complement of herbivorous damselfish and schooling grunts. Live corals can be seen throughout the site.

Name:	*San Pedro*	Last owner:	Gaspar de Larrea Berdugo
Type:	Wooden galleon	Sunk:	July 15, 1733
Previous names:	n/a		
Length:	n/a		
Tonnage:	287t		
Construction:	Holland		

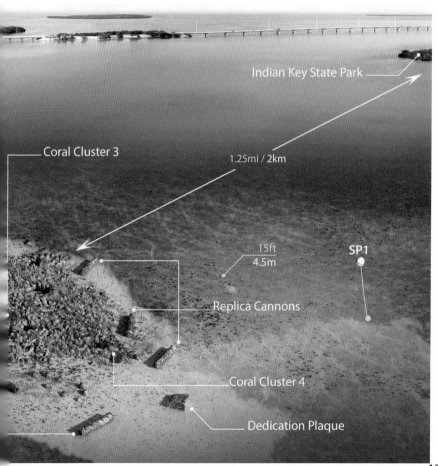

Indian Key State Park

Coral Cluster 3

1.25mi / 2km

15ft
4.5m

SP1

Replica Cannons

Coral Cluster 4

Dedication Plaque

CALOOSA ROCKS

Difficulty ● ○ ○
Current ● ○ ○
Depth ● ○ ○
Reef ★★☆
Fauna ★★☆

Access
1mi (1.6km) from Lower Matecumbe Key

Level Open water

Location Islamorada
GPS   24° 50.200'N, 80° 43.683'W

Getting there
Caloosa Rocks are located just a mile (1.6 kilometers) off the southern tip of Lower Matecumbe Key. Getting there involves a boat, canoe or kayak trip of just a few minutes from shore.

Access
Despite their proximity to shore, the patch reefs at Caloosa Rocks are only accessible by boat. The seabed has a maximum depth of just 20 feet (6 meters), making this site more suitable for snorkelers and novice divers. There are no mooring buoys at this site, so visitors should anchor with care in sandy areas to not damage the fragile corals. Current is generally low, and visibility can be poor when the weather stirs up the sediment in Hawk Channel.

Description
Caloosa Rocks gets its name for its position directly seaward of the Caloosa Cove Marina. The site measures nearly 0.3 miles (450 meters) across and is scattered with coral patches surrounded by rubble and sand. As with other patch reefs in Hawk Channel, the site is alive with marine life, including gray and Queen angelfish, yellowtail snapper, blue tangs and rainbow parrotfish. Lobsters and the occasional nurse shark can be found hiding beneath the overhanging corals at this site.

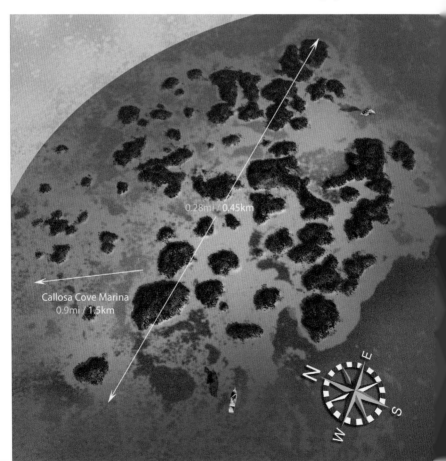

0.28mi / 0.45km

Callosa Cove Marina
0.9mi / 1.5km

SCIENTIFIC INSIGHT

Invasive lionfish pose a real threat to marine ecosystems in the Western Atlantic. Lionfish are indigenous to the Indo-West Pacific and came to Caribbean as an invasive species. They were first spotted near Dania Beach in southeastern Florida in 1985. No one knows exactly how they came to be there, but it is suspected that the first individuals were aquarium fish that were intentionally released into local waterways. Since then, the lionfish population has expanded south throughout the Caribbean and north into the Carolinas, as well as west into the Gulf of Mexico. Initial genetic testing suggested that the current Caribbean-wide population originated from just 10 individuals, but more recent studies place the original number of colonists at closer to 120, likely released over multiple instances.

The main threat posed by lionfish is that they are voracious predators. Although they feed almost exclusively on fish and crustaceans, they are not picky about what species they target. According to a 2018 study by Peake et al. published in the Journal of Applied Ecology, an adult lionfish's diet includes 167 species, of which many are ecologically or economically important. They also reproduce incredibly rapidly, producing thousands of eggs in just a few days. And with few natural predators outside of the Indo-Pacific region, they keep expanding their range and increasing their numbers. As a result, they are causing serious damage to local reef ecosystems.

Lionfish are unlikely to ever be fully removed from the Western Atlantic at this point – there are just too many of them and they are too well established. However, there are many long-term efforts underway to help control their numbers. Divers have become particularly effective at removing lionfish through spearfishing. Lionfish derbies (fishing competitions) have become popular in the Florida Keys, as well as throughout the Caribbean, and many restaurants are now serving lionfish dishes, sometimes using fish that customers have caught themselves.

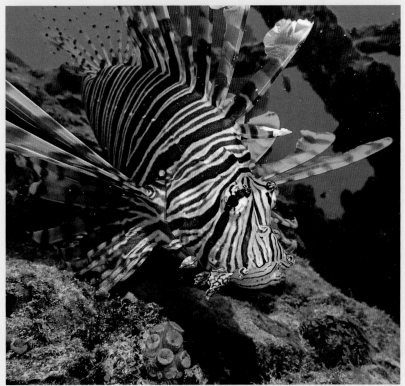

Bed Edmonds ©

MIDDLE KEYS DIVE SITES
Marathon

Marathon anchors a region referred to as the Middle Keys. With more than 8,500 residents, Marathon can hold its own against its more well-known neighbors to north and south, namely Key Largo and Key West. Marathon consists of 13 islands in total and boasts sandy beaches and incredible diving, both at the deeper reef line and within the shallower patch reefs of Hawk Channel.

The region has both natural and artificial reefs and even boasts a world-famous lighthouse, making this reef system an important stop in the dive and snorkel itinerary of any Florida Keys visitor.

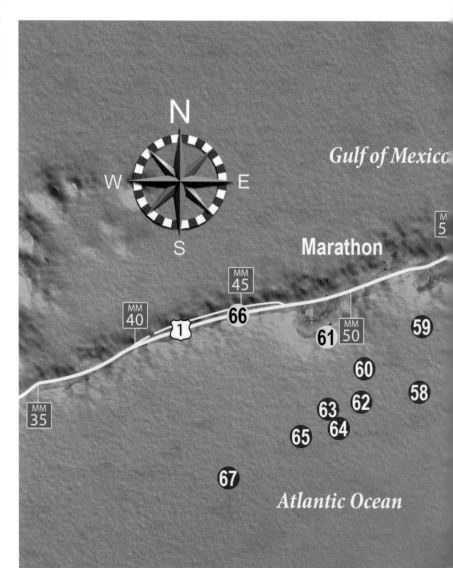

Dive and snorkel sites

47	Long Key State Park	
48	Tennessee Reef	Research Only
K	*Nuestra Señora de las Angustias*	
L/49	*Sueco de Arizón* (#1 and #2)	
50	*Adelaide Baker* ClusterA	
51	*Adelaide Baker* ClusterB	
52	East Turtle Shoal	
53	West Turtle Shoal	
54	Curry Hammock State Park	
55	Coffins Patch	
56	*Thunderbolt*	
57	Samantha's Reef	
58	Herman's Hole	
59	Marker 48	
60	East Washerwoman Shoal	
61	Sombrero Beach	
62	*Flagler's Barge*	
63	*North America wreck*	
64	Delta Shoal	
65	Sombrero Reef	
66	Pigeon Key	
67	7-Mile Bridge Rubble	

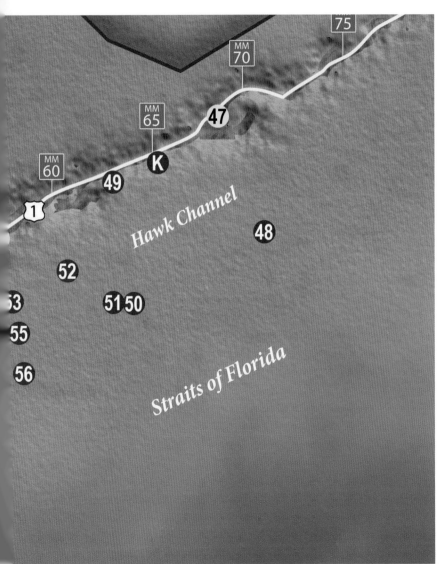

LONG KEY STATE PARK

Difficulty	● ○ ○
Current	● ○ ○
Depth	● ○ ○
Reef	★★☆
Fauna	★☆☆

Access
15mi (24km) from Islamorada

Level n/a

Location Long Key
GPS   24° 49.000'N, 80° 49.428'W

Getting there
Long Key is located just southwest of Lower Matecumbe Key and Islamorada. When arriving from the north, drive southbound on the Overseas Highway. Exactly 0.62 miles (1 kilometer) after the town of Layton, turn left into the state park entrance. From the south, the entrance is on the right, 6.3 miles (10.1 kilometers) after Duck Key. There is ample parking located just 550 feet (170 meters) past the fee station. Parking is more limited near the beach, which is located another 0.25 miles (410 meters) southwest of the main parking lot. The official address is 67400 Overseas Hwy, Layton, FL 33001 or at mile marker 67.5.

Access
There is a fee to access the state park. The park features multiple nature trails, an observation tower, restrooms and showers. The primary snorkeling access is along the main beach located at the southern edge of the Atlantic side of the park.

Description
Long Key was originally a fishing camp for the rich and famous in the early 1900s. Today, snorkelers can access rocky reefs directly from the beach, where they are likely to see grunts, butterflyfish, parrotfish and surgeonfish, along with damselfish and wrasses.

Long Key State Park has sandy beaches that offer the chance to snorkel and swim near seagrass and small rocky reefs

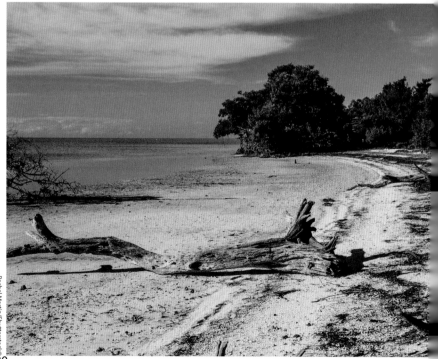

Rachel Martin/Shutterstock©

TENNESSEE REEF

Difficulty ● ○ ○
Current ● ● ○
Depth ● ○ ○
Reef ★★☆ Access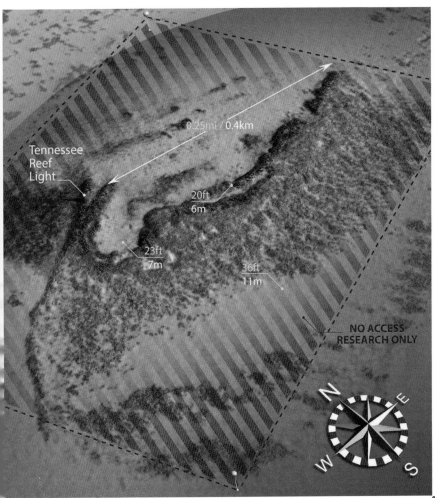
Fauna ★★☆ 19mi (30.5km) from Marathon

Level Open water

Location Long Key
GPS 24° 44.741'N, 80° 46.878'W

Getting there
Tennessee Reef is a small reef located just over 4.5 miles (7.5 kilometers) south southeast of Long Key. Getting there involves a boat trip of

just over an hour from Marathon.

Access
As of the publication date of this book, access to Tennessee Reef is restricted for research purposes only. Visitors require a permit from Florida Keys National Marine Sanctuary to access the site, which is marked by four yellow Research-Only buoys at the corners of the site.

Description
The shallow reef and well-defined spur and groove formations in the deeper reef feature many slow-growing corals and sponges. Scientists study this site to see how changing environmental conditions are impacting coral reefs in the Keys. By restricting access to the site, researchers can differentiate between changes caused by diving and fishing pressure on reefs and those due to the influence of environmental factors.

Tennessee Reef Light

0.25mi / 0.4km

20ft
6m

23ft
7m

36ft
11m

NO ACCESS
RESEARCH ONLY

N E S W

SUECO DE ARIZÓN

Difficulty ● ○ ○
Current ● ○ ○   **Access** 🛥️
Depth ● ○ ○   12mi (19km) from Marathon
Reef ★★★   **Access** 🚙
Fauna ★☆☆   11mi (17.7km) from Marathon

Level n/a

Location Conch Key
GPS   (#1) 24° 46.625'N, 80° 53.372'W
        (#2) 24° 46.728'N, 80° 53.480'W

Getting there

Sueco de Arizón is a historic shipwreck located in very shallow waters just 0.6 miles (1 kilometer) south of Conch Key. Getting there involves a boat ride of about 30 to 40 minutes from Marathon.

Snorkelers with access to a kayak may be able to access the site from shore via the Florida Keys Heritage Trail parking located just north of Conch Key near mile marker 63. There is no beach along the shore adjacent to the parking lot, but experienced kayakers should be able to enter the water here and paddle out to the site.

Access

The shallow water makes this site only suitable for snorkelers.

Description

Sueco de Arizón was a Spanish merchant ship that ran aground off Conch Key in July 1733, when a hurricane caught its convoy by surprise (for more on the story of the ill-fated Spanish Fleet of 1733, see page 12.) Officially named *Nuestra Señora del Rosario Santo Domingo, San Antonio y San Vincente Ferrer*, she was generally referred to by her shorter name, *Sueco de Arizón*, which means the Swede from Arizón.

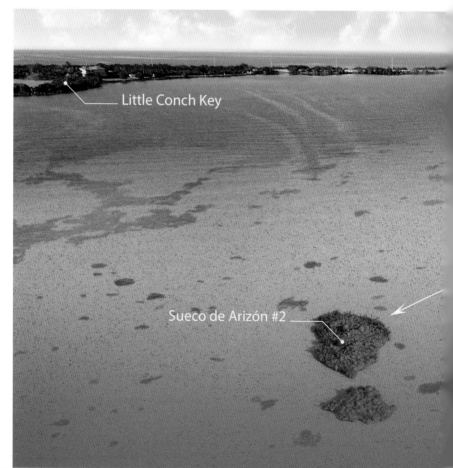

Little Conch Key

Sueco de Arizón #2

The nickname suggested that she was built in Sweden for her owner, Jacinto de Arizón and her captain, Juan José de Arizón.

She was one of the smaller ships of the fleet, which is possibly why the storm carried her so much deeper into the reef than the other galleons that were wrecked in this same storm – she ultimately grounded in just 9 feet (2.5 meters) of water. Her hull remained intact during the grounding, which allowed her crew to reach safety and her cargo of silver, porcelain, leather hides, tobacco and precious dyes to be safely recovered. She lost her masts and her rudder, however, and was solidly wedged in the sand and seagrass beds.

The wooden hull rotted away over the years, and all that remains today are two separate piles of ballast stones, one at the initial grounding site and another lying 830 feet (250 meters) closer to shore. These piles of river stones are colonized with hard and soft corals, and plenty of marine life, including juvenile angelfish, drums and various crustaceans. The currents here are generally mild, although they can vary based on tide. Visibility can be limited given the shallowness of the site and the proximity to the channel leading into Florida Bay.

Name:	*Sueco de Arizón*	**Tonnage:**	n/a
Type:	Wooden galleon	**Construction:**	Unknown, possibly Sweden
Previous names:	*Nuestra Señora del Rosario*	**Last owner:**	Jacinto Arizón
	Santo Domingo, San Antonio	**Sunk:**	July 15, 1733
	y San Vincente Ferrer		
Length:	n/a		

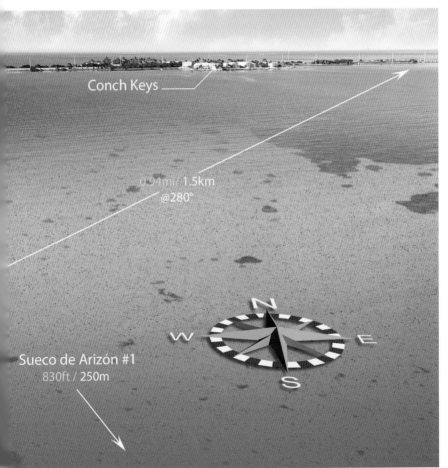

Conch Keys

0.94mi / 1.5km
@280°

Sueco de Arizón #1
830ft / 250m

ADELAIDE BAKER

Difficulty ● ○ ○
Current ● ○ ○
Depth ● ○ ○
Reef ★★☆
Fauna ★★☆

Access 🚤 9.6mi (15.5km) from Marathon

Level Open Water

Location Marathon
GPS (Cluster A) 24° 42.140'N, 80° 53.560'W
(Cluster B) 24° 42.179'N, 80° 53.676'W

Getting there
The wreck site of the *Adelaide Baker* sits just inside of the outer reef line, roughly 4.3 miles (7 kilometers) offshore of Duck Key. Getting there involves a boat ride of approximately 30 to 40 minutes from Marathon.

Access
The site is only accessible by boat given its distance from shore. This site is suitable for divers and snorkelers of all experience levels given the maximum depth is just 25 feet (7.5 meters). There is currently a mooring buoy on the secondary site, known as Cluster B, but typically there is also one on Cluster A. If no mooring buoy is present, be sure to anchor at a distance from the site to avoid damaging or disturbing the historic debris.

Description
Adelaide Baker was a three-masted, iron-rigged bark built in Bangor, Maine, in 1863. Originally named *F.W. Carver*, this 153-foot (46.6-meter) sailing ship was carrying timber up the coast to Savannah, Georgia, when she ran aground just north of Coffins Patch. Apparently the captain mistook Sombrero Light for Cape Florida Light (located up near Miami) and turned his vessel to the north to follow what he believed to be the coastline. Thankfully local wreckers were able to help rescue the ship's crew and her captain with no loss of life.

Sometimes known locally as the *Conrad*, the remains of the *Adelaide Baker* are spread across nearly 0.25 miles (0.85 kilometers) of reef in a roughly north-northwest direction, with two main clusters of debris. Cluster A is believed to be the initial grounding site, and includes ballast stones, a water tank and a lower portion of the mizzen mast, among other elements. Cluster B is thought to represent a secondary site created by early salvagers. The main feature of Cluster B is the 77-foot

(23.5-meter) iron main mast, along with remains of a bilge pump, knee-riders and miscellaneous rigging and tackle, among other items.

The wreckage is well encrusted by gorgonians, tube sponges and encrusting corals. The small amount of relief still provides enough structure to attract plenty of reef fish, including blue tangs, hogfish, porkfish and Bermuda chub. Stingrays and nurse sharks are known to frequent the site, while a green moray eel can often be spotted in the pile of ballast stones in Cluster A. Schools

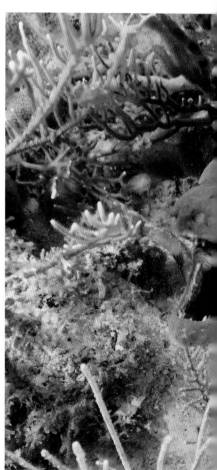

ADELAIDE BAKER

of bluestriped, French and white grunts are common on both sites, along with yellowtail snapper and a host of damselfish species, such as bicolor damselfish and sergeant majors.

Authorities have not definitively identified the site as the resting place of the *Adelaide Baker*, but they remain confident that this is where the British bark ran aground. The site is one of

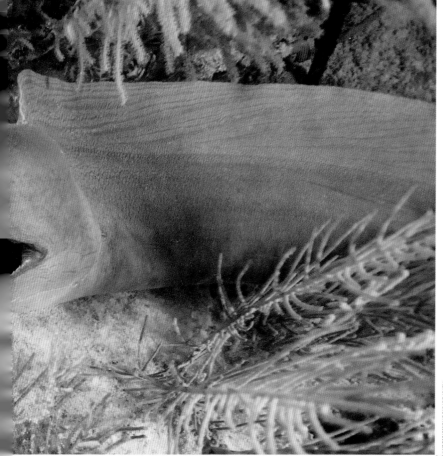

Karel Bartik/Shutterstock©

green moray eel is commonly seen hiding in the pile of ballast rocks found in Cluster A.

ADELAIDE BAKER

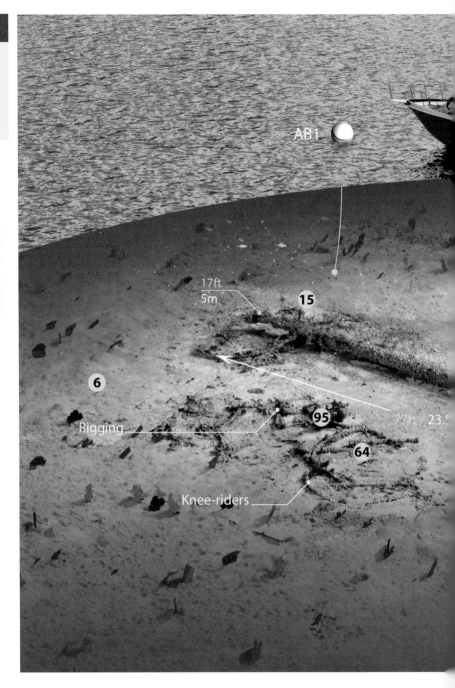

AB1

17ft
5m

15

6

Rigging

95

64

Knee-riders

nine shipwrecks that make up the Florida Keys
National Marine Sanctuary Shipwreck Trail.

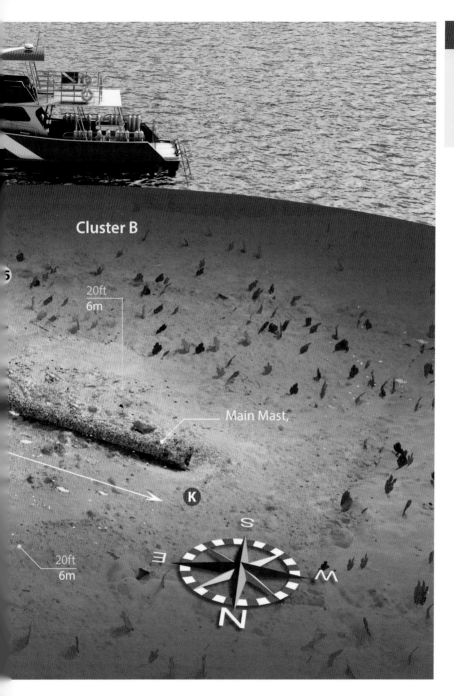

Cluster B

20ft
6m

Main Mast,

K

20ft
6m

Name:	*SV Adelaide Baker*	**Last owner:**	Barrie Charles & Sons
Type:	Transport bark	**Sunk:**	Jan. 28, 1889
Previous names:	*F.W. Carver*		
Length:	153ft (46.6m)		
Tonnage:	n/a		
Construction:	Bangor, Maine, 1863		

EAST TURTLE SHOAL

Difficulty	● ○ ○
Current	● ○ ○
Depth	● ○ ○
Reef	★★☆
Fauna	★☆☆

Access
8.3mi (13.5km) from Marathon

Level Open water

Location Marathon
GPS 24° 43.279'N, 80° 55.698'W

Getting there
East Turtle Shoal sits in the middle of Hawk Channel, 3 miles (5 kilometers) south of Duck Key. Getting there involves a 30-minute boat ride from Marathon.

Access
This site is more suitable to snorkelers and novice divers given it has a maximum depth of just 20 feet (6 meters). There are no mooring buoys at the site, so visitors should anchor in the sand to avoid disturbing the fragile coral reef. Visibility can be reduced during wind and wave events, which can stir up the sediment in Hawk Channel. Currents are often mild.

Description
East Turtle Shoal is a section of raised bedrock in Hawk Channel that has been colonized by clusters of coral heads. The loose collection of patch reefs only offers approximately 3 to 6.5 feet (1 to 2 meters) of relief above the surrounding sand and rubble bottom. Divers and snorkelers are likely to see plenty of juvenile reef fish, including grunts and snapper. Seagrass beds surround the shoal, making this a popular site for green turtles.

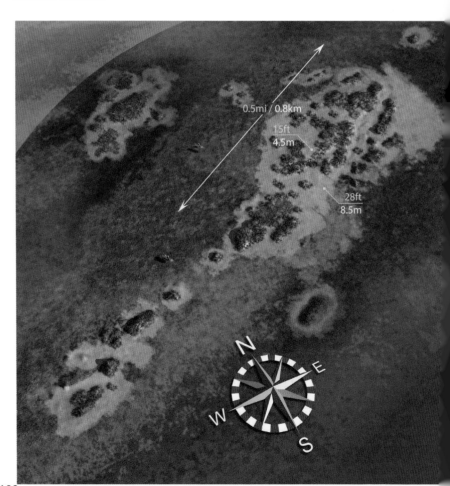

0.5mi / 0.8km

15ft
4.5m

28ft
8.5m

WEST TURTLE SHOAL

Difficulty ● ○ ○
Current ● ○ ○
Depth ● ○ ○
Reef ★★☆ Access 🚤
Fauna ★☆☆ 5mi (8km) from Marathon

Level Open water

Location Marathon
GPS 24° 42.012'N, 80° 57.968'W

Getting there

West Turtle Shoal sits in the middle of Hawk Channel, 3 miles (5 kilometers) south of Curry Hammock State Park. Getting there involves a boat ride of approximately 10 to 15 minutes from Marathon.

Access

This site is more suitable to snorkelers and novice divers given it has a maximum depth of just 26 feet (8 meters). There are no mooring buoys at the site, so visitors should anchor in the sand to avoid disturbing the fragile coral reef. Visibility can be reduced during wind and wave events which can stir up the sediment in Hawk Channel. Currents are often mild.

Description

West Turtle Shoal is slightly more popular than East Turtle Shoal given its proximity to Marathon. Like its neighbor to the northwest, West Turtle Shoal consists of a section of raised bedrock within Hawk Channel, which has been colonized by clusters of corals. The loose collection of patch reefs offers nearly 10 feet (3 meters) of relief from the seabed, particularly around the sand and reef interface. The site is surrounded by dense seagrass beds, offering snorkelers and divers the chance to explore multiple ecosystems on a single visit. In addition to seeing bluestriped grunts, yellowtail snapper, bicolor damselfish and a variety of parrotfishes on the reef, visitors to West Turtle Shoal may also encounter green turtles foraging in the seagrass beds. Snorkelers may wish to spend time at the pilings for channel marker 47, which are heavily encrusted with fire corals and host many small reef fish, such as sergeant majors and various blennies and gobies.

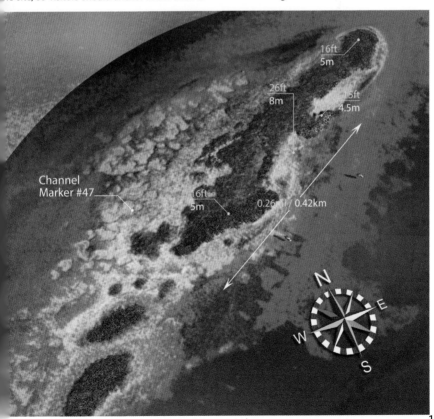

CURRY HAMMOCK STATE PARK

Difficulty ● ○ ○
Current ● ○ ○
Depth ● ○ ○
Reef ★★★
Fauna ★☆☆

Access 🚚 5mi (8km) from Marathon

Level n/a

Location Little Crawl Key
GPS 24° 44.414'N, 80° 58.886'W

Getting there

Curry Hammock State Park is located at the northern end of Marathon. It represents a stretch of undeveloped land right in the middle of one of the more developed areas of the Keys. When arriving from the north, drive southbound on the Overseas Highway, continuing 3.5 miles (5.6 kilometers) after first entering Vaca Key. Turn left into the state park entrance just after passing through Crawl Key. From the south, the entrance is on the right, 4 miles (6.5 kilometers) after the Marathon airport. There is ample parking located just 0.2 miles (320 meters) past the fee station. The official address is 56200 Overseas Hwy, Marathon (near mile marker 56).

Access

There is a fee to access the state park. The park features multiple hiking and paddling trails, picnicking areas, restrooms and showers. Snorkeling is possible from the beach located just a few steps from the parking lot. The water is very shallow, which makes this less suited for diving.

Description

The water right off the beach at Curry Hammock State Park is protected by a large sand bar farther offshore. While this makes navigating slightly trickier for kayakers and kiteboarders who like to use the beach as a launching point, it does mean that snorkelers will typically find calm water to explore. The area is dominated by a large, 15-acre seagrass bed whose shallow waters provide shelter for a variety of marine creatures. Snorkelers may see conch hidden among the seagrasses, as well as sea anemones and small crabs and other crustaceans. Many commercially important fish species including snapper spend part of their lives among seagrass beds. Juvenile Nassau grouper are also known to shelter in this important ecosystem.

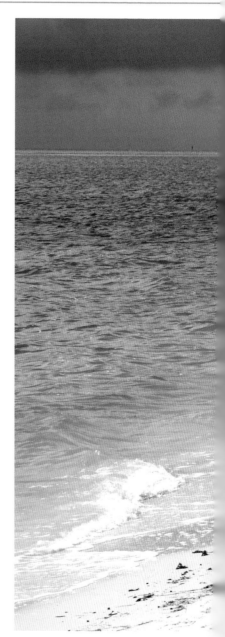

Snorkelers willing to swim slowly and take their time will likely see damselfish and goatfish as well as many different species of wrasse in the seagrass bed just off the beach. Sea breams and silversides are also commonly found among seagrasses, as are green sea turtles and even manatees. Turtles and manatees feed on the seagrasses themselves while many other species feed on the algae and invertebrates found on the grasses.

The water reaches a depth of just a few feet (less than a meter) in some places making it important to avoid standing or otherwise crushing the seagrasses where possible. Seagrass beds are an important ecosystem, and they need to be protected for them to continue to fulfill their role providing shelter for marine creatures and for acting as the lungs of the sea.

Visitors can snorkel right from the shoreline at Curry Hammock State Park.

CURRY HAMMOCK STATE PARK

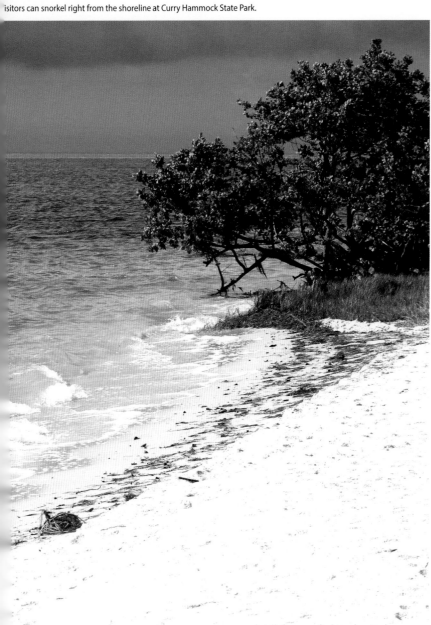

COFFINS PATCH

Difficulty	● ○ ○	
Current	● ○ ○	
Depth	● ○ ○	
Reef	★★☆	Access 🚤
Fauna	★★☆	5.5mi (9km) from Marathon

Level Open Water

Location Marathon
GPS
CP0 24° 41.129'N, 80° 57.784'W
CP1 24° 41.164'N, 80° 57.740'W
CP2 24° 41.153'N, 80° 57.768'W
CP3 24° 41.131'N, 80° 57.808'W
CP4 24° 41.144'N, 80° 57.839'W
CP5 24° 41.124'N, 80° 57.841'W
CP6 24° 41.141'N, 80° 57.865'W
CP7 24° 41.108'N, 80° 57.872'W

Getting there

Coffins Patch sits on the edge of Hawk Channel just inside of the outer reef line, 4 miles (6.5 kilometers) southeast of Key Colony Beach. Getting there involves a boat ride of about 15 to 20 minutes from Marathon.

Access

These shallow patch reefs are only accessible by boat given their distance from shore. They are suitable to divers and snorkelers of all levels. Eight mooring buoys provide access to the set of reefs within the Sanctuary Preservation Area (SPA). Access to the patch reefs outside of the SPA require careful anchoring in the sand. Currents are rarely strong on the inside edge of the outer reef line, and visibility is generally good, although it can deteriorate rapidly when the wind and waves stir up the sediment. There is no harvesting of any kind allowed within the boundaries of the SPA.

Description

Coffins Patch includes six separate aggregations of shallow patch reefs that stretch in a line roughly parallel to shore. Two of the patch reef sections located in the middle of the set of reef are contained within the SPA. These represent the primary focus of the site and are the mo

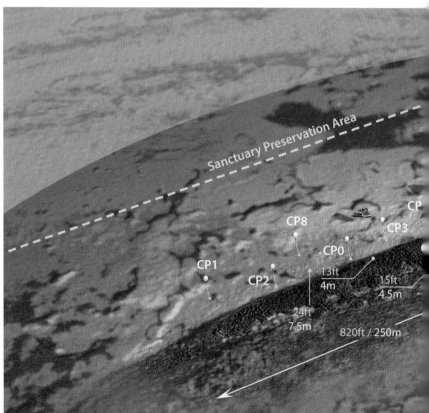

DID YOU KNOW? ❓

The wreck of the *San Ignacio de Urguijo* is believed to be located just off the northeastern edge of the northernmost patch reef in Coffins Patch. This Spanish galleon was another member of the ill-fated convoy that was caught in a hurricane off the coast of the Keys in July 1733. The British-built vessel was carrying 12,000 pesos in silver and bullion. By all reports, most of her crew did not survive the violent grounding. However, the Florida Keys National Marine Sanctuary has not positively identified the wreck located near Coffins Patch as that of the *San Ignacio*. And because the wreck lies within the Florida Keys National Marine Sanctuary, it is illegal to disturb or remove any artifacts from the site, regardless of the wreck's actual identity.

easily accessed from the established mooring buoys. A third and smaller reef (called Shoal Reef) is located in the southwestern corner of the SPA and shelters some pillar corals in the region at a depth of 25 feet (7.5 meters). This reef is too far to reach by swimming from the mooring buoys, however.

The reef patches near the mooring buoys are shallow, with the tops reaching just 10 feet (3 meters) in some places, and the sand bottoming out at 24 feet (7.5 meters). They support a variety of hard and soft corals, including boulder corals measuring up to 3 feet (1 meter) across. Nurse sharks, grouper and moray eels are often seen here, along with stingrays and sea turtles. The vibrant color of the corals and fish species are on full display in the shallow water, which makes this a popular site with macro photographers.

Three other sections of patch reef are located just under a mile (1.6 kilometers) to the northeast of the SPA. These reefs are harder to access as they require anchoring in the sand but offer plenty of coral and marine life for snorkelers and divers to enjoy.

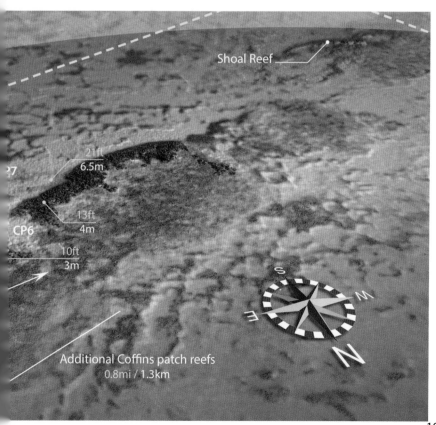

Shoal Reef

21ft
6.5m

13ft
4m

10ft
3m

CP6

Additional Coffins patch reefs
0.8mi / 1.3km

Difficulty ● ● ○
Current ● ● ○
Depth ● ● ●
Reef ★★★
Fauna ★★☆

Access 🚤 7mi (11.5km) from Marathon

Level Advanced

Location Marathon
GPS   24° 39.665'N, 80° 57.794'W

Getting there
Thunderbolt rests just offshore of the central cut in Marathon, on a sandy seafloor just beyond the outer reef line. Getting there involves a boat ride of about 25 to 30 minutes from Marathon.

Access
Thunderbolt is best suited to advanced divers because of its depth. The top of the wheelhouse reaches a depth of 79 feet (24 meters) while the seafloor bottoms out at a maximum depth of 119 feet (36 meters). Two submerged buoys provide access to the wreck. Currents can be strong when the Gulf Stream runs closer to shore. Visibility is generally good.

Description
Thunderbolt was originally a U.S. Army minelayer built in West Virginia during World War II. Commissioned as the *USAMP Major General Wallace F. Randolph*, she and her 15 sister ships were built to manage the coastal minefields for the Army's Coastal Artillery Corps. At the end of the war, the U.S. Navy took over those operations, and Randolph was transferred into the Naval reserve fleet. She was renamed *USS Nausett* in May 1955. In 1961 she was stripped and sold to an oilfield exploration company called Caribbean Enterprises, based in Miami, Florida, and renamed *Sea Searcher*.

She was eventually sold to the Florida Power & Light Company in the early 1980s for use in researching the effects of lightning strikes on power systems (Florida sustains more lightning strikes than any other state in the United States). Part of her work involved researchers firing wired rockets into a storm system to encourage lightning strikes that would then surge down the length of the conductive wire to register on the onboard equipment. The work meant she sustained multiple lightning strikes over the course of her duties, and she was rechristened *Thunderbolt*. Her new line of work took its toll, however, and she ended up sinking while docked in Miami in the mid-80s. Eventually, she was donated to the Florida Keys Artificial Reef Association and was cleaned and prepped for

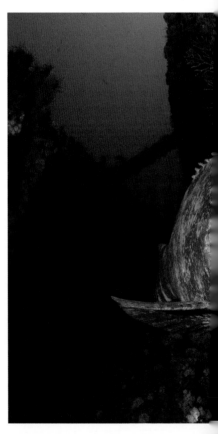

deployment as an artificial reef off the coast of Marathon. She is one of nine wrecks that a part of Florida Keys National Marine Sanctua Shipwreck Trail.

As part of the preparation, the entire aft end the superstructure was removed, which expose the interior of the vessel and its engineeri space for easy access by divers. Although mo of her equipment was removed, the large cab reel on the forecastle, as well as the shi rudder and propellers, were left in place. Tod

RELAX & RECHARGE

Keys Fisheries (3502 Gulfview Ave, Marathon) is a restaurant with a killer sundown view and some of the freshest fish in the Keys. Located within the Keys Fisheries Marina, the restaurant and its upstairs bar serve a wide range of seafood from baked grouper and conch fritters to seasonal stone crab and their famous lobster reuben. They even have a "cook your catch" option, where diners are invited to bring their own fish for preparation by the restaurant's chefs. The ambiance at Keys Fisheries is electric and the view of the setting sun from the upstairs bar cannot be beat. Visit at sundown and enjoy a complimentary group sundowner shot. Visit: **Keysfisheries.com**

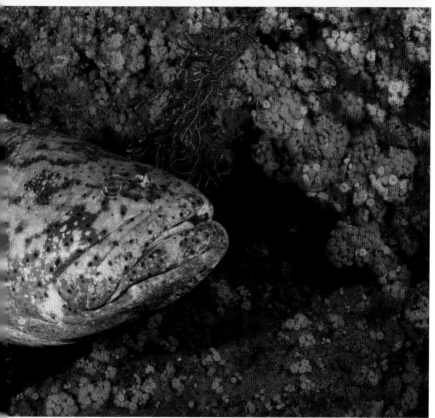

Matt9122/Shutterstock©

oliath grouper are commonly found on the colorfully encrusted wreck of the *Thunderbolt*, along with the invasive orange p corals depicted here.

e entire wreck is well colonized by colorful onges and encrusting algae and corals.

vers will encounter plenty of marine life on *underbolt*, including angelfish, butterflyfish d creolefish. Blue chromis and bar jacks are mmonly seen schooling near the cable reel ar the bow while Spanish hogfish are often en on the main deck closer to the stern. The wreck attracts many large fish species as well, including goliath grouper, which are often found around the propellers and within the engine room. Black grouper, Nassau grouper, dog snapper, gray snapper and barracuda are also found here. Large amberjacks and almaco jacks are also commonly seen at *Thunderbolt*, attracted by large schools of baitfish. The size of the fish on *Thunderbolt* makes it a popular dive

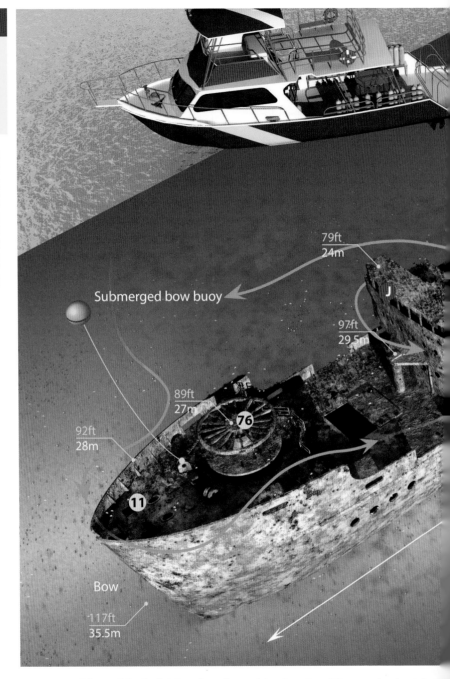

Submerged bow buoy

79ft
24m

J

97ft
29.5m

89ft
27m

76

92ft
28m

11

Bow

117ft
35.5m

among spearfishers while the bright colors of the corals and sponges make it a must-dive for underwater photographers.

Route

Although deep, the wreck is ideal for exploration by divers, with the engineering compartments

and the aft section of the superstructure left wi open to encourage access. Many divers start descending the lines attached to the submerg buoys at the bow and stern of the wreck, the current can be strong at times. Divers w experience at depth may want to start th dive by exploring the propellers to look for t

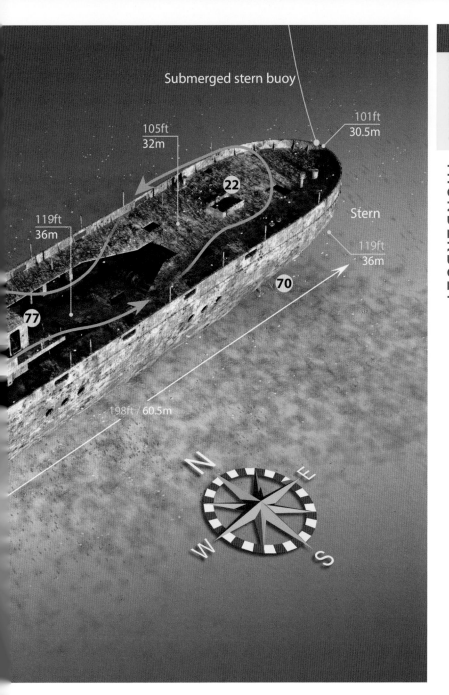

Submerged stern buoy

101ft
30.5m

105ft
32m

22

Stern

119ft
36m

119ft
36m

70

77

198ft / 60.5m

ident goliath grouper. Others may wish to
plore the main deck, which is slightly shallower
a depth of 105 feet (32 meters). The cable reel
the forecastle and the open observation deck
well worth investigating during the latter
ges of the dive.

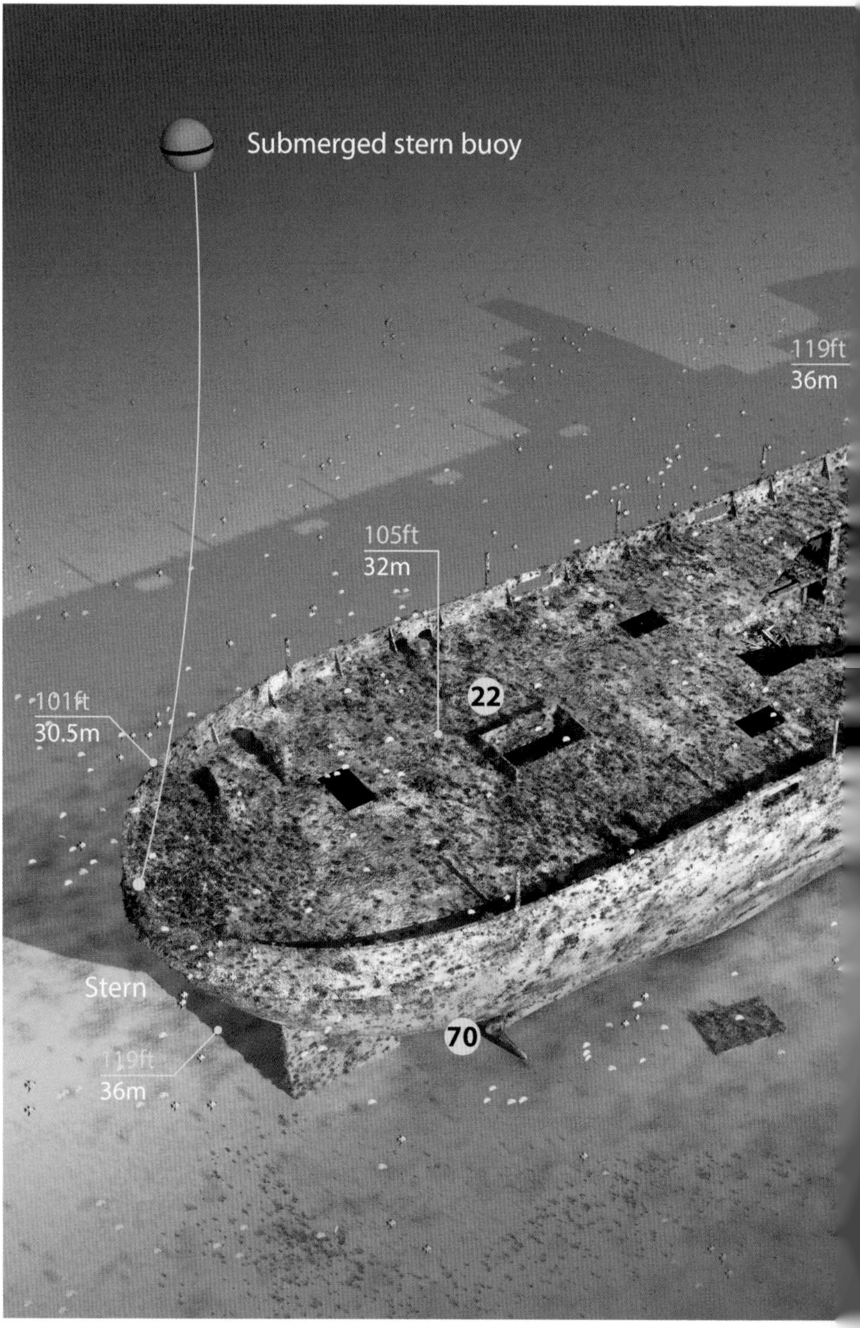

Submerged stern buoy

119ft
36m

105ft
32m

101ft
30.5m

22

Stern

119ft
36m

70

THUNDERBOLT

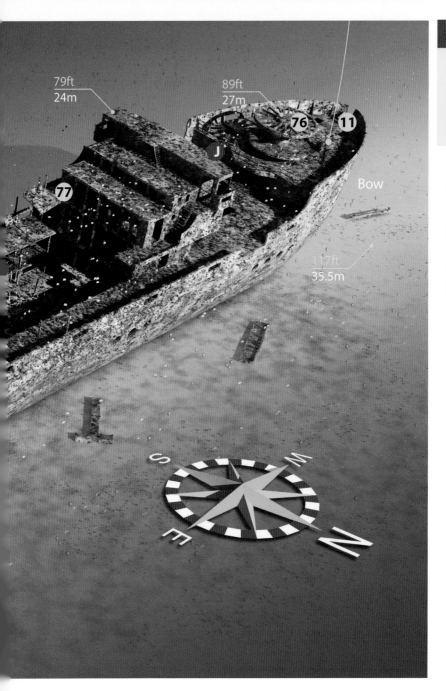

79ft
24m

89ft
27m

76

11

J

Bow

77

117ft
35.5m

me:	SS Thunderbolt	Tonnage:	920grt
e:	Minelayer	Construction:	Marietta Manufacturing
vious names:	USAMP Major General		Company, Point Pleasant,
	Wallace F. Randolph,		West Virginia
	Nausett, Sea Searcher	Last owner:	Florida Power & Light
gth:	189ft (56m)	Sunk:	March 6, 1986

SAMANTHA'S REEF

Difficulty	● ○ ○
Current	● ○ ○
Depth	● ○ ○
Reef	★★☆
Fauna	★★☆

Access 🛥
5mi (8km) from Marathon

Level Open Water

Location Marathon
GPS   24° 39.508'N, 81° 00.314'W

Getting there

Samantha's Reef sits on the plateau just behind the outer reef line, around 5 miles (8 kilometers) south of Key Colony Beach. Getting there involves a boat ride of approximately 15 to 20 minutes from Marathon.

Access

Divers and snorkelers of all levels can enjoy th fragmented ledge that runs roughly parall to shore at this site. Samantha's Reef is on accessible by boat, but there are no moorin buoys, so visitors must anchor in the sand clos by. The location of this site on the outer re line means visibility is often better than at site

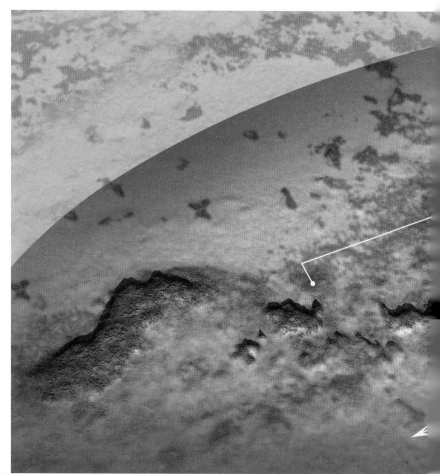

ocated closer to shore, but it can sometimes experience stronger currents.

Description

The site goes by a few names, including Samantha's Ledge and Sam's Reef. The ledge tops out at a depth of 20 feet (6 meters) with the seabed at around 26 feet (8 meters). Locals also call it Shark Reef because of the many nurse sharks seen here. In the past, dive operators have fed the sharks, which has made them relatively unafraid of divers and snorkelers and more likely to approach. The practice is now discouraged as it can be dangerous for both divers and sharks (see the Eco Tip). It is also common to see stingrays, blue tangs, sergeant majors, stoplight parrotfish, bluehead wrasses, clown wrasses and graysbies at this reef.

ECO TIP

Some dive operators believe feeding sharks can enhance the diver experience. This practice is not allowed within Florida's state waters, which extend 3 miles (5 kilometers) from the shore. The practice is generally discouraged by most biologists as sharks have been known to become more aggressive in areas where feeding occurs, which can result in injury to divers and snorkelers. Moreover, sharks habituated to feeding at a chum station are no longer exhibiting natural behavior. We strongly encourage divers and snorkelers to seek out more natural experiences and avoid the potentially dangerous encounters that can occur through chumming, unless it is part of a well-organized educational experience.

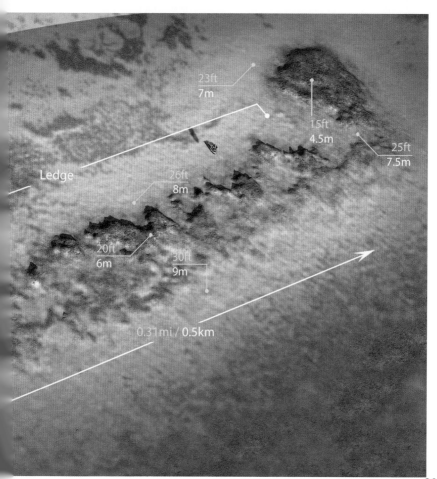

Ledge

23ft
7m

15ft
4.5m

25ft
7.5m

26ft
8m

20ft
6m

30ft
9m

0.31mi / 0.5km

HERMAN'S HOLE

Difficulty	● ○ ○
Current	● ○ ○
Depth	● ● ○
Reef	★★★
Fauna	★★★

Access 🚤
6.2mi (10km) from Marathon

Level Open water

Location Marathon
GPS   24° 39.031'N, 81° 01.830'W

Getting there
Herman's Hole sits along the outer reef line, around 5 miles (8 kilometers) south of Key Colony Beach. Getting there involves a boat ride of approximately 15 to 20 minutes from Marathon.

Access
Herman's Hole is suitable for divers and snorkelers of all levels, although the seabed, which average around 28 feet (8.5 meters) may be a little too deep for some snorkelers. The site is only accessible by boat, and there are no mooring buoys, which means visitors must anchor in the sand nearby. The location of this site on the outer reef line means visibility is often better than at sites located closer to shore, but it can sometime experience stronger currents.

Description
Herman's Hole gets its name from the fact that the site features a large, shallow "hole" in the reef and for the green moray eel, named Herman, that once lived here. Herman is long since gone, but the low profile ledge that encircles the sand and rubble bottomed center is still present. Divers may have sense of being in the center of an arena when the explore this site, which is why another name for the site is Arena. Other green moray eels are present this site, along with goldentail morays, stingray nurse sharks and even a resident goliath group has been reported. Many other reef fishes are also common here, such as gray angelfish, schoolmast snapper, striped parrotfish and Spanish grunts.

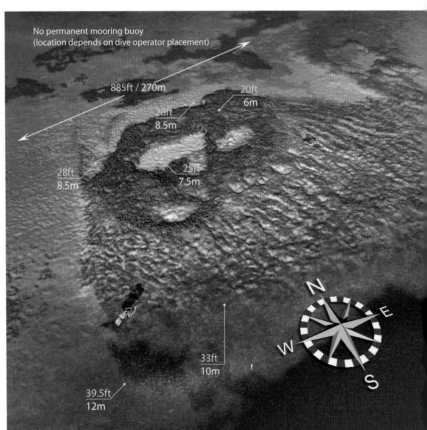

No permanent mooring buoy
(location depends on dive operator placement)

885ft / 270m

20ft
6m

28ft
8.5m

28ft
8.5m

25ft
7.5m

33ft
10m

39.5ft
12m

N
E
S
W

MARKER 48

Difficulty	● ○ ○
Current	● ○ ○
Depth	● ○ ○
Reef	★★★
Fauna	★☆☆

Access 🚤
2.5mi (4km) from Marathon

Level n/a

Location

Marathon
GPS   M481 24° 41.486'N, 81° 04.522'W
      M482 24° 41.390'N, 81° 01.773'W
      M483 24° 41.388'N, 81° 01.822'W

Getting there

Marker 48 sits in the middle of Hawk Channel just
2.5 miles (4.5 kilometers) south of Key Colony Beach.
Getting there involves a boat ride of approximately
10 minutes from Marathon.

Access

Marker 48 is more suitable to snorkelers than
divers, as the maximum depth is just 14 feet
(4.3 meters). The site is only accessible by boat,
and with three mooring buoys to choose from,
visitors should have no trouble tying up. Current
is rarely an issue at this site, but visibility can be
poor when waves stir up the sediment.

Description

The site gets its name from its proximity to
the red daymarker 48, which is located at the
northern end of the series of patch reefs. Each
cluster of aggregated coral heads is surrounded
by a distinct halo of dense seagrass in the
surrounding area. Snorkelers will see plenty
of reef fish among the coral heads, including
parrotfishes, grunts, damselfishes and wrasses.
Barracuda are often seen here, as are nurse
sharks. Stingrays often settle in the seagrass
beds along with various crustaceans and green
sea turtles.

MARKER 48

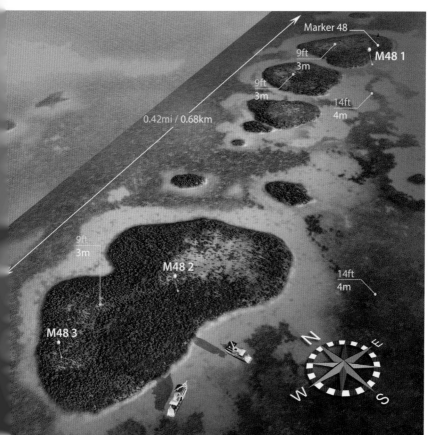

EAST WASHERWOMAN SHOAL

Difficulty ● ○ ○
Current ● ○ ○
Depth ● ○ ○
Reef ★★☆ Access
Fauna ★☆☆ 6mi (9.5km) from Marathon

Level Open Water

Location Marathon
GPS 24° 39.943'N, 81° 04.331'W

Getting there

East Washerwoman Shoal sits in the middle of Hawk Channel just under 2 miles (3 kilometers) south of Sombrero Beach. Getting there involves a boat ride of approximately 20 to 25 minutes from Marathon. The site is easy to identify as it is marked by a 36-foot-tall (11-meter) lighted tower.

Access

East Washerwoman Shoal is more suitable to snorkelers and novice divers as the maximum depth is just 21 feet (6.5 meters). The complexity of the patch reef provides plenty for visitors to explore. There are no mooring buoys at the site, so boats should anchor in the sand to avoid disturbing the fragile reef system. Visibility can be reduced when wind and waves stir up the sediment in Hawk Channel. Currents are often mild.

Description

East Washerwoman Shoal is a section of raised bedrock in Hawk Channel that has been colonized by aggregated clusters of coral heads. The main part of the site is bisected by a sand channel that opens to the south and measures 180 feet (55 meters) across. The channel bottom sits at 20 feet (6 meters) and provides a suitable anchoring spot – the GPS coordinates mark the northern end of this channel. The channel is roughly southeast of the lighted tower that sits shoreward of the reef.

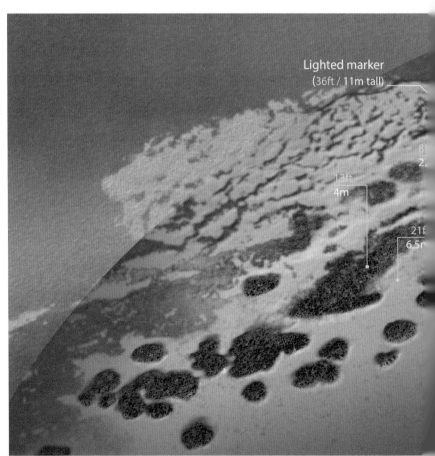

Lighted marker
(36ft / 11m tall)

13ft
4m

8f
2.

21f
6.5r

RELAX & RECHARGE

Burdines Waterfront (1200 Oceanview Avenue, Marathon) combines a wonderful old-style Keys vibe with a deliciously unpretentious menu packed with comfort food favorites ranging from mahi mahi sandwiches to poke bowls and salads. There are plenty of burger options, including classics like the bacon Swiss burger, and more unique creations like the shrimp burger, the Florentine chicken burger, which is served with creamy feta cheese, and the mammoth Italian Stallion, which has Italian sausages resting on top of the burger. Wrap up the meal with their famous fried key lime pie and enjoy the relaxed waterfront views as the sun sets over the ocean.

Visit: **Burdineswaterfront.com**

From the sand channel, clusters of patch reefs fan out to the east, west and to the north at depths that vary between 8 and 16 feet (2.5 and 4 meters). The site is marked by rose, brain and star corals, while staghorn corals do well in the shallow water here. The structure supports a variety of marine life, including bar jacks, and the ubiquitous yellowtail snapper and bluestriped grunts. Colorful Spanish hogfish frequent the corals at this site, along with sharpnose puffers, beaugregory damselfish and blue tangs. Snorkelers have even reportedly seen nurse sharks and stingrays resting on the sand bottom while barracuda may patrol above the reef.

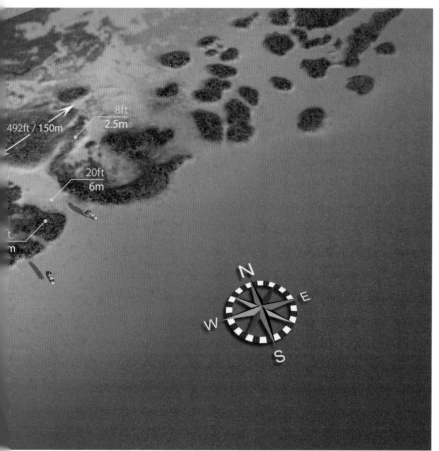

SOMBRERO BEACH

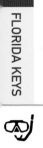

Difficulty ● ○ ○
Current ● ○ ○
Depth ● ○ ○
Reef ★★☆
Fauna ★★☆

Access 🛻
4.1mi (6.6km) from Marathon

Level n/a

Location Marathon
GPS   24° 41.500'N, 81° 05.067'W

Getting there

Driving south on Overseas Highway through the center of Marathon, turn left on Sombrero Beach Road near mile marker 50. The turn is at the traffic lights 1.6 miles (2.6 kilometers) south of the entrance to the Marathon airport. When driving north on Overseas Highway, turn right into Sombrero Beach Road 2.5 miles (4 kilometers) after leaving Hog Key and entering Marathon. Once on Sombrero Beach Road, follow it for 2 miles (3.2 kilometers) as it curves south-southwest all the way to the beach. There is ample free parking at the beach along with bathroom and shower facilities. The official address is 2150 Sombrero Beach Road, Marathon

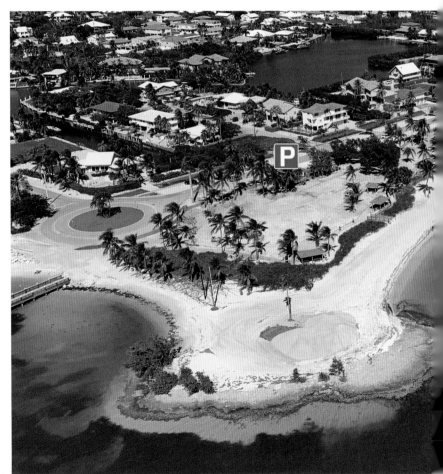

Access

The beach, which sits just 130 feet (40 meters) from the parking lot, and the associated pavilions are fully accessible thanks to the city's 2001 redevelopment efforts. The paved walkways and ramps now vastly improve access to the beach for persons with disabilities, as well as the families with children in strollers. The beach is open 365 days a year from 7am to dusk.

Description

Sombrero Beach is roughly 0.2 miles (350 meters) of white sand beach with a limestone outcropping in the middle that divides the beach into two crescents. The shallow waters just off the beach are great for snorkeling and swimming, with plenty of marine life to see, including Bermuda chub, damselfish and wrasses, French and bluestriped grunts, gray and lane snapper, and sergeant majors. The beach is a sea turtle nesting beach, primarily for loggerhead sea turtles. Nesting season stretches from April through October, and it is not uncommon for a nesting turtle to crawl up the sandy beach during the night to lay their eggs above the high-water mark. Authorities regularly monitor the beach for nesting activity and mark out the nests to prevent daytime beach goers from disturbing them. The city may opt to close a portion of the beach if there is a concentration of nests, but this typically represents just a small percentage of the total beach area at any given time. (For more on sea turtles, check out the sea turtle ecology section on page 310.)

Along with the sandy beach and gentle surf, Sombrero Beach also boasts a children's playground and a beach volleyball court. Dogs are allowed in the park and on the beach, provided they remain on leash. The spot is a well-kept secret among locals and is rarely overwhelmed by visitors.

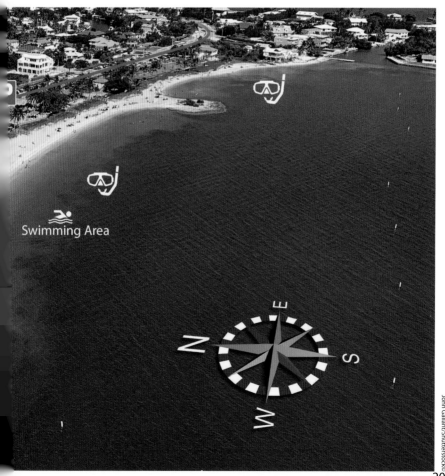

Swimming Area

John Gallant/Shutterstock©

FLAGLER'S BARGE

Difficulty	● ○ ○	
Current	● ○ ○	
Depth	● ○ ○	
Reef	★★★☆	Access
Fauna	★☆☆	7.1mi (11.5km) from Marathon

Level Open Water

Location Marathon
GPS   24° 38.642'N, 81° 04.308'W

Getting there

Flagler's Barge sits in shallow water on a wide sand berm located just north of Delta Shoal. Getting there involves a boat ride of 25 to 30 minutes from Marathon.

Access

There are no mooring buoys at this site, so boats will need to anchor in the sand well away from the wreck to avoid damaging the site. The wreck itself has deteriorated so care is needed when exploring the site. The site's shallow depth means it is suitable to both snorkelers and divers looking for a shallow second dive.

Description

The 100-foot (30.5-meter) barge was one of many used to carry the equipment and supplies necessary to build the Overseas Railway constructed by Henry Flagler between 1905 and 1912. The project was challenging from an engineering point of view and required many innovations to successfully connect Key West to Miami. However, nature also provided its own challenges, with three hurricanes hitting the region during the construction period. It is believed that the barge that currently sits near Delta Shoal broke free from its moorings during one of the storms and drifted out to the shoal where it eventually sank.

Today, the barge (which is also sometimes called *Delta Shoal Barge*) remains upright but most of the deck plates have corroded away. The sandy seabed sits at a maximum depth of 23 feet (7 meters) while the top of the barge reaches a depth of 16 feet (5 meters). The internal structural reinforcements remain, but it is not clear how much longer the barge will remain intact. The bow section has broken off and rests in place on the

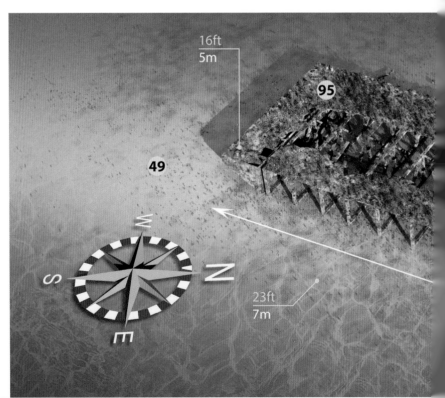

DID YOU KNOW?

The Overseas Railroad was called the 8th Wonder of the World when it was completed in 1912, but it fell well short of financial expectations and later earned the nickname Flagler's Folly. The project cost over $50 million ($1.25 billion in 2019 dollars) to complete, but the heavy volume of trade

Henry Flagler anticipated would arrive in Key West from the construction of the Panama Canal did not materialize. After a 1935 Hurricane caused tremendous damage to the Keys and the railroad, Flagler's company sold it to the state of Florida and Monroe County for $640,000. The railroad and its bridges were then used to help build the Overseas Highway.

sand. Penetration of the wreck is possible, but care should be taken as there is a risk of entanglement from the bent metal reinforcing bars.

The wreck is heavily encrusted in hard and soft corals including a dense covering of sea fans and other gorgonians. As the only structure in the area, the wreck supports a lot of marine life, including French grunts, gray angelfish, yellowtail snapper and plenty of bar jacks. Spotfin butterflyfish are common at the site as are Atlantic trumpetfish. The usual complement of yellowtail, schoolmaster and mahogany snapper are joined by barracuda who often hang out in the water column just off the wreck.

Name:	Flagler's Barge	Last owner:	Henry Flagler
Type:	Deck barge	Sunk:	c. 1905-1912
Previous names:	n/a		
Length:	100ft (30.5m)		
Tonnage:	n/a		
Construction:	n/a		

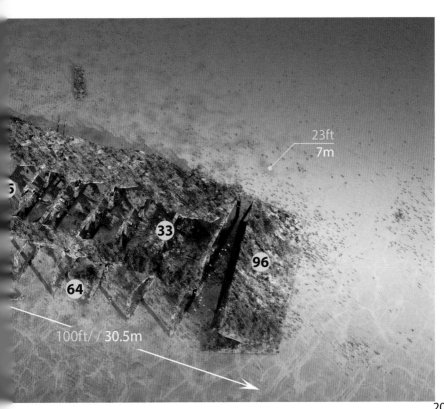

DELTA SHOAL & NORTH AMERICA WRECK

Difficulty ● ○ ○
Current ● ○ ○
Depth ● ○ ○
Reef ★★☆
Fauna ★☆☆

Access 🚤 8.5mi (13.5km) from Marathon

Level Open Water

Location Marathon
GPS (Delta Shoal) 24° 37.916'N, 81° 05.435'W
(NA1) 24° 38.265'N, 81° 05.607'W

Getting there
Delta Shoal sits 3.8 miles (6 kilometers) south of Boot Key at the southern end of Marathon. Getting there involves a boat ride of 25 to 30 minutes from Marathon.

Access
There are no mooring buoys near the reef on Delta Shoal, so boats will need to anchor in the sand well clear of the coral spurs and rubble-bottom grooves found along the seaward edge of the shoal. The shoal hosts multiple historical wrecks, including what is believed to be the wreck of the *North America*, which sits on a shallow sand berm 0.4 miles (0.7 kilometers) north of the reef. There is a mooring buoy near the wreck for convenient access. The shallow depths make the wreck site and nearby reef more suitable to snorkelers, but divers can still enjoy the reef as a shallow second dive. Currents are typically mild at these sites.

Description
Delta Shoal consists of a long stretch of spur and groove reef backed by a broad, shallow sand berm. The shoal helps mark the entrance to the open stretch of water crossed by the famous Seven-Mile Bridge of the Overseas Highway. The location of this reef helps explain why there are so many wrecks on the slope that extends seaward of the shallow spurs and grooves.

One such wreck is called *Ivory Wreck* by locals, after ivory tusks were found in the wreckage when it was first discovered along the western edge of the shoal in the late 1940s. Although authorities have so far been unable to confirm the vessel's identity, shackles and a cannon were also discovered at the site which, along with the ivory, suggests that the wreck was involved in the slave trade. The wreck is difficult to identify as it has become incorporated into the reef, and there are no visible remains at this site today.

Another wreck in this area is known locally as the *Delta Metal Wreck*. It too is difficult to locate, near the middle of the shoal, as the debris has largely become incorporated into the surrounding reef, but you can still look for metal structures in the sand patches between the reef spurs. It gets its name from the fact that the wreckage is dominated by metal debris.

Perhaps the most famous wreck site on Delta Shoal is the wreck of the *North America*

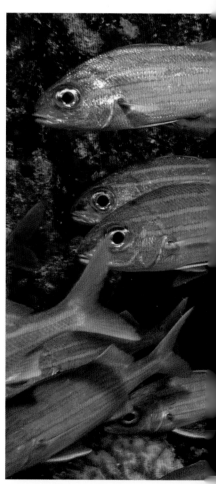

The identity of the wreck has not yet been conclusively confirmed. However, the tentative identification is based on passenger reports, which state that the three-mast, square-rigged *North America* first ran aground on the Bahama Banks on its way from New York to Mobile, Alabama. The ship, which was carrying dry goods and furniture, as well as passengers, apparently lost its rudder while it was being pulled off the reef and had to be fitted with a replacement before continuing on to Mobile. Later reports from wreckers in the area indicated that *North America* ran into more trouble off Vaca Key (one of the islands of Marathon) and eventually grounded for good on Delta Shoal.

The wreckage currently lies in just 14 feet (4.5 meters) of water north of the reef. The remains are consistent with the size and build of the *North America*, including the nature of the ballast stones. Most of the hull remains hidden under the sand, however, with only the pile of ballast remaining consistently visible. A section of floors and futtocks – the curved timber pieces that form the lower part of a ship's frame – are sometimes visible just north of the ballast stones. The wreck is part of the Florida Keys National Marine Sanctuary Shipwreck Trail and represents one of the easiest sites on the Trail for snorkelers to visit.

Visitors to Delta Shoal are likely to see a wide range of marine life at the site. The shallow spurs and grooves support bluehead wrasses, slippery dicks and yellowhead wrasses. Redband and stoplight parrotfish are commonly seen feeding on the algae that covers the coral reef, while schools of French and white grunts can be seen among the spurs and grooves.

Moray eels and nurse sharks are often seen sheltering at the base of spurs, while stingrays are a common sight out on the sandy sections of reef. Divers have reported seeing green sea turtles here, often feeding in the seagrass beds

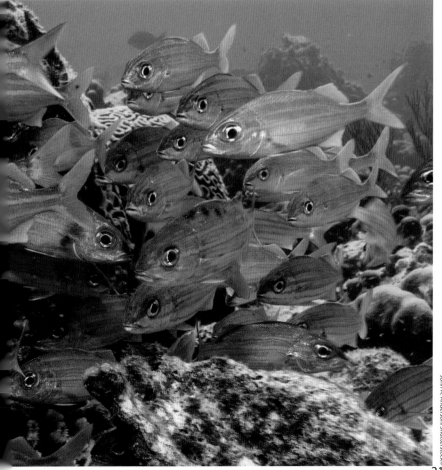

Schools of grunts, such as these smallmouth grunts, are common on bank reefs in the Keys.

DELTA SHOAL & NORTH AMERICA WRECK

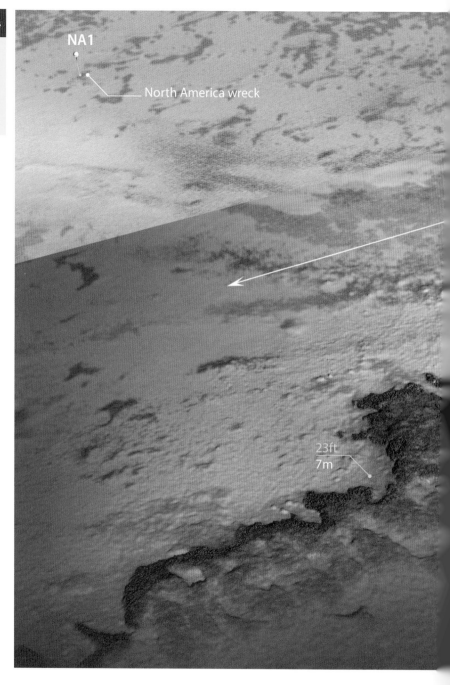

NA1

North America wreck

23ft
7m

that surround the northern section of the *North America* wreck site.

DELTA SHOAL & NORTH AMERICA WRECK

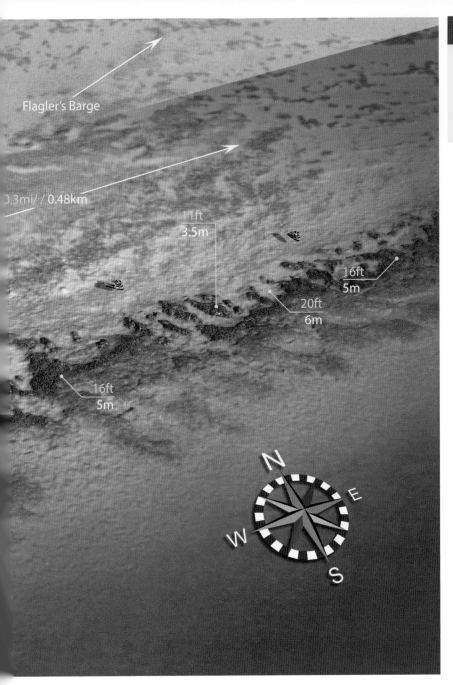

Flagler's Barge

0.3mi/ / 0.48km

11ft
3.5m

16ft
5m

20ft
6m

16ft
5m

Name:	SV North America	**Construction:**	Bath, Maine, 1833
Type:	Three-mast, square-rigged vessel	**Last owner:**	James B. Hall and George S. Hall
Previous names:	n/a	**Sunk:**	Nov. 25, 1842
Length:	130ft (39.6m)		
Tonnage:	n/a		

SOMBRERO REEF

Difficulty	● ○ ○
Current	● ○ ○
Depth	● ● ○
Reef	★ ★ ☆
Fauna	★ ★ ☆

Access 🚤 10mi (16km) from Marathon

Level Open Water

Location Marathon

GPS
SR0 24° 37.628′N, 81° 06.501′W
SR1 24° 37.607′N, 81° 06.494′W
SR2 24° 37.595′N, 81° 06.516′W
SR3 24° 37.613′N, 81° 06.522′W
SR4 24° 37.585′N, 81° 06.530′W
SR5 24° 37.582′N, 81° 06.564′W
SR6 24° 37.571′N, 81° 06.590′W
SR7 24° 37.556′N, 81° 06.578′W
SR8 24° 37.563′N, 81° 06.555′W
SR9 24° 37.559′N, 81° 06.592′W
SR10 24° 37.535′N, 81° 06.633′W
SR11 24° 37.567′N, 81° 06.621′W
SR12 24° 37.553′N, 81° 06.645′W
SR13 24° 37.525′N, 81° 06.674′W
SR14 24° 37.536′N, 81° 06.655′W
SR15 24° 37.546′N, 81° 06.687′W
SR16 24° 37.515′N, 81° 06.700′W
SR17 24° 37.555′N, 81° 06.720′W
SR18 24° 37.540′N, 81° 06.750′W
SR19 24° 37.510′N, 81° 06.731′W
SR20 24° 37.381′N, 81° 06.626′W
SR21 24° 37.382′N, 81° 06.661′W
SR22 24° 37.327′N, 81° 06.733′W

Getting there

Sombrero Reef sits 4.5 miles (7.2 kilometers) south of Boot Key at the southern end of Marathon, 1.2 miles (2 kilometers) west of nearby Delta Shoal. The reef is easily identified by the 142-foot-tall (43-meter) lighthouse that looms over the sand berm behind the spur and groove section of the reef. Getting there involves a boat ride of 30 to 35 minutes from Marathon.

Access

Access to Sombrero Reef is only possible by boat. There are 20 mooring buoys anchored along the shallow spur and groove section of the reef, with three additional moorings anchored along the deeper reef slope. The shallow spur and grooves section of the reef is ideal for snorkelers and novice divers given its maximum depth of just 26 feet (8 meters). The deeper reef slope bottoms-out at 60 feet (18 meters) making it suitable to divers of all levels.

Description

Sombrero Reef is one of the largest and best examples of a spur and groove coral reef in the Middle Keys. It was originally named Cayo Sombrero by the Spanish in the early years of Florida's history and was sometimes referred to as Dry Bank because part of the reef is known to break the surface of the water at low tide. Today, the reef is protected within the boundaries of a Sanctuary Preservation Area (SPA). Fishing and other extractive activities are not permitted, and visitors must tie into a mooring buoy if one is available.

The dominant feature of the site is the metal-frame lighthouse that towers above the reef. Sombrero Light is the tallest of Florida's six reef lighthouses and was built by George Meade, who was a engineer in his early days, but went on to become the Union General who defeated Robert E. Lee at Gettysburg. The lighthouse was completed in 1858 and helped reduce the frequent shipwrecks that occurred along this stretch of reefs, drawing to a close the lucrative salvaging industry in the area. Rumors state that Gustave Eiffel was traveling by boat along the coast of the Keys during a trip to the Americas and was struck by the lines and form of the towering metalwork. He apparently requested the captain return to the lighthouse so that he could make sketches and take notes on the architecture. It is believed that the lighthouse provided some inspiration to the young engineer who went on to design and oversee the construction of the Eiffel Tower, which has much in common in terms of the design with the remarkable Sombrero Light.

In addition to the brain and branching corals that divers and snorkelers will see at Sombrero Reef, the site is teeming with reef fishes of all kinds. Barracuda are regularly seen here, along with black grouper and even goliath grouper. Nurse sharks are common along the shallow reef, while reef sharks and scalloped hammerheads have been seen deeper on the reef slope. Stoplight parrotfish, foureye butterflyfish and ocean surgeonfish are common along the coral spurs while spotted and yellow goatfish patrol the sandy areas. Divers who look closely may even spot yellowhead jawfish sticking their heads out of holes in the rubble-bottomed grooves.

RELAX & RECHARGE

Bongo's Botanical Beer Garden and Cafe (59300 Overseas Highway, Marathon) is located on the Lagoon in Grassy Key. The eclectic café with its 2,000-square foot (186-square meter) beer garden right on the edge of the lagoon serves brunch on the weekends and is a favorite among locals as a venue for live music. It has 20 craft beers on tap to accompany its light and local fare that showcases the organic fruits and herbs grown right there on Grassy Key. The menu has some unique offerings which are unlikely to be found elsewhere, like coconut shrimp curry, Hawaiian BBQ chicken and jerk chicken sandwiches. After dining, consider taking a stroll through the botanical gardens or for those looking for a little more excitement, try a tow through the lagoon on the Keys Cable.
Visit: **Ridethelagoon.com/bongos-cafe**

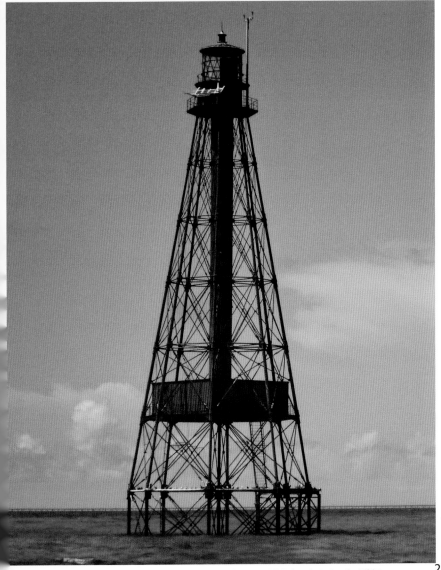

The iconic Sombrero Reef Lighthouse is believed to have inspired Gustave Eiffel when designing the Eiffel Tower.

J. Skoway/Shutterstock©

SOMBRERO REEF

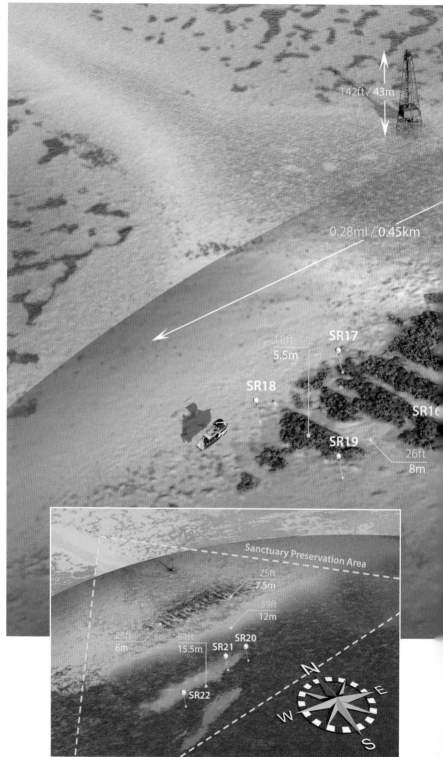

142ft / 43m

0.28mi / 0.45km

18ft
5.5m

SR17

SR18

SR16

SR19

26ft
8m

Sanctuary Preservation Area

25ft
7.5m

39ft
12m

26ft
8m

51ft
15.5m

SR20

SR21

SR22

N

E

W

S

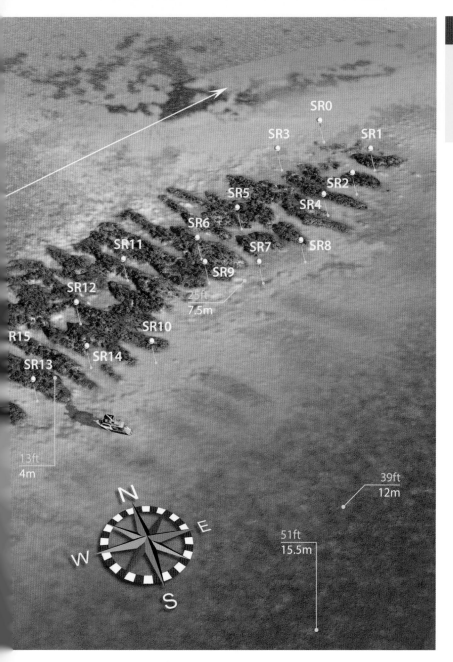

SR0

SR3

SR1

SR2

SR5

SR4

SR6

SR7

SR8

SR11

SR9

SR12

25ft
7.5m

R15

SR10

SR13

SR14

13ft
4m

N

E

W

S

39ft
12m

51ft
15.5m

217

PIGEON KEY

Difficulty	● ○ ○
Current	● ● ●
Depth	● ○ ○
Reef	★ ☆ ☆
Fauna	★ ☆ ☆

Access
2mi (3.1km) from Marathon

Access
2mi (3.1km) from Marathon

Level n/a

Location Pigeon Key
GPS   24° 42.233'N, 81° 09.333'W

Getting there

Pigeon Key is connected to Vaca Key by the old Seven Mile Bridge that was recently refurbished. The bridge is only open to foot and bike traffic, however, although a tram ride will be added

soon. Visitors can also get to the island via a short 10-minute ferry ride from Marathon. The visitor's center for the island is located at 2010 Overseas Highway in Marathon, which is the bay-side of the highway, located near mile marker 47.5.

Access

Access to the refurbished bridge is free, but access to the island itself involves an entry fee of $15 for adults, $12 for children aged 6 to

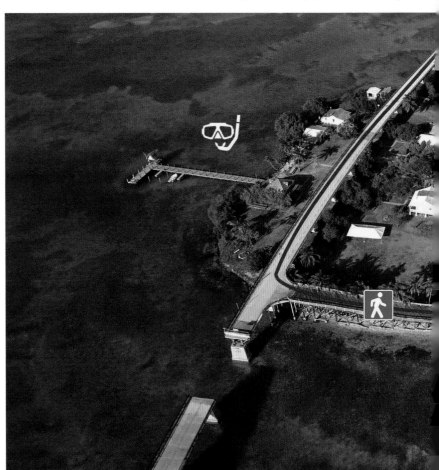

12 years, and $5 for those aged five years and under. Visitors must first register at the visitor's center in Marathon.

Description

Pigeon Key once housed a work camp for the Florida East Coast Railway company, starting in 1909 as Henry Flagler began the massive undertaking of extending the railroad south to Key West. Originally named Cayo Paloma (Spanish for pigeon), supposedly after the many large flocks of pigeons that once roosted here, the small 5.3-acre (2.1-hectare) island is now run by the Pigeon Key Foundation and Marine Science Center. The island has been transformed into a world-class education center, focusing on the cultural and natural resources of the Florida Keys. Aside from the guided historical tours available on the island, visitors can opt for a self-led tour to wander the grounds. Catch-and-release fishing is allowed from the dock and families often bring picnics to the island.

Swimming and snorkeling are popular activities at the island. Visitors looking to snorkel will need to bring their own gear along with their own dive buoy as rental gear is not available on the island. The best snorkel areas are near the dock, directly off the beach and by the opening of the saltwater pool – there is no swimming in the pool itself. The island is largely surrounded by hard-bottom habitat with seagrass beds beyond that. Visitors may see gray snapper, scrawled cowfish, cocoa damselfish and plenty of sergeant majors in the shallow waters around the island. Barracuda are known to hang out in the waters off the beach, while southern stingrays and nurse sharks are often spotted resting on the seabed.

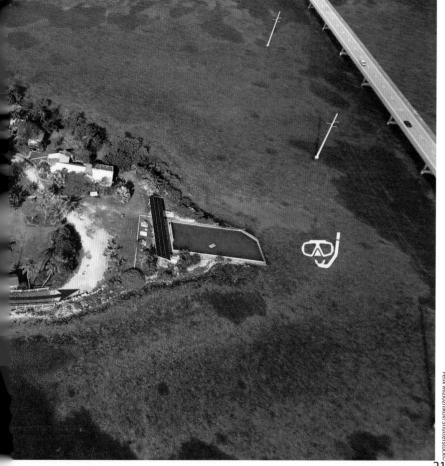

SEVEN-MILE BRIDGE RUBBLE

Difficulty ● ● ○
Current ● ● ○
Depth ● ● ●
Reef ★★★☆
Fauna ★★★

Level Advanced

Location Marathon
GPS   (Swingspan Rubble)
         24° 36.062'N, 81° 09.808'W

Getting there
The Seven-Mile Bridge Rubble dive site includes multiple artificial reef deployments in a general area located roughly 7 miles (11.3 kilometers) south of the existing Seven-Mile Bridge, due south of Moser Channel. It involves a boat ride

of around 45 to 50 minutes from Marathon.

Access
The site is only accessible by boat. The maximum depth of the seabed ranges from 90 to 115 feet (27.5 to 35 meters) across the broader deployment site, making it more suitable to advanced divers. There are no mooring buoys at the site so divers will need to anchor in the sand.

Description
The new Seven Mile Bridge opened for traffic

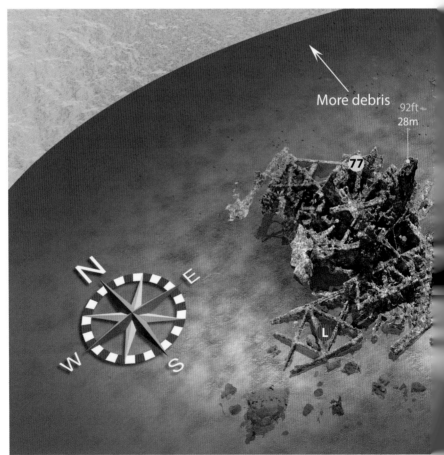

More debris

92ft
28m

77

SAFETY TIP ❗

The dive site is very popular with spearfishers due to its depth and the presence of large grouper and snapper. Over the years, there have been numerous reports of aggressive bull shark encounters, most likely because of the spearfishing that occurs at the site. Non-spearfishing divers have little to worry about from the bull sharks but might want to reconsider visiting the site if other divers are actively involved in spearfishing there at the same time.

n 1982, replacing the old roadway built on the foundation of Henry Flagler's Oversea Railroad Bridge that spanned the seven-mile gap between Marathon and Bahia Honda Key. The old roadway was lower than the new bridge, and it included a metal swing bridge that could rotate to allow tall ships to transit from the Atlantic into the waters of Florida Bay, and vice versa. This swing bridge and the concrete and steel rubble debris created from its removal now make up the bulk of the artificial reefs deployed in this area. In all, a reported 4,500 tons of concrete and steel debris were deployed across the region from 1980 through 1984 to create habitat for marine life.

The rubble and metal spans that make up the Swingspan rubble are heavily encrusted with soft corals and sponges. The artificial reef offers more than 25 to 30 feet (7.5 to 9 meters) of relief in some places and hosts a wide variety of reef creatures, including some large pelagic species. Goliath grouper and large black grouper, cubera snapper and red snapper all can be found here, along with bull sharks. Plenty of smaller reef fish are also found here, including bar jacks, yellowtail snapper, grunts and damselfish.

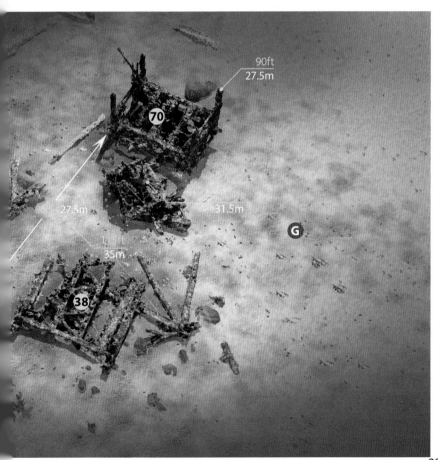

LOWER KEYS DIVE SITES
Big Pine Key to Key West

If Key Largo is the gateway to the Florida Keys, Key West is its hot and humid beating heart. The rich history of pirates, authors, musicians and poets plays out across every corner of this 7 square-mile (18 square-kilometer) island that accommodates more than 24,000 residents.

The region known as the Lower Keys extends northeast from Key West through Sugarloaf Key, Cudjoe Key, Big Pine Key and even Bahia Honda Key, but Key West is where the Conch Republic has its roots. It is the magnet that draws visitors down the 100 miles (160 kilometers) of narrow, often single-laned highway that stretches south from Key Largo.

Tourists come for the atmosphere but also for the diving and snorkeling. The famous

Vandenberg artificial reef is located just offshore from Key West, while the impressive *Adolphus Busch* is found at the northern edge of the Lower Keys, just off Big Pine Key. The region can hold its own when it comes to natural reefs too, with Western Sambo and Eastern Dry Rock being among the most popular reefs in the area. And the snorkeling is hard to beat, particularly in the Dry Tortugas at Fort Jefferson.

Many operators offer visitors the option for a sunset snorkel cruise that cannot be beat. Since Key West is located at the western end of the chain of islands that make up the Florida Keys, the sunsets truly are a thing of beauty whether you are enjoying them out on the water or sipping a delicious drink on land.

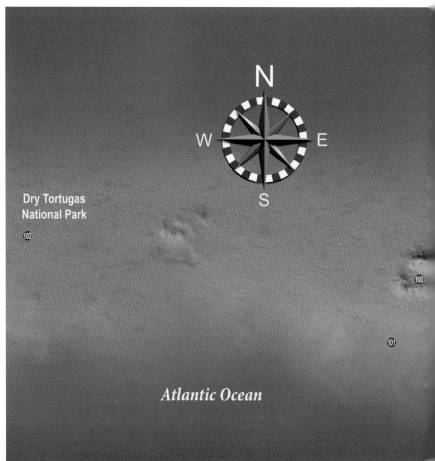

Dry Tortugas
National Park

102

100

101

Atlantic Ocean

Dive and snorkel sites

8	Bahia Honda State Park		
9	Horseshoe Beach		
0	Big Pine Shoal (aka G Marker)		
1	Newfound Harbor		
2	Looe Key		
3	Looe Key Deep		
4	*Adolphus Busch Sr*		
5	American Shoal		
6	Maryland Shoal		
7	*Wilkes-Barre*		
8	Pelican Shoal		
9	Speculator shoal		
0	Eastern Sambo	Research Only	
1	Middle Sambo		
2	Western Sambo		
	• Haystacks		
3	10 Fathom Ledge		
4	*General H.S. Vandenberg*		

85	*Joe's Tug*	
86	Toppino's Buoy (aka Marker 32)	
87	9' Stake	
88	*Cayman Salvager*	
89	*Curb*	
90	Key West Marine Park	
91	Fort Zachary Taylor Snorkel Reefs	
92	Eastern Dry Rocks	
93	Rock Key	
94	Sand Key Reef	
95	Archer Key	
96	Cottrell Key	
97	Western Dry Rocks	
98	Lost Reef	
99	*Amesbury* (aka *Alexander's Wreck*)	
100	Marquesas Keys	
101	Cosgrove Shoal	
102	Fort Jefferson	

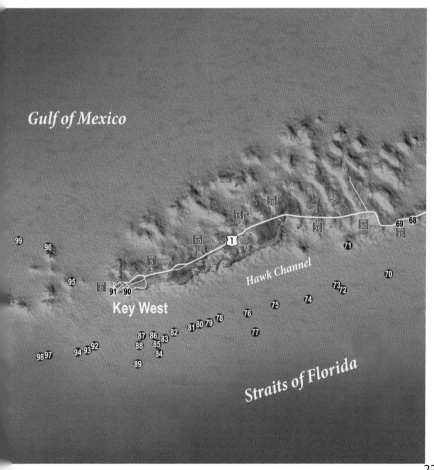

Gulf of Mexico

Hawk Channel

Key West

Straits of Florida

BAHIA HONDA STATE PARK

Difficulty ● ○ ○
Current ● ○ ○
Depth ● ○ ○
Reef ★★☆
Fauna ★★☆

Access 🚗 12mi (19km) from Marathon
🚗 35mi (56km) from Key West

Level n/a

Location Bahia Honda
GPS 24° 39.333'N, 81° 16.679'W

Getting there

Bahia Honda State Park is on Bahia Honda Key at the southwestern end of the famous Seven Mile Bridge. To get there, head south from Marathon across the Seven Mile Bridge, and then cross through Little Duck Key, Missouri Key and Ohio Key, in that order. The entrance to the state park is on the left side of the road (ocean side) just 1.57 miles (2.5 kilometers) after passing over the short bridge that provides access to Bahia Honda Key. The park is located between mile markers 36 and 37.

When arriving from the south, drive east from Big Pine Key along the Overseas Highway, which makes a sharp turn south along the eastern edge of Big Pine Key before turning east again toward West Summerland Key. A 1.25-mile (2-kilometer) stretch of bridge separates East Summerland from Bahia Honda Key, and the entrance to the state park is the first right after arriving on Bahia Honda. Once in the park, follow the road past the ranger station at the entrance and stay right to reach the snorkeling beaches. The official address is 36850 Overseas Highway, Big Pine Key.

Access

There is a fee to enter the park. There are showers, restrooms and ample parking in the southwestern end of the park, next to the two snorkel beaches, as well as the park's main concession building and nature center. A third beach at the southeastern end of the park was closed for reconstruction at the time of publication. The park is open from 8am to sundown every day of the year, however this spot is very popular and may be closed to new visitors once capacity is reached in its day-use areas. There is very little shade, so plan accordingly. And though technically accessible to divers, the shallowness of the waters off Bahia Honda State Park makes it more suitable for snorkeling.

Description

Bahia Honda State Park features 524 acres

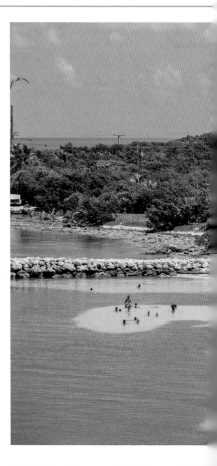

of Florida wilderness with hiking and biking trails, a boat ramp, two beaches and overnight accommodations in the form of tent camping cabins and an RV campground. The two main snorkeling areas are adjacent to the northwest facing Calusa Beach that opens to Florida Bay and the southeast facing Loggerhead Beach which opens to the Atlantic Ocean. The beaches are either side of the narrow spit of land that houses the parking lot and the park's day-use buildings.

Calusa Beach is sheltered from the currents and offers snorkelers the opportunity to explore

SAFETY TIP ❗

Florida law requires that divers and snorkelers display a red and white diver down flag whenever they are in the water to help warn nearby boaters. One exception to this rule is when snorkeling in an area specifically reserved for swimming, such as a beach with a boundary line of buoys. When diving or snorkeling from a boat, the boat can fly its own flag. Divers and snorkelers just need to remain within 300 feet (90 meters) of their boat when it is flying the diver down flag. If exploring without a boat, floating dive buoys with the same markings or a floating flag must be towed by one of the divers or snorkelers in the group.

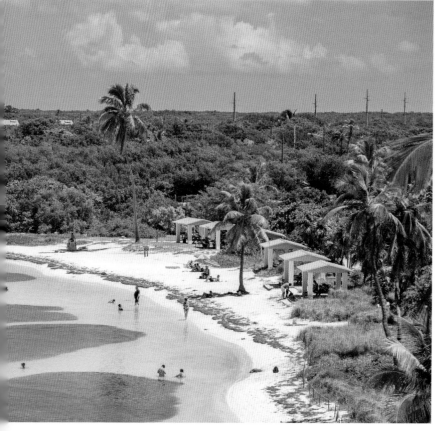

Simon Dannhauer/Shutterstock©

BAHIA HONDA STATE PARK

hallow seagrass beds that extend more than 00 feet (90 meters) from the beach. Visitors can ee many different reef fish species, including rgeant majors, hogfish and grunts, while xploring this area. Calusa is ideal for novice norkelers because it is better protected than oggerhead Beach, but the marine life is less verse here than on the Atlantic side.

ggerhead Beach is much longer than the ore sheltered Calusa Beach and stretches m the channel to the park entrance, and yond. Loggerhead is often subject to stronger rrents at the western end of the beach, near the channel, particularly at or near high tide. But this beach is widely considered to offer the best shore-entry snorkeling experience in the Florida Keys. Snorkelers have reported seeing stingrays, scrawled cowfish, gray snapper, highhats, Queen conch, spiny lobsters and pinfish. Manatees are not commonly encountered here, but it does happen on occasion.

The park also offers a snorkeling tour that departs from the small dock located next to the concession building. The tour visits the deeper waters at nearby Looe Key Reef.

HORSESHOE BEACH

Difficulty	● ○ ○
Current	● ○ ○
Depth	● ○ ○
Reef	★★☆
Fauna	★★☆

Access 🚙 14mi (22.5km) from Marathon
🚙 34mi (55km) from Key West

Level Open Water

Location West Summerland Key
GPS 24° 39.320'N, 81° 18.108'W

Getting there
Horseshoe Beach is on Summerland Key just east of Big Pine Key. To get there, head south from Marathon across the Seven Mile Bridge and Bahia Honda Key. The entrance to the beach is on the northern, bay side, of the highway and is the first right after crossing the Bahia Honda Bridge. From the south, drive east from Big Pine Key along the Overseas Highway. The highway makes a sharp turn south along the eastern edge of Big Pine Key before turning east again to cross over to West

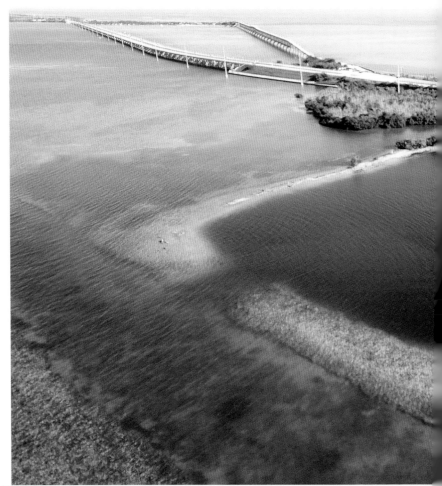

Summerland Key. The entrance to the beach is on the left, just a mile (1.7 kilometers) after the bridge onto West Summerland. The entrance is located near mile marker 35, and the official address is 1969 Overseas Highway, Big Pine Key.

Access

The access road to the beach runs parallel to the highway and ends in a narrow parking area. A dirt track leads from the parking lot to the water. The path is just under 400 feet (120 meters) in length and is easy to navigate unless it has just rained. There are no facilities at the beach and no parking or access fees.

Description

Horseshoe Beach (also called Horseshoe Pit) gets its name from its resemblance to a horseshoe. It was excavated back when limestone was needed to build the Overseas Railway. The sides of the quarry offer easy shore access to snorkelers and divers, and the depth in the middle of the pit maxes out at 30 feet (9 meters). The bottom at the center is a mix of sand and mud with little relief other than what remains of an old ambulance that was dropped as an artificial reef. Divers often visit here when the wind is blowing hard enough to render the offshore sites inaccessible.

Divers and snorkelers may see stoplight, blue and rainbow parrotfishes, schoolmaster and gray snapper, gray angelfish, Bermuda chub and barracuda. Rays are commonly spotted along the seabed here along with the occasional nurse shark.

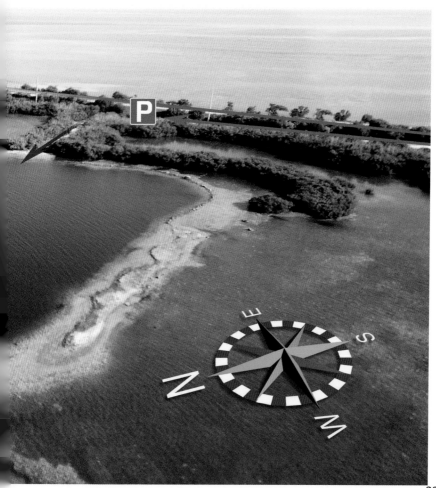

BIG PINE SHOAL

Difficulty	● ● ○	
Current	● ○ ○	
Depth	● ● ○	
Reef	★☆☆	
Fauna	★★☆	

Access
12mi (19km) from Big Pine Key

Level Open Water

Location Big Pine Key
GPS   24° 34.102'N, 81° 19.538'W

Getting there
Big Pine Shoal is located 5 miles (8 kilometers) south of the southeastern corner of Big Pine Key. Located on the outer reef line, it takes 35 to 40 minutes to get there by boat from Big Pine Key.

Access
Due to its distance from shore, this reef is only accessible by boat. At its shallowest point, the reef reaches only 18 to 20 feet (5.5 to 6 meters) in depth, making it more suitable for divers than snorkelers. There are no mooring buoys so boats must anchor in the sand. Visibility can be poor here, so boaters should double check their position relative to the reef before dropping anchor. The site is marked by red navigational marker 22.

Description
Big Pine Shoal, also sometimes called G Marker, is a standard shoal along the coast of the Florida Keys. The shoal boasts a small ledge of

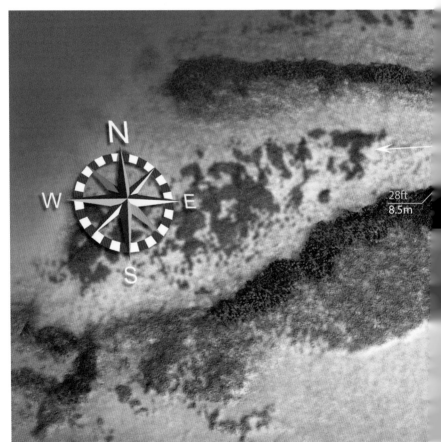

SCIENTIFIC INSIGHT

Big Pine Shoal is located near a Florida Keys National Marine Sanctuary Water Quality Monitoring Program site. Big Pine Shoal is part of a network of sites throughout the United States that monitor a range of water quality variables, including biological, physical and chemical metrics. These data are critically important for proper management of ocean resources where local runoff can put nutrient-rich waste and other pollutants into coastal waters. This runoff represents one of the greatest threats to coral reefs not just in the Florida Keys, but elsewhere in the world too. Corals have evolved to thrive in clear, nutrient-poor waters, and they are in constant competition for space with macroalgae. The input of nutrient-rich runoff into coastal water can shift an ecosystem toward one dominated more by algae, which can impact the entire system. It is critically important for the health and long-term survival of corals that coastal development and nutrient-rich waste is limited in coastal waters.

s shoreward side and a deeper ledge along s seaward side where it meets a narrow sand hannel at a depth of 34 feet (10.5 meters). The nannel is 200 feet (60 meters) wide and runs oughly parallel to shore. It separates the shoal om a deeper reef slope that descends to 50 feet 5 meters).

he reef here is well colonized with soft corals and sponges, along with a scattering of hard corals including brain and star corals. The hard bottom is host to a variety of marine life, including bluestriped grunts, yellowtail snapper and barracuda. Angelfish can often be seen patrolling the reef in pairs while damselfish defend their territories from grazing schools of ocean surgeonfish and blue tangs.

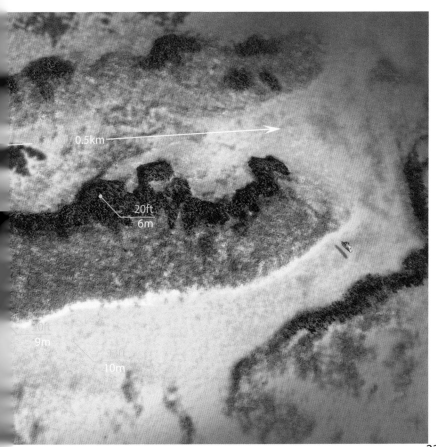

NEWFOUND HARBOR

Difficulty ● ○ ○
Current ● ○ ○
Depth ● ● ○
Reef ★★☆
Fauna ★★☆

Access 🚤
5mi (8km) from Big Pine Key

Level n/a

Location Big Pine Key
GPS
NH1 24° 36.899'N, 81° 23.631'W
NH2 24° 36.926'N, 81° 23.639'W
NH3 24° 36.938'N, 81° 23.627'W
NH4 24° 36.943'N, 81° 23.608'W
NH5 24° 36.977'N, 81° 23.485'W
NH6 24° 36.988'N, 81° 23.460'W

Getting there

Newfound Harbor is located just 0.4 miles (0.
kilometers) south of Big Munson Island, which i
at the southwestern corner of Big Pine Key. It is
shallow patch of reef that involves a boat ride
about 15 minutes from nearby Big Pine Key.

Access

Despite its proximity to shore, this site is on
accessible by boat. The shallow, inshore patc
reefs are suitable for snorkelers of all levels b

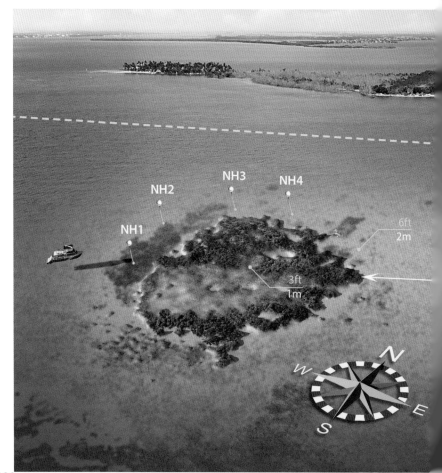

the shallowness of the reef – at less than 12 feet (3.5 meters) across most of the site – makes it less suitable to divers. A total of six mooring buoys spread across two large sections of reef provide easy access to the site. Visibility can be poor when winds push the cloudier water from Hawk Channel onto the reef, so the best time to visit is during a northeasterly wind, which is more common during the winter. Most of the local snorkel tour operators include a visit to Newfound Harbor on their schedules, particularly when wind and waves limit access to the popular Looe Key barrier reef.

Description

The inshore patch reefs at Newfound Harbor are protected within the boundaries of a Sanctuary Preservation Area (SPA), so fishing and the removal of marine life is not permitted. Touching or standing on living or dead coral is also not allowed here, which can require careful attention even the reef is as shallow as 3 feet (1 meter)

in many spots. In fact, the reef is so shallow in this area that there is evidence of multiple boat groundings from inexperienced boaters navigating into the nearby harbor.

The site consists of two largely circular patches of reef separated by a 510-foot (155-meter) stretch of sand and seagrass. The reefs support a variety of marine life, including many boulder corals, along with star and brain corals, as well as a variety of soft corals and gorgonians, including sea fans. Snorkelers will see blue tangs, porkfish, and both French and bluestriped grunts on the reef. Yellowtail snapper and schoolmaster snapper are also relatively common here. The biodiversity on the reef is evident in the presence of larger predators, including black grouper and Nassau grouper, and large barracuda. Nurse sharks are common in the shallow waters and are often seen resting next to a coral head or small ledge.

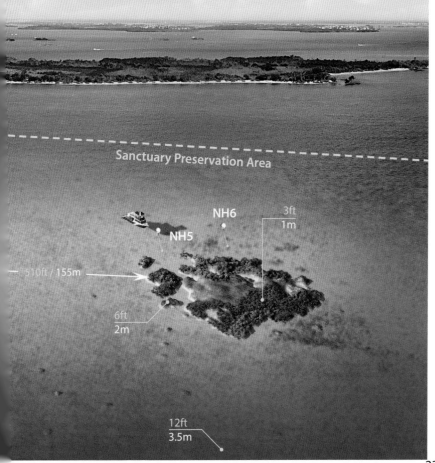

LOOE KEY REEF & LOOE KEY DEEP

Difficulty	● ○ ○
Current	● ● ○
Depth	● ● ○
Reef	★★★
Fauna	★★☆

Access 🚤 9mi (14.5km) Big Pine Key

Level Open Water

Location Ramrod Key

Looe Key Reef

GPS
LK1 24° 32.796'N, 81° 24.079'W
LK2 24° 32.792'N, 81° 24.118'W
LK3 24° 32.808'N, 81° 24.180'W
LK4 24° 32.781'N, 81° 24.185'W
LK5 24° 32.788'N, 81° 24.212'W
LK6 24° 32.765'N, 81° 24.212'W
LK7 24° 32.770'N, 81° 24.236'W
LK8 24° 32.742'N, 81° 24.258'W
LK9 24° 32.771'N, 81° 24.282'W
LK10 24° 32.744'N, 81° 24.293'W
LK11 24° 32.759'N, 81° 24.318'W
LK12 24° 32.743'N, 81° 24.342'W
LK13 24° 32.743'N, 81° 24.347'W
LK14 24° 32.749'N, 81° 24.382'W
LK15 24° 32.736'N, 81° 24.416'W
LK16 24° 32.694'N, 81° 24.494'W
LK17 24° 32.695'N, 81° 24.428'W
LK18 24° 32.703'N, 81° 24.456'W
LK19 24° 32.671'N, 81° 24.485'W
LK20 24° 32.693'N, 81° 24.545'W
LK21 24° 32.678'N, 81° 24.522'W
LK22 24° 32.666'N, 81° 24.560'W
LK23 24° 32.680'N, 81° 24.568'W
LK24 24° 32.723'N, 81° 24.595'W
LK25 24° 32.701'N, 81° 24.618'W
LK26 24° 32.687'N, 81° 24.639'W
LK27 24° 32.714'N, 81° 24.642'W
LK28 24° 32.690'N, 81° 24.690'W
LK29 24° 32.720'N, 81° 24.619'W
LK30 24° 32.596'N, 81° 24.651'W
LK31 24° 32.553'N, 81° 24.762'W
LK36 24° 32.882'N, 81° 24.357'W
LK37 24° 32.888'N, 81° 24.387'W
LK38 24° 32.869'N, 81° 24.413'W
LK40 24° 33.825'N, 81° 24.140'W
LK41 24° 33.864'N, 81° 24.220'W
LK42 24° 33.756'N, 81° 24.327'W

Looe Key Deep
LK32 24° 32.554'N, 81° 24.838'W
LK33 24° 32.511'N, 81° 24.917'W
LK34 24° 32.451'N, 81° 24.930'W
LK35 24° 32.499'N, 81° 24.971'W
LK39 24° 32.869'N, 81° 24.412'W

LK43 24° 32.275'N, 81° 25.745'W
LK44 24° 32.263'N, 81° 25.813'W
LK45 24° 32.243'N, 81° 25.820'W
LK46 24° 32.268'N, 81° 25.913'W

Getting there

Looe Key Reef is a well-developed spur and groove reef system along the outer edge of the Keys reef line just under 7 miles (11 kilometer) offshore from Ramrod Key. It is the marquee reef system along this stretch of the Florida Key and all the local dive and snorkel operato make regular trips out to the site. Getting there involves a boat ride of around 30 minutes from Ramrod Key.

Access

Looe Key Reef is accessible to divers an snorkelers of all levels. The reef is peppered wi 46 mooring buoys, the vast majority of which a anchored along the spurs and grooves section the reef. A total of nine buoys are anchored f to the west of the main site in deeper waters these are often collectively referred to as Loo Key Deep. Three buoys are anchored to the nor of the main site (LK40, LK41, and LK42) along line of shallow patch reefs on the seaward ed of Hawk Channel. These inshore buoys fall rig next to the Looe Key Research Only area, which only accessible by permit.

Description

Looe Key Reef is contained within the Lo Key Existing Management Area. The 5 square nautical mile (18.3 square kilometre management area includes the Sanctua Preservation Area (SPA) that covers the ma site, and the research-only area located d east of the northernmost buoys (LK40, LK and LK42). The reef has been under spec protection since 1981.

The reef gets its name from the British friga HMS Loo, which ran aground here in 17 Historical records vary greatly around the deta of the vessel's final days, but most agree th Loo had captured and was towing the Billan Betty believed to be a British ship captured a operated by the Spanish at the time. On her v

RELAX & RECHARGE

No Name Pub (30813 Watson Blvd, Big Pine Key) is real Keys institution known for its pizza and burgers (particularly its massive pork burger). But the real attraction is the history of this place. Established in 1931, the building was originally a general store and bait-and-tackle shop with an upstairs brothel. The bar and restaurant opened in 1936. And in the wild-west heydays of the 1970s and 80s, the establishment was known for being a hangout for drug-runners and other shady customers. The tradition of stapling dollar bills to the ceiling began soon after opening, and continues today, although little room remains. The establishment estimates there is close to $100,000 worth of currency stuck to the ceiling. No Name Pub can be hard to find, however. At Mile Marker 30.2, turn onto Key Deer Boulevard at the Big Pine Key traffic light, which is the gateway to Big Pine Key and the National Key Deer Wildlife Refuge. After 1.7 miles (2.7 kilometers) turn right onto Watson Boulevard and follow that for another 1.5 miles (2.5 kilometers) as it twists and turns through residential neighborhoods until you arrive at the pub. This area is the only place in the world where you'll find the endangered Key deer, so drive slowly and keep your eyes peeled.
Visit: **Nonamepub.com**

Charleston, South Carolina, with her prize, *Loo* ot caught in the Florida current and was pushed against the reef in the early hours of February smashing rudder-first into the shallow coral urs. Caught against the corals with no way to er, the pounding waves soon made quick work her wooden hull, and the ship sank. Thankfully, r crew managed to salvage enough food and unitions to survive.

e wreck was first discovered in 1950 on the st end of the reef. The addition of an "e" at the d of the name was apparently a clerical error ade during the report on the ship's loss, which why the reef's name differs slightly from the ginal frigate. Little remains of the wrecked

vessel today, aside from her name on the reef, and by far the star attraction of this dive site is the long stretch of well-defined coral spurs.

The main section of this reef stretches 0.7 miles (1.1 kilometers) from east to west. Like many of the large reefs further north, off Key Largo, each buoy on Looe Key reef represents its own unique dive or snorkel experience. Local operators have given names to the various sites, including the Gardens (LK1 and LK2), the Nursery (LK3 to LK8), The Looe (LK9 to LK15), Shark Alley (LK16 to LK24) and the West End (LK25 to LK31). Each of these areas feature corals spurs that run north to south and top out at just 10 feet (3 meters) below the surface. The rubble and sand grooves bottom out

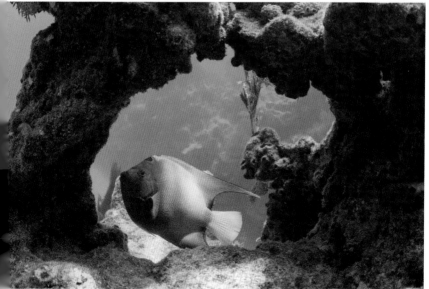

Peter Douglas Clark/Shutterstock©

ueen angelfish swims below a coral arch on Looe Key Reef.

233

LOOE KEY REEF & LOOE KEY DEEP

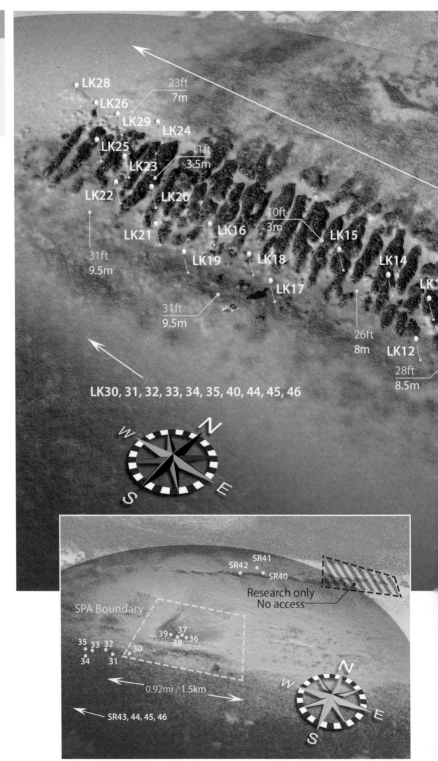

LK28
LK26
23ft
7m
LK29
LK24
LK25
11ft
3.5m
LK23
LK22
LK20
10ft
3m
LK21
LK16
LK15
31ft
9.5m
LK19
LK18
LK14
LK
LK17
31ft
9.5m
26ft
8m
LK12
28ft
8.5m

LK30, 31, 32, 33, 34, 35, 40, 44, 45, 46

SR41
SR42
SR40
Research only
No access
SPA Boundary
39 37
35 33 32 38 36
34 31 30
0.92mi / 1.5km
SR43, 44, 45, 46

LOOE KEY REEF & LOOE KEY DEEP

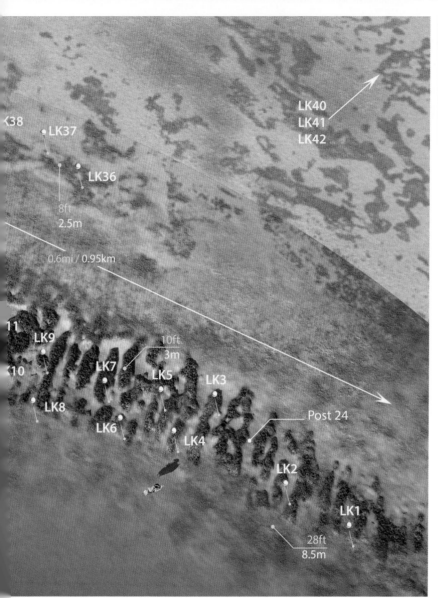

depth of approximately 26 feet (8 meters). ...oughout the entire reef, divers and snorkelers ...see a wide variety of marine life. Barracuda ...bar jacks are common along the shallower ...ions of the reef, while French and bluestriped ...nts, along with yellowtail snapper, sergeant ...ors and foureye butterflyfish are common ...nd down the spurs and grooves around the ...crest. Stoplight, midnight and blue parrotfish ...regularly seen here, grazing on the algae ...grows on the reef. Rock beauties, Queen ...elfish and other angelfish species can be seen ...olling the reef, while schools of blue chromis ...n above the reef.

The density of reef fishes makes this site popular with larger predators, including reef sharks, blacktip sharks and even the occasional bull shark. Spotted eagle rays are also a common occurrence in the deeper waters of the reef.

Looe Key Deep is located outside of the boundaries of the SPA. Here the hard-bottom reef slope tracks to the west at a depth of around 46 feet (14 meters) and deeper. This area of the reef tends to be more popular among fishers.

235

ADOLPHUS BUSCH SR

Difficulty ● ● ○
Current ● ● ○
Depth ● ● ●
Reef ★★★☆
Fauna ★★★

Access 🚤 9mi (15km) from Ramrod Key

Level Advanced

Location Ramrod Key
GPS   24° 31.814'N, 81° 27.710'W

Getting there

Adolphus Busch Sr rests in deep water, just 8 miles (13 kilometers) south of Cudjoe Key, just beyond the outer reef line. Getting there involves a boat ride of 30 minutes from Ramrod Key.

Access

The wreck is only accessible by boat given its distance from shore, and it is only suitable for advanced divers given its depth. The seabed bottoms out at 115 feet (35 meters) while the main deck sits at 96 feet (29.5 meters). There are typically two buoys on the wreck, one attached to the bow and one attached to the stern, which provide convenient access to the site. Visibility is generally good, but currents can be strong.

Description

Adolphus Busch Sr was built in Burntisland, Scotland, in 1951. The 210-foot (64-meter) short-haul island freighter was originally named *MV London*. Over her decades-long career she changed ownership and names seven times, including making a brief appearance as a movie prop in the 1957 movie, Fire Down Under. Her final name before becoming a wreck was *Ocean Alley*.

In September 1998, she struck a pier in the harbor of Port-au-Prince, Haiti, and partially sank. She was refloated and subsequently purchased by the Looe Key Artificial Reef Association with the financial assistance of Adolphus Busch IV, an avid diver and fisherman, and the grandson of Adolphus Busch Sr., founder of the Anheuser-Busch brewery. The purchase marked the culmination of a long search for a suitable vessel to deploy as an artificial reef to enhance the diving in the area between American Shoal and Looe Key Reef.

Ocean Alley was towed to Florida where she was cleaned and prepared for sinking. She was renamed *Adolphus Busch Sr* in honor of the Busch brewing company's patriarch. She

was eventually scuttled on December 5, 1998 without the use of explosives. She settled upright and intact on a sandy seabed at a depth of 115 feet (35 meters) and remains in excellent condition today. The holes cut in her superstructure and hull prior to her deployment allow penetration for divers with suitable training and experience. Her superstructure tops out at a depth of 77 feet (23.5 meters), which puts her out of reach of many divers. But aside from her depth, she is an easily explored wreck that represents a great introduction to wreck diving.

RELAX & RECHARGE

The Square Grouper Bar and Grill (22658 Overseas Highway, Cudjoe Key) is a great place to enjoy quality, fresh seafood. Specialties include the Square Grouper seafood stew, almond encrusted grouper, and seared sesame encrusted tuna. There are also mouth-watering appetizers like flash-fried conch, buffalo shrimp with blue cheese dressing, and coconut shrimp with spicy mango sauce. It's not all seafood at Square Grouper though, there are salads, steaks, burgers and sandwiches too, along with a boutique wine list and rotating selection of microbrews that will quench your thirst. The Square Grouper is environmentally friendly, which means corn products have replaced plastic. Visit: **Squaregrouperbarandgrill.com.**

The wreck plays host to a variety of marine life, both large and small. Goliath grouper, black grouper and cubera snapper are all regularly seen around the wreck. Reef butterflyfish, sharpnose puffers and bicolor damselfish are often seen flitting above the coral and sponge encrusted exterior of the wreck, while bar jacks, permits and yellowtail snapper form loose schools in the water column above. Everything from Atlantic trumpetfish to green morays can be found here, making this site popular with locals and visitors alike.

Route

Divers often descend the bow line to start their swim into the prevailing currents, which typically run from the southwest. The depth of the main deck means there is not a lot of time to spend exploring the bulk of the wreck, but a doorway in the lower levels offers an interesting swim-through opportunity between the two cargo holds. Another swim-through from the funnel down to an exit hole on the starboard side at the funnel's base will be of interest to

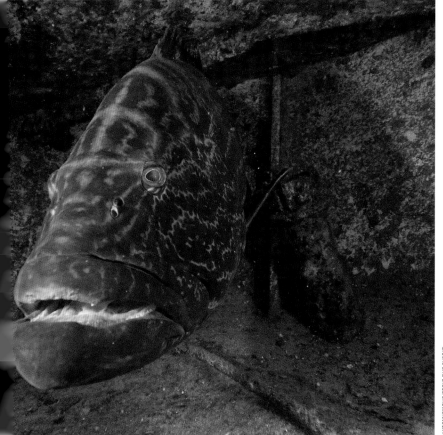

Black grouper and other large pelagic fish species are common on the *Adolphus Busch Sr.*

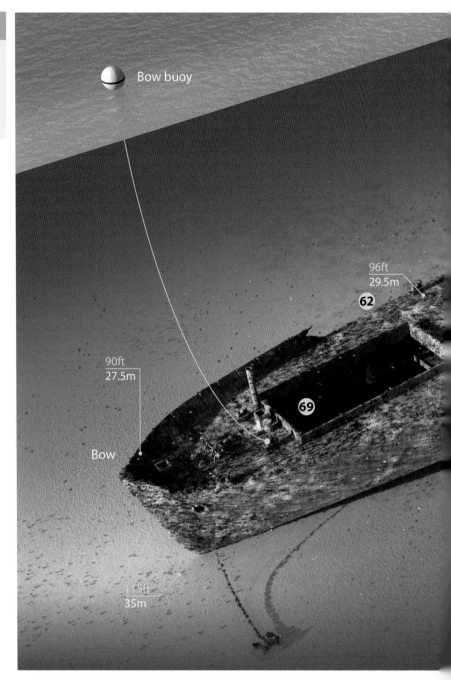

Bow buoy

96ft
29.5m

62

90ft
27.5m

69

Bow

115ft
35m

divers with experience in confined spaces. The front of the wheelhouse was completely removed, offering easy access to all divers, while other strategic holes allow divers limited and full penetration opportunities, depending on their level of experience.

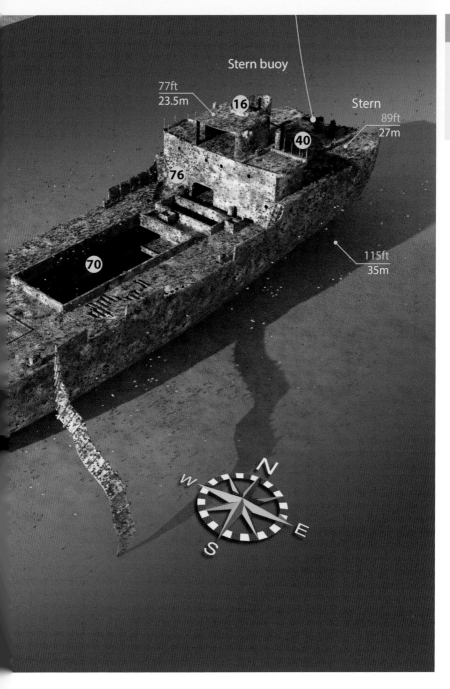

Stern buoy

77ft
23.5m

16

40

76

70

Stern

89ft
27m

115ft
35m

N
W
E
S

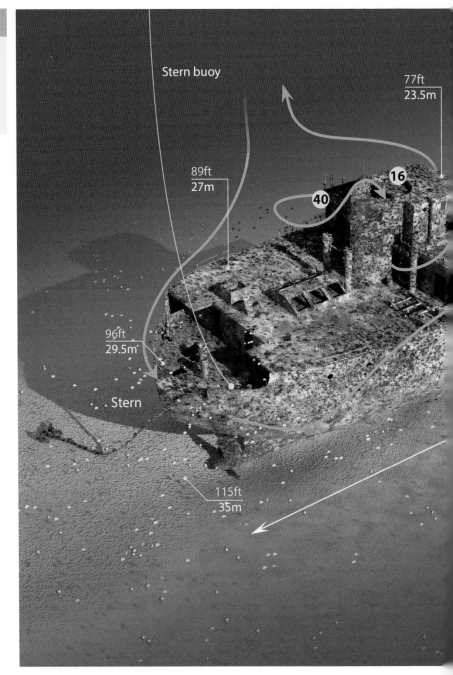

Stern buoy

77ft
23.5m

89ft
27m

16

40

96ft
29.5m

Stern

115ft
35m

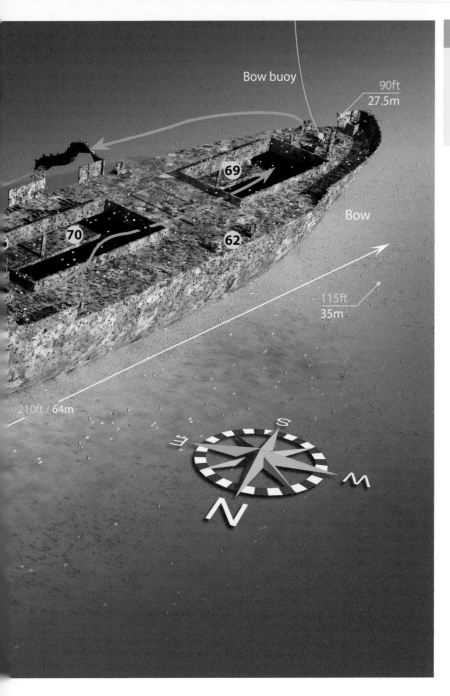

Bow buoy

90ft
27.5m

69

70

62

Bow

115ft
35m

210ft / 64m

ame:	*MV Adolphus Busch Sr*	**Tonnage:**	706grt
ype:	Freighter	**Construction:**	Burntisland Shipbuilding Co,
revious names:	*London, Windsor Trader,*		Scotland
	Topsail Star, Sophie Express,		Looe Key Artificial
	Princess Tarrah, Ocean Alley	**Last owner:**	Reef Association
ength:	210ft (64m)	**Sunk:**	Dec. 5, 1998

AMERICAN SHOAL

Difficulty ● ○ ○
Current ● ○ ○
Depth ● ○ ○
Reef ★★☆   Access 🚤
Fauna ★★☆   20mi (32km) from Key West

Level Open water

Location Sugarloaf Key
GPS   24° 31.373′N, 81° 31.079′W

Getting there

American Shoal is located 6.2 miles (10 kilometers) south of Sugarloaf Key, along the outer reef line. Getting there involves an hour-long boat ride from Key West, but few Key West operators visit this site. Operators based in Summerland and Cudjoe Keys may make special trips, however. A 110-foot (33.5-meter) lighthouse makes this site easy to find.

Access

The site is suitable for divers and snorkelers of all levels. There are no mooring buoys at this site, so boats must anchor in the sand well clear of the reef to avoid damaging the fragile corals.

Description

This site features a short ledge that tops out at a depth of 16 feet (5 meters) and runs nearly the full length of the shoal. The ledge is only broken in a few places, including a large v-shaped sand patch marked by the GPS coordinates provided. A handful of shallow coral spurs extend from the ledge toward the lighthouse, while the hard bottom reef slope descends gradually seaward to a depth of more than 80 feet (24.5 meters). This site plays host to a variety of reef creatures, including damselfishes, angelfishes and butterflyfishes. Loose schools of ocean surgeonfish and blue tangs forage on turf algae while French and bluestriped grunts are a common sight among the spurs and grooves. Visitors are likely to see nurse sharks along the base of the ledge, while green moray eels often stick their heads out of nooks and crannies in the reef.

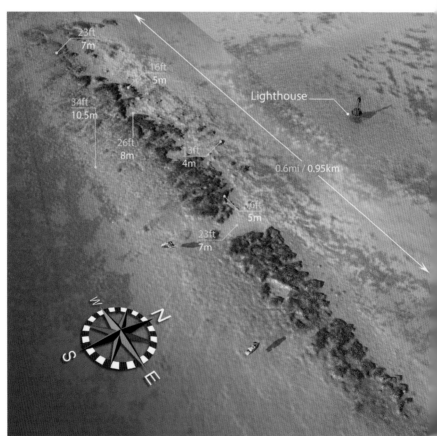

MARYLAND SHOAL

Difficulty ● ○ ○
Current ● ○ ○
Depth ● ○ ○
Reef ★★★☆
Fauna ★★★☆

Access 🚤
16.5mi (26.5km) from Key West

Level Open Water

Location Saddlebunch Keys
GPS 24° 30.680′N, 81° 33.968′W

Getting there
Maryland Shoal is located 5.5 miles (9 kilometers) south of Saddlebunch Keys, along the outer reef line. Getting there involves a boat ride of 50 to 60 minutes from Key West, but few Key West operators visit this site. Operators based out of Sugarloaf and Big Pine Keys may be more likely to schedule trips here.

Access
The site is suitable for divers and snorkelers of all levels. There are no mooring buoys at this site, so boats must anchor in the sand well clear of the reef to avoid damaging the fragile corals.

Description
Maryland Shoal was formed by the same processes as nearby Pelican and American Shoals. The reef here features a shallow ledge much like American Shoal but far more broken up than its neighbor to the east. Poorly defined coral spurs extend seaward from the ledge, breaking up the otherwise hard bottomed slope that descends to a depth of more than 60 feet (20 meters). The slope and ledge support plenty of soft corals and sea fans, while large barrel sponges pepper the deeper slope. The lack of frequent visits by dive operators means the reef receives fewer visitors than the more popular Looe Key Reef to the east and the Sambo Reefs to the west. There are plenty of reef fish to see, including highhats, hogfish, rainbow parrotfish and foureye butterflyfish. The usual complement of grunts and snapper can be found here, along with French and gray angelfish.

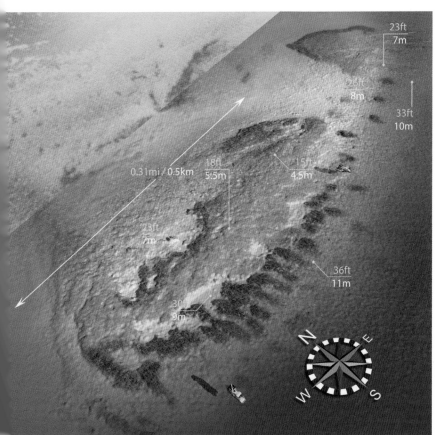

23ft / 7m
25ft / 8m
33ft / 10m
18ft / 5.5m
15ft / 4.5m
0.31mi / 0.5km
23ft / 7m
36ft / 11m
30ft / 9m

WILKES-BARRE

Difficulty ● ● ●
Current ● ● ●
Depth ● ● ●
Reef ★★☆
Fauna ★★☆

Access 🚤 17mi (27.5km) from Key West

Level Technical

Location Saddlebunch Keys
GPS   (Bow) 24° 29.094'N, 81° 33.202'W
          (Stern) 24° 29.069'N, 81° 33.138'W

Getting there

The wreck of the *Wilkes-Barre* is located 8 miles (13 kilometers) south of Saddlebunch Keys. Getting there involves an hour-long boat ride from Key West, but few Key West operators visit this site except for specially scheduled trips or charters.

Access

The site is only accessible by boat and only suitable for technical divers as it sits at a depth of 250 feet (76 meters). There are no mooring buoys on this site. The current can be strong this far off the reef line.

Description

The 610-foot (186-meter) Cleveland Class Light Cruiser was built in Camden, New Jersey, in the final year of World War II. She saw action in Iwo Jima and Okinawa, earning herself the nickname of Willie Bee. She received four battle stars before she was decommissioned in October 1947. A total of 52 ships of this class were ordered, but just 29 were completed as cruisers with another nine converted to light aircraft carriers. The rest were canceled due to the war ending. Each of the completed vessels were named after a city in the United States – Wilkes-Barre is named after the city in Pennsylvania.

In 1972, the vessel was brought out from retirement so that she could be used as a target for undersea explosives testing. On May 12, 1972, these explosions tore the ship in two; the stern section sank almost immediately, while the bow section remained afloat. The latter section was scuttled the following day with the help of additional explosives. Today, the stern sits upright on a sandy seabed oriented along an east-west axis. The stern's superstructure rises to a depth of 145 feet (44 meters) placing it at depths suitable only for technical diving.

The bow section settled on its starboard side

over 400 feet (120 meters) southeast of the stern. The fact that the bow section lies on its side means it only rises to a depth of 200 feet (61 meters). The difference in orientation and depth means that most divers typically focus their exploration on the stern section.

Penetration is possible in both the stern and the bow sections. Much of the equipment including phones, monitors and radar equipment are still in place, along with gun emplacements and gun turrets and anti-aircraft gun stations. The explosion caused significant damage to the wreck sections, however, and caution is warranted when approaching, and especially when entering, the wreck. Some divers refer to this wreck by another nickname: Lethal Lady.

The ship was not properly prepared for

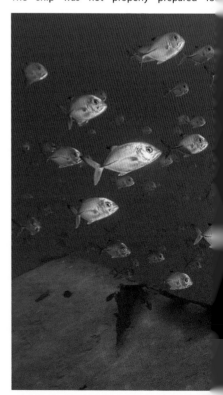

DID YOU KNOW? ❓

Wilkes-Barre was just one of four vessels sunk off the cost of the Florida Keys during underwater explosives tests in the late 1960s and early 70s. The U.S. Navy hypothesized that a small charge could sink a massive ship if it was placed in the right spot along the keel, but it needed to both test the process

and collect data on the results to make future warships less susceptible to this kind of attack. The *USS Fred T Berry, USS Kendrick* and *USS Saufley* were all subjected to the same tests, with largely the same result. The three other wrecks now sit at depths greater than 300 feet (91 meters) but within the same general vicinity of *Wilkes-Barre.*

deployment as an artificial reef prior to the explosives test, which is why there are so many pipes, cables and other clutter on the wreck. Research into the importance of properly cleaning and stripping vessels before their sinking had not yet been conducted in the 1970s, when converting wartime ships into artificial reefs was still a relatively new concept. Despite being the result of military testing first, and artificial reef second, the two sections of

wreck have created incredible reef habitat for a variety of large fish species.

Divers will be rewarded with a chance to see anything from sharks to massive snapper, grouper and barracuda. Mahi mahi are also plentiful along with amberjacks, cero and horse-eye jacks. Divers have even reportedly seen manta rays and even a sperm whale at the site.

Name:	USS Wilkes-Barre		Camden, NJ, 1942
Type:	Light cruiser	**Last owner:**	U.S. Navy
Previous names:	n/a	**Sunk:**	May 12 and 13, 1972
Length:	610ft (186m)		
Tonnage:	11,800grt		
Construction:	New York Shipbuilding Corp,		

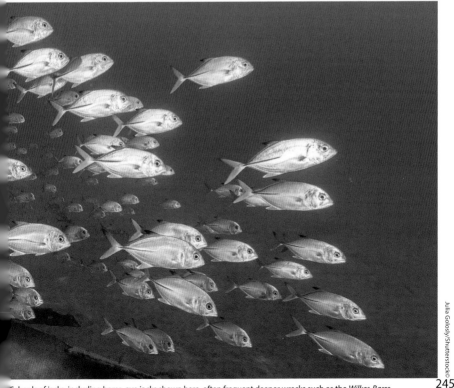

Julia Golosiy/Shutterstock©

Schools of jacks, including horse-eye jacks shown here, often frequent deeper wrecks such as the *Wilkes-Barre.*

PELICAN SHOAL

Difficulty ● ○ ○
Current ● ○ ○
Depth ● ● ○
Reef ★★☆ Access
Fauna ★★☆ 12.5mi (20km) from Key West

Level Open water

Location Boca Chica Key
GPS   PS1 24° 30.043'N, 81° 37.704'W
        PS2 24° 30.008'N, 81° 37.763'W
        PS3 24° 29.987'N, 81° 37.884'W
        PS4 24° 30.085'N, 81° 37.954'W

Getting there
Pelican Shoal is located 5.2 miles (8.5 kilometers) south of the Key West Naval Air Station. Getting there involves a boat ride of 35 to 40 minutes from Key West, but few Key West operators visit sites this far east of Key West.

Access
The site is suitable for divers and snorkelers of all levels. There are four mooring buoys at this site. The area is part of the Pelican Shoal Wildlife Management Area and includes a 165-feet (50-meter) no access buffer from the island between April 1 and August 31 by order of the Florida Fish and Wildlife Commission.

Description
Pelican Shoal originally received protection as an important nesting site for birds. It consisted of an island and surrounding reef, but recent hurricanes washed away much of the sand, leaving only a long, thin strip of dry sand and rubble. The strip remains closed year-round, while access to the waters immediately surrounding the dry land is restricted between the start of April and the end of August. That period marks a peak in the nesting activity of the roseate tern, and the site has historically hosted the only ground-nesting colony of roseate terns in Florida.

Divers and snorkelers can explore the shoal's ledge that runs parallel to shore throughout the year. However, the northern end of the shallow coral spurs found next to the ledge are close to the outer edge of the buffer so visitors should be careful to maintain their distance during the late spring and summer months. There are plenty of reef fishes at this site, including ocean surgeonfish, blue tangs and stoplight parrotfish. French and bluestriped grunts are also common here, as are Spanish hogfish and yellowhead wrasses. Barracuda regularly hang out in the water column, while nurse sharks are frequently seen resting at the bottom of the ledge.

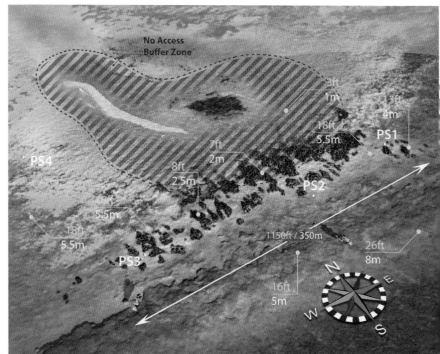

SPECULATOR SHOAL

Difficulty ● ○ ○
Current ● ○ ○
Depth ● ○ ○
Reef ★★☆   Access 🚤
Fauna ★★☆   10mi (16km) from Key West

Level Open Water

Location Boca Chica Key
GPS   24° 29.730'N, 81° 38.887'W

Getting there
Speculator Shoal is located 5 miles (8 kilometers) south of the Key West Naval Air Station. Getting there involves a boat ride of 35 minutes from Key West, but few Key West operators venture farther east than Western Sambo, except by special request.

Access
The site is suitable for divers and snorkelers of all levels. There are no mooring buoys here, and boats will need to anchor in the sand well clear of the fragile reef. The GPS coordinates provided mark a large patch of sand in the middle of the ledge, just south of the coral spurs, which should provide access to most of the site with limited risk of causing damage with an anchor.

Description
Speculator Shoal is similar in form to many of the shoals along this stretch of the Lower Keys. There is a 3- to 6.5-foot (1- to 2-meter) ledge that runs parallel to shore and zig zags back and forth. The ledge sits adjacent to a series of poorly defined spurs and grooves. The reef here provides habitat for a variety of marine reef life. Nearly the full complement of Caribbean parrotfish is on display here, including stoplight, redband, rainbow, midnight and Queen parrotfish. Snapper are well represented as well, with yellowtail, schoolmaster, gray and mahogany snapper regularly spotted on the ledge and along the coral spurs. Spotted goatfish and yellowhead jawfish are found along the rubble and sand-bottomed grooves. As with nearby Pelican Shoal, nurse sharks are often seen here along with the occasional stingray.

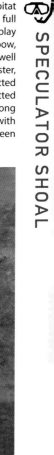

EASTERN SAMBO & MIDDLE SAMBO REEFS

Difficulty	● ○ ○	
Current	● ○ ○	
Depth	● ○ ○	
Reef	★★★	Access 🚤
Fauna	★★☆	12mi (19km) from Key West

Level Open Water

Location Boca Chica Key
GPS   (Eastern) 24° 29.524'N, 81° 39.718'W
           (Middle) 24° 29.323'N, 81° 40.385'W

Getting there

Middle Sambo and Eastern Sambo are two of three sets of reefs that bear the name Sambo. They lie just 4.6 miles (7.5 kilometers) due south of the Key West Naval Air Station. Getting there involves a boat ride of 35 minutes from Key West, but few Key West operators venture past the more popular Western Sambo Reef, except by special request.

Access

Middle Sambo is suitable for divers and snorkelers of all levels while access to Eastern Sambo is restricted by permit and only accessible for research purposes. There are no mooring buoys at either reef site, so boats visiting Middle Sambo will need to anchor in the sand well clear of the fragile reef. The GPS coordinates provided mark a patch of sand just south of the well-defined spur and groove formations that dominate Middle Sambo.

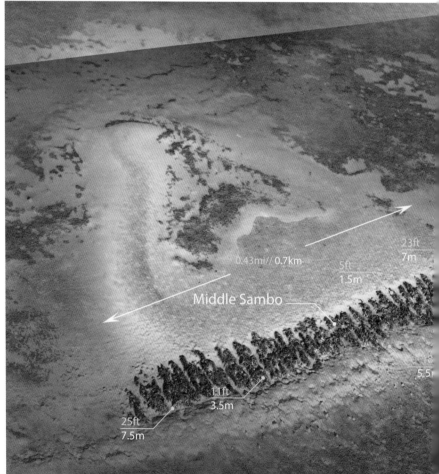

0.43mi// **0.7km**

5ft
1.5m

23ft
7m

Middle Sambo

18
5.5

11ft
3.5m

25ft
7.5m

Description

Middle and Eastern Sambo reefs are classic examples of the spur and groove reefs that dominate this stretch of the Florida Keys coastline. The two reefs sit slightly apart from their larger and more popular neighbor to the west, Western Sambo, each separated from the other by a stretch of sand. The no-access boundary around Eastern Sambo is clearly marked with four yellow buoys labeled "Research Only." The reef here is one of several locations in the Keys that are set aside for research and monitoring. Scientists use these sites to better gauge the effect of environmental influences on corals compared to the effect of human activities, such as diving, snorkeling and fishing. Please respect these boundaries.

Although Middle Sambo has no mooring buoys, it is well worth the visit. The well-defined spurs support healthy corals including both hard and soft species. The spurs are shallow, topping out at between 5 and 12 feet (1.5 to 3.5 meters) while the grooves bottom out at 23 feet (7 meters) in many places. In all, the spurs stretch across an area over 0.4 miles (700 meters) wide, offering plenty for divers and snorkelers to explore during multiple trips. A short ledge sits just seaward of the spurs, which leads in to a hard-bottomed slope that descends to a depth of more than 65 feet (20 meters).

The reef habitat here supports a variety of marine life, including dense congregations of bluehead wrasses, yellowhead wrasses, bicolor damselfish and blue tangs. Stoplight, redband, striped and Queen parrotfish are also seen here at relatively high densities. Larger species are also present, with regular sightings of barracuda, black grouper and nurse sharks. Goliath grouper and spotted eagle rays occasionally visit the deeper waters off the reef slope.

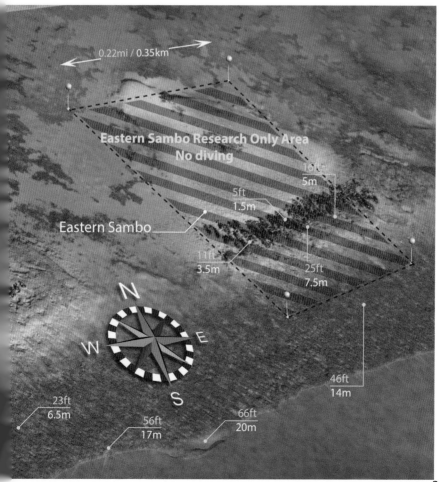

WESTERN SAMBO

Difficulty ● ○ ○
Current ● ○ ○
Depth ● ○ ○
Reef ★★★
Fauna ★★☆

Access 🚤 8mi (13km) from Key West

Level Open Water

Location Boca Chica Key

GPS	
WS0	24° 29.007'N, 81° 42.225'W
WS1	24° 28.965'N, 81° 42.206'W
WS2	24° 28.929'N, 81° 42.230'W
WS3	24° 28.925'N, 81° 42.303'W
WS4	24° 28.902'N, 81° 42.345'W
WS5	24° 28.934'N, 81° 42.440'W
WS6	24° 28.954'N, 81° 42.455'W
WS7	24° 28.840'N, 81° 42.630'W
WS8	24° 28.830'N, 81° 42.715'W
WS9	24° 28.814'N, 81° 42.797'W
WS10	24° 28.782'N, 81° 42.873'W
WS11	24° 28.761'N, 81° 42.973'W
WS12	24° 28.749'N, 81° 43.006'W
WS13	24° 28.758'N, 81° 43.043'W
WS14	24° 28.821'N, 81° 43.149'W
WS15	24° 28.753'N, 81° 43.078'W
WS16	24° 28.833'N, 81° 43.134'W
WS17	24° 28.858'N, 81° 43.146'W
WS18	24° 28.873'N, 81° 43.134'W
WS20	24° 29.010'N, 81° 42.915'W
WS21	24° 29.014'N, 81° 42.851'W
WS22	24° 29.050'N, 81° 42.741'W

Getting there

Western Sambo is a bank reef located just 5 miles (8 kilometers) due south of the Key West Naval Air Station. Getting there involves a boat ride of 30 minutes from Key West.

Access

Western Sambo is suitable for divers and snorkelers of all levels. There are a total of 22 mooring buoys spread across two sections of adjacent reef that are separated by a narrow stretch of sand. Most of the buoys are anchored along the well-defined spur and groove sections of reef, although some are anchored along the sides of the reef and across the landward side.

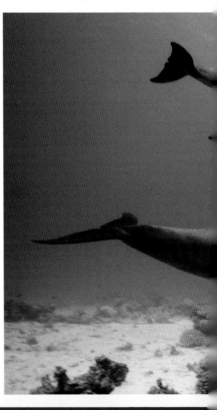

DID YOU KNOW?

In deeper waters off the reef slope between Western Sambo and Middle Sambo lie the remains of the *Aquanaut*. This 55-foot (16.5 meter) wooden tugboat sits at a depth of 75 feet (23 meters) and was originally owned by Chet Alexander, the marine salvager responsible for sinking the *USS Amesbury* west of Key West and renamed the *Alexander* wreck. As the story holds, *Aquanaut* sank but was refloated. Alexander decided it would cost too much to repair and refurbish her, so he towed the vessel into deeper water and sank her as an artificial reef. Unfortunately, her wooden hull soon broke apart and little is left today apart from some debris that has now been incorporated into the surrounding reef.

RELAX & RECHARGE

Matt's Stock Island Kitchen & Bar (7001 Shrimp Rd Suite 200, Key West) located in Perry Hotel Key West on Stock Island, serves "American coastal comfort food" using simple ingredients and innovative twists. Dine inside or outside on the patio while overlooking the marina – you can't go wrong with either choice. Matt's won the OpenTable Diner's Choice Award for ambiance in 2018. The only thing that might overshadow the atmosphere here is the quality of the food. From the tuna tacos and crab beignet appetizers to the grouper gnudi and swordfish skewers, there is plenty to choose from on the menu. And don't forget the incredible sides, featuring crispy smash potato. Since Key West is the capital city of Key limes, Matt's offers a unique twist on key lime pie with their deconstructed version, along with Key lime martinis. There's also a gooey and deliciousness skillet brownie. Matt's serves breakfast and dinner daily, with happy hour from 5pm to 7pm.
Visit: **Perrykeywest.com/stock-island-restaurants/matts-stock-island-kitchen-and-bar**

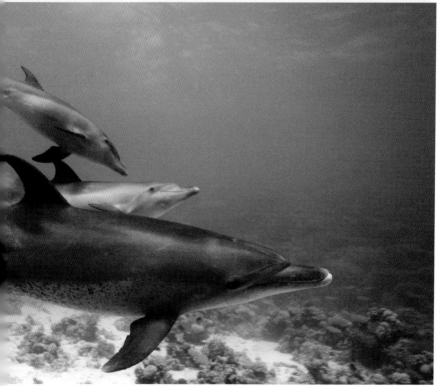

Dolphins often visit the reefs along the Keys, including Western Sambo, to hunt and play.

Dray van Beeck/Shutterstock©

Most local area operators visit Western Sambo as part of their regular scheduled trips.

Description

Western Sambo is one of the premier reef dives the Key West area. It is contained within the boundaries of the Western Sambo Ecological Reserve, which extends from the shore of Boca Chica Key out to beyond the reef line of Western Sambo reef. Large yellow buoys mark the boundary line of the management area, including three that run along the southern edge of the reef. The management area contains the greatest habitat diversity in the entire Lower Keys.

The spur and groove formations support healthy coral populations including stands of elkhorn coral. Boulder and scroll corals (sometimes referred to as sheet corals) are also found here, as are anemones, sea fans and a variety of sponges. The complex habitat supports a variety of fish species and crustaceans, including lobsters

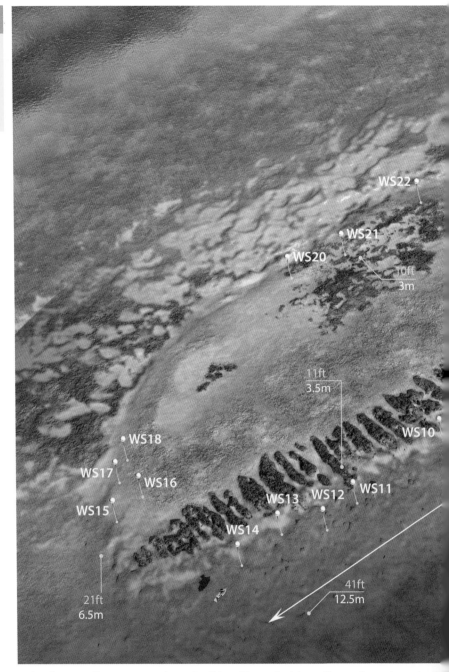

and crabs, as well as sea cucumbers, star fish and sea urchins. Visitors to the site commonly encounter foureye butterflyfish, rock beauties and gray angelfish, while French and Queen are present at lower densities. The reef supports the full complement of parrotfish as well, including stoplight, redband, Queen, striped, princess, blue and rainbow. Barracuda regular cruise th shallow water above the reef, while Caribbea reef sharks are commonly spotted in the deep grooves and along the reef slope. Nurse shar are also seen resting along the rubble botto grooves while pods of Atlantic bottlenos dolphins may come in to explore and hunt alor

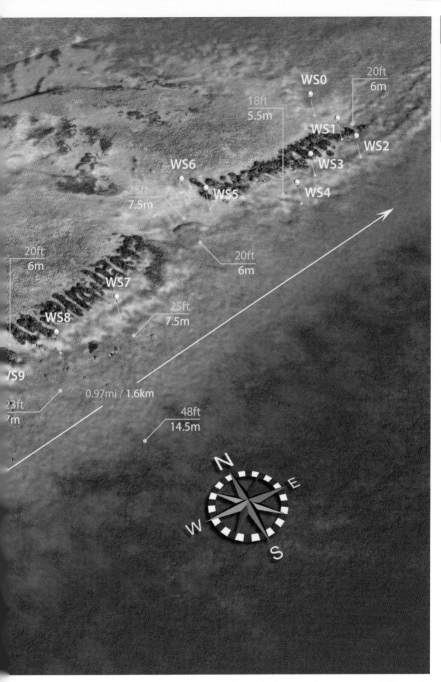

WS0

20ft
6m

18ft
5.5m

WS1

WS2

WS6

WS3

WS4

25ft
7.5m

WS5

20ft
6m

20ft
6m

WS7

25ft
7.5m

WS8

/S9

0.97mi / 1.6km

23ft
7m

48ft
14.5m

e deeper reef slope.

ach like the reefs off Key Largo, Western Sambo s many named sites that are often associated th individual regions of the reef. For instance, e popular Cannonball Cut is located at the far stern end of Western Sambo, whereas Haystacks is located closer to the eastern end. Haystacks gets its name from the large coral mounds that rise-up from the reef slope just south of the spurs and grooves. The coral mounds can reach as high as 15 to 20 feet (4.5 to 6 meters) off the seafloor, crowned with sea fans and a variety of hard coral heads, typically star coral.

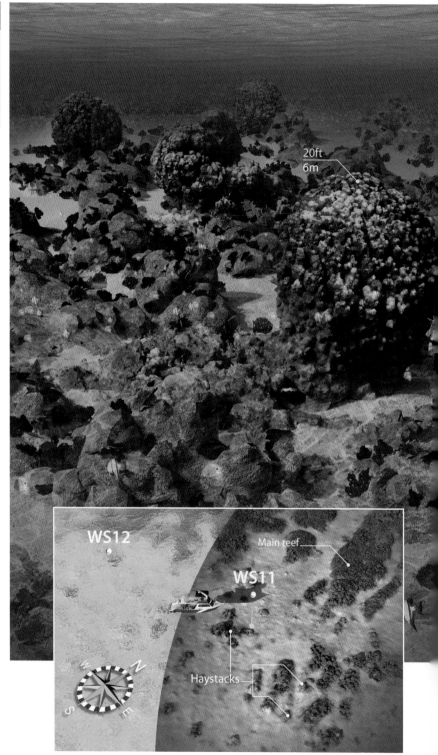

20ft
6m

WS12

Main reef

WS11

Haystacks

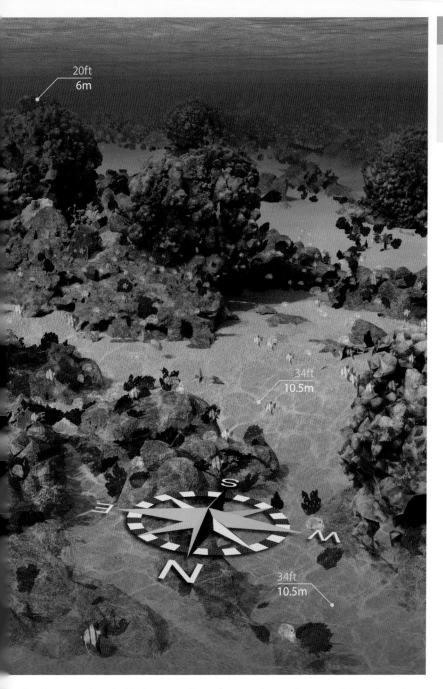

20ft
6m

34ft
10.5m

34ft
10.5m

ere is a large area dotted with these towering al haystacks. It is primarily associated with oys WS11, WS12 and WS13. To find them, head th from the main section of spur and groove nations that constitute the main reef. The area lotted with low-profile, broken up spurs and ble grooves, with individual coral towers and large coral mounds scattered throughout. It can be easy to get disoriented exploring the haystacks, so divers should be sure to get their bearings when they enter the water so they can return to their mooring buoy.

10 FATHOM LEDGE

Difficulty	● ● ○
Current	● ● ○
Depth	● ● ○
Reef	★★☆
Fauna	★★☆

Access
7.5mi (12km) from Key West

Level Open Water

Location Key West
GPS   24° 28.152'N, 81° 43.579'W

Getting there

10 Fathom Ledge is a barrier reef located just south of the southwest corner of the Western Sambo boundary line. Getting there involves a boat ride of 30 minutes from Key West.

Access

10 Fathom Ledge is suitable to divers of all levels but the reef slope descends to depths that are more suitable for advanced divers. There are no mooring buoys at this site, so visitors must anchor in the sand, taking care not to damage the fragile coral reef. The GPS coordinate provided mark a sand patch adjacent to the shallower spur and groove section of the reef. Currents can be strong at this site given the proximity of the Gulf Stream, so divers should plan their dives accordingly, and may want to consider exploring the site as a drift dive.

Description

10 Fathom Ledge represents a series of coral spurs and associated grooves found at a depth of between 40 and 50 feet (12 and 15 meters). From this shallower plateau, a reef slope descends to sand at a depth of 115 feet (35 meters). The reef

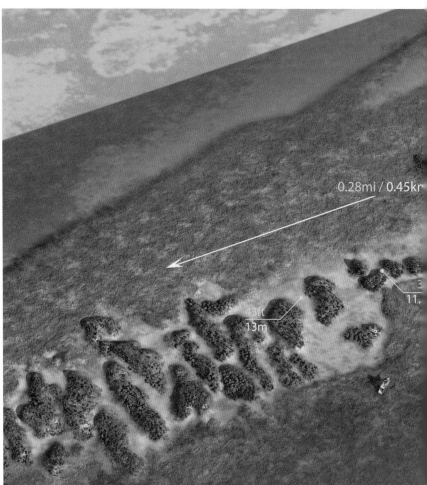

DID YOU KNOW? ❓

The *All-Alone* tugboat rests at a depth of 90 feet (27.5 meters) on 10 Fathom Ledge. Very little is known about the history of this 75-foot (23-meter) wreck, and after the hull split years ago, most of the wreckage has dispersed or been incorporated into the reef. Very little remains of the original wreck, although the surrounding reef is healthy and supports plenty of marine life, including hard and soft corals and a variety of parrotfishes, grunts, snapper and damselfishes, among others.

sits offshore of the main reef line, which is what allows the slope to reach depths not typically found on the other reefs in the area. The site gets its name from this reef slope and its starting depth of 60 feet (18 meters).

The complex habitat of the seabed here includes ledges, overhangs and even some caverns and swim-throughs. Lobsters and grouper like to hide out in the caves and under ledges, while French angelfish, foureye butterflyfish, butter hamlets and Queen angelfish patrol the reef. Barracuda are commonly seen in the water column above the reef, while hogfish root around in the sand rubble grooves. The deeper sections of the site pull in some larger pelagics, including reef sharks from time to time.

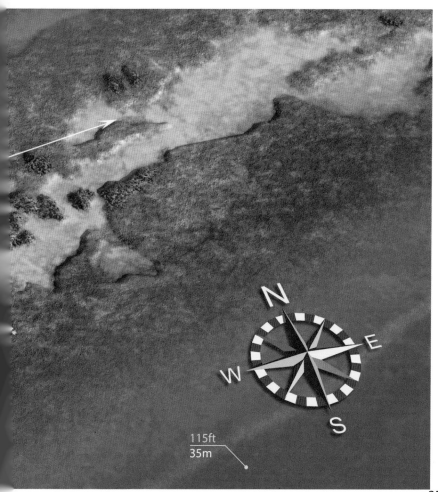

115ft
35m

GENERAL HOYT S. VANDENBERG

Difficulty ● ● ●
Current ● ● ○
Depth ● ● ●
Reef ★★☆
Fauna ★★☆

Access 🚤 9mi (14.5km) from Key West

Level Advanced

Location Key West
GPS   24° 27.027'N, 81° 43.992'W

Getting there

Vandenberg is located 7.5 miles (12 kilometers) southwest of Key West. It is the most popular dive site in the region and is visited by most local operators. Getting there involves a boat ride of about 20 to 25 minutes.

Access

The wreck is only suitable for advanced divers due to her depth. The seabed sits at a depth of 148 feet (45 meters) while the main deck level is at 104 feet (31.5 meters). There are five mooring buoys attached to the wreck that provide easy access to the artificial reef. There is one at the bow, one at the bridge, one each on the two towers placed midships, and one at the stern. The currents on the wreck can be strong since the artificial reef sits in the path of the Gulf Stream, so most divers access the ship by descending and ascending the mooring lines.

Description

USS General Hoyt S. Vandenberg (or simply *Vandenberg* for short) was originally a transport ship, built in 1943. She was commissioned by the U.S. Navy in 1944 as a U.S. General G.O. Squire Class transport ship under the name *USS General Taylor*. She saw service during World War II, carrying passengers in both the Pacific Theater and in European and Middle Eastern operations. She was decommissioned in 1946 and transferred to the U.S. Army Transport Service, before being reacquired by the Navy in 1950. Over the next five years, she served in the Occupation Service in Europe. Her final operation ended in April 1955, and she was subsequently removed from service in 1957 before being transferred to the Maritime Commission and placed in the reserve fleet in 1958.

The U.S. Air Force acquired her in 1961 and she underwent a conversion to a missile range instrumentation ship. Two massive radar dishes were added to her main deck during this conversion. Her new fit allowed her to support NASA in tracking the space program's launches from Cape Canaveral, Florida. She was once

again reacquired by the Navy in 1964 and placed in the service of the Military Sealift Command. She continued her work monitoring American defense missile test launches in the Pacific, as well as spying on Russia and its Cold War missile tests. Her secret mission monitoring Soviet launches was leaked in a May 1969 edition of the Space Coast weekly newspaper.

She spent some time in the Pacific during the early 1970s before returning to the Atlantic Ocean in 1976, once again operating out o

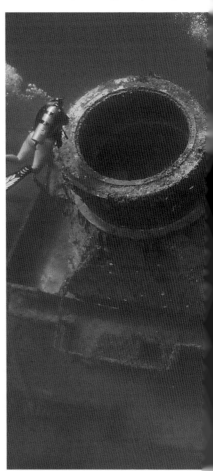

RELAX & RECHARGE

Kermit's Kitchen (200 Elizabeth Street, Key West) is perfectly located adjacent to the Key West Bight which serves as the departure spot for many of the local dive boats. It is a popular place to pick up a delicious breakfast sandwich or burrito before heading out for a day on the water. Kermit's also has lunch and light dinner options for later in the day. There are burgers, hotdogs, salads and a slew of wraps and sandwiches to choose from.

House specials include Kermit's BBQ ribs, wings, buffalo shrimp and spicy grouper. If you have the time, their shaded patio with its tropical plants and tranquil koi pond is a great place to eat, relax and unwind. Kermit's is also home to the Key West Lime Shoppe, which has been serving killer key lime pies for over a quarter of a century at the same spot. Their gift store is packed full of treats from sauces and salsas, to jellies and candies. They also have a range of soaps, shampoos and lotions. Visit: **Keylimeshop.com.**

Port Canaveral, Florida. She continued her space-tracking duties for NASA launches until 1983 when she was moved to the James River in Virginia for storage. She was eventually struck from the naval register in April 1993. In 1996, she was used in the shooting of the 1999 sci-fi

horror movie, Virus, where *Vandenberg* stood in as a Russian science ship, the *Akademik Vladislav Volkovs*. Some of the Cyrillic letters painted on interior walls for the movie are still visible.

In 1996, *Vandenberg* was picked from a list of

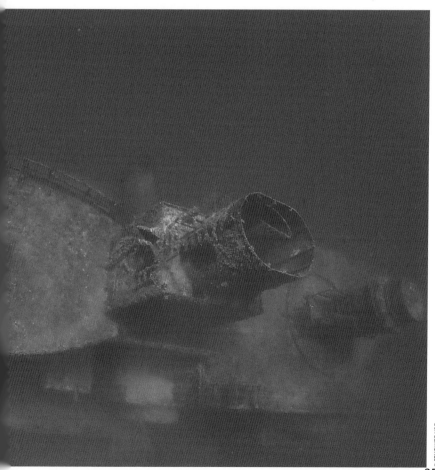

Ben Edmonds ©

GENERAL HOYT S. VANDENBERG

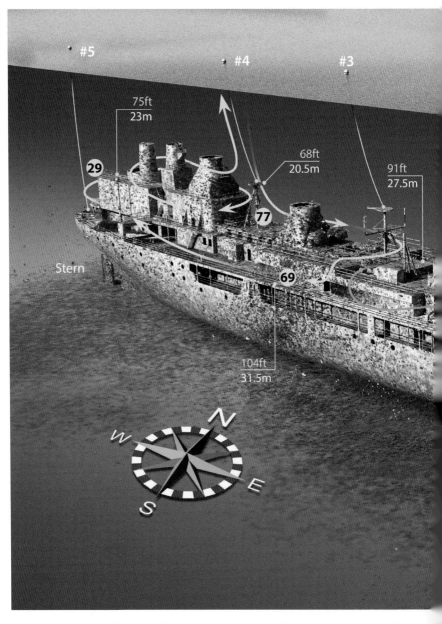

#5

#4

#3

75ft
23m

68ft
20.5m

91ft
27.5m

29

77

Stern

69

104ft
31.5m

400 ex-military vessels for potential deployment as an artificial reef. Her title transferred to the State of Florida in 2007 and she was towed to the Colonna Shipyard in Norfolk, Virginia, for stripping and cleaning in preparation for reefing. However, the contractor failed to make full payments and a federal court intervened, forcing her into an auction to pay off the lien. In December 2008, Key West's First State Bank of the Florida Keys made the winning bid, and they subsequently transferred the rights to the City of Key West. After final preparation for reefing, she

was towed down to the Keys in April 2009 a tied up to the East Quay Pier in Key West Harb On May 27, 2009, she was towed beyond t outer reef line and sunk. Accounts from the d of the deployment report that it took just un two minutes to send the massive ship to her fi resting place. The demolition crew lined the bi area with explosives that cracked open the sh hull below the waterline. She settled with lit fuss onto a sandy seabed at a depth of 148 f (45 meters) and continues to remain upright.

GENERAL HOYT S. VANDENBERG

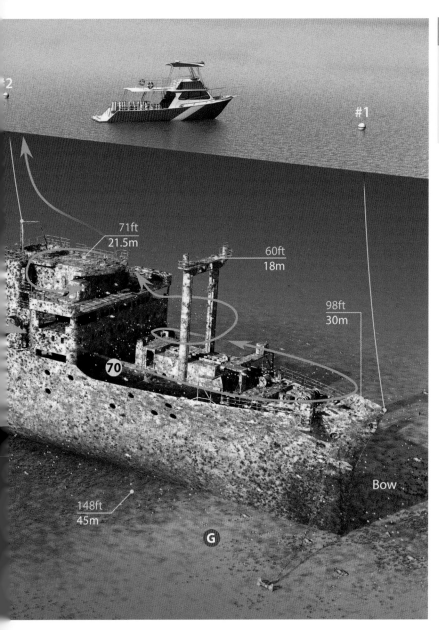

71ft
21.5m

60ft
18m

98ft
30m

70

#1

148ft
45m

G

Bow

...*ndenberg* is the second largest artificial reef ...Florida waters behind the mighty *Oriskany*, ...ated near Pensacola. The wreck has proven ...redibly resilient over the years, with the most ...ticeable change being the collapse of the ...ssive radar dishes on her main deck, which ...curred during Hurricane Irma in 2017 after ...eral years of gradual decline. The powerful ...rm also rotated the massive ship and scoured ...d out from under her hull to where divers can ...w see evidence of the fractures that occurred ...m the scuttling charges near the bow.

As she weathers gracefully, *Vandenberg* continues to be an incredible resource for both the diving and fishing communities of the Lower Keys. As an artificial reef, she supports a wide variety of reef and pelagic fish species, from large bull sharks and goliath grouper to tiny sharpnose puffers and bluehead wrasses. Barracuda are a constant sight on this artificial reef, hanging out in the current and observing divers as they explore the wreck. Yellowtail and gray snapper are plentiful on the wreck, as are schools of bar jacks, horse-eye jacks and greater amberjacks.

261

GENERAL HOYT S. VANDENBERG

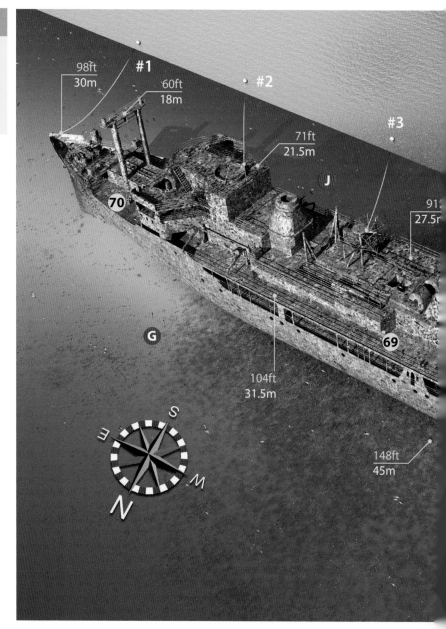

98ft
30m

#1

60ft
18m

#2

#3

71ft
21.5m

J

70

91
27.5m

G

104ft
31.5m

69

148ft
45m

Route

Given the wreck's depth and size, recreational divers will not be able to fully explore the site on a single tank. Most operators opt for back-to-back dives on the wreck so that divers can take the time necessary to fully appreciate this incredible artificial reef. Prevailing currents and the availability of mooring buoys will determine how divers plan their dive, whether starting at the stern or the bow. The main deck and side passageways offer ample opportunity for exploration, including the two massive radar dishes. There are numero limited and full penetration opportunities divers with the right experience. And with ne 50 feet (15 meters) of relief from the main dec the tallest point on the wreck, there is plenty structure for divers to explore even as they exte their bottom time by finishing at shallower dept Divers should pay close attention to the b that their boat is tied to, as it is easy to beco disoriented when exploring the wreck and asce the wrong line.

GENERAL HOYT S. VANDENBERG

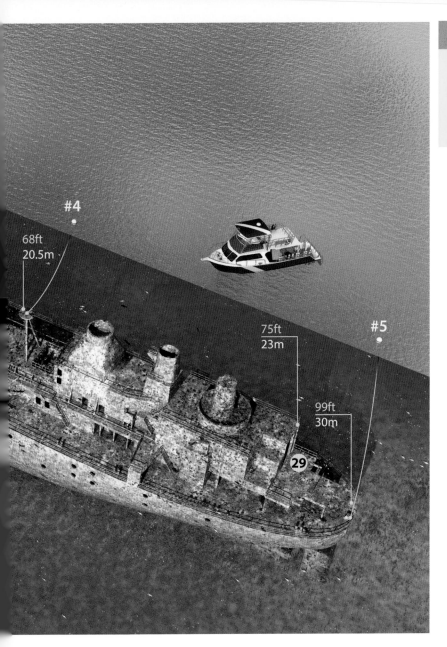

#4

68ft
20.5m

75ft
23m

#5

99ft
30m

29

me:	USAFS General H.S. Vandenberg	Tonnage:	14,300grt
pe:	Missile Range Instrumentation Ship	**Construction:**	Kaiser Co, Richmond, CA, 1943
		Last owner:	First State Bank of the Florida Keys
vious names:	General Taylor		
ngth:	522ft (159m)	**Sunk:**	May 27, 2009

JOE'S TUG

Difficulty ● ○ ○
Current ● ○ ○
Depth ● ● ○
Reef ★☆☆
Fauna ★★☆

Access 🛥
8mi (13km) from Key West

Level Open Water

Location Key West
GPS 24° 27.843'N, 81° 44.262'W

Getting there

Joe's Tug sits just outside the outer reef line, around 6 miles (10 kilometers) south of Key West. Getting there involves a boat ride of about 25 to 30 minutes from Key West.

Access

Joe's Tug is suitable for divers of all levels and is particularly popular with novice divers given its open nature and shallower depths relative to other wrecks in the Key West area -- it sits in just 65 feet (20 meters) of water. There are no mooring buoys at this site so boats need to anchor in the sand nearby or tie into the wreck

Description

Joe's Tug (also known locally as *Joe's Wreck* is not, in fact, a tug. The 75-foot (23-meter steel-hulled vessel was a shrimper back in the day, and she has quite the backstory. As loca lore holds, the boat originally sank next to the pier in Stock Island's Safe Harbor. Althoug the owner successfully refloated her, she wa deemed too expensive to refurbish, so she wa earmarked for reefing off the coast of Miam Her hull was reinforced with metal braces, an she was cleaned and prepped for reefing in lat January 1989.

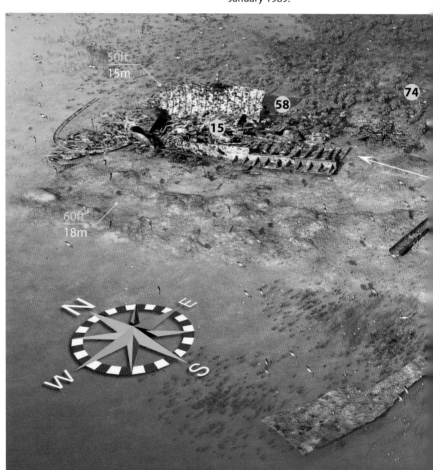

On the night before she was scheduled to leave for Miami, however, she was stolen from the wharf (some allege by pirates in keeping with Key West's lawless past). Under cover of darkness, she was towed out to the reef line outside of Key West and scuttled in an area of sand at a depth accessible to all divers.

She remained upright and in good condition until a pair of hurricanes tore her apart. Hurricane Georges stripped the wheelhouse off the main deck and smashed it to pieces in the summer of 1998, while Hurricane Irene broke the wreck in two the following year. Since then, the wreck has further degraded in various storms – even to the point of being moved along the reef from its original position. While the wreck no longer offers visitors the structure that it once did, it still provides a valuable artificial reef for the surrounding marine life. The metal hull and debris are heavily encrusted with hard and soft corals as well as sponges. Divers will see foureye butterflyfish, sergeant majors and yellowtail snapper on the wreck, along with schools of French and bluestriped grunts. Nurse sharks are common here, as are barracuda.

Name:	Joe's Tug	**Last owner:**	n/a
Type:	Steel-hulled shrimp boat	**Sunk:**	January 21, 1989
Previous names:	n/a		
Length:	75ft (23m)		
Tonnage:	n/a		
Construction:	n/a		

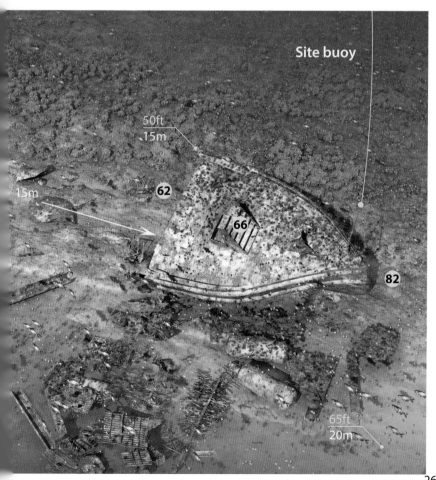

Site buoy

50ft
15m

15m

62

66

82

65ft
20m

TOPPINO'S BUOY (AKA MARKER 32)

Difficulty	● ○ ○
Current	● ○ ○
Depth	● ○ ○
Reef	★★★
Fauna	★★☆

Access
7.2mi (11.5km) from Key West

Level Open Water

Location Key West
GPS   T1 24° 28.457'N, 81° 44.561'W
         T2 24° 28.432'N, 81° 44.610'W
         T3 24° 28.429'N, 81° 44.657'W

Getting there
Toppino's Buoy sits just inside of the reef line, around 5.3 miles (8.5 kilometers) south of Key West. Getting there involves a boat ride of about 20 to 25 minutes from Key West.

Access
This site is suitable to divers and snorkelers of all levels. There are three mooring buoys that provide easy access to the short corals spur that represent the focus of this site. The ease of access also makes this site popular as a night dive, assisted by the lighted marker that dimly illuminates the area at night.

Description
Toppino's Buoy is also known as Marker 32 as is located just to the west of the red navigation marker of that number. The site bottoms out i sand and rubble at a depth of 28 feet (8.5 meter while the tops of the coral spurs rise to a dept of just 15 feet (4.5 meters). Each of the 15 or s

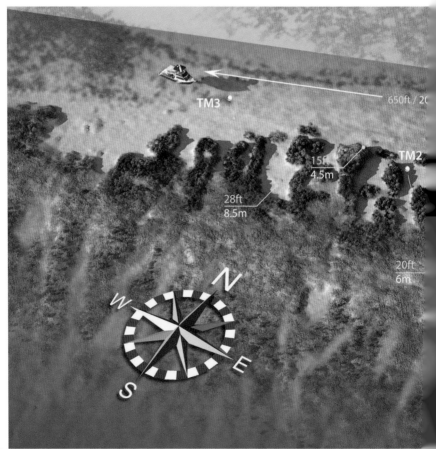

SCIENTIFIC INSIGHT

Divers and snorkelers may notice hundreds of evenly spaced staghorn corals growing along the top of the ledge. Toppino's Buoy is one of nearly a dozen out-planting sites managed by The Coral Restoration Foundation™. These corals were raised in nurseries and out-planted by the team between 2018 and 2020. Actively propagating staghorn and elkhorn corals, raising them in nurseries and then out-planting them on the reef can help the reef maintain the structural integrity important to support a biodiverse ecosystem. This work is an important component in the fight to ensure coral reefs are here for future generations.

owering spurs is heavily colonized by a mix of ard and soft encrusting corals, including star orals, sea fans and other gorgonians. South of he coral spurs is a shallow ledge that backs onto hard-bottomed reef slope. A field of young ransplanted staghorn corals from a local coral estoration project sits atop this ledge (see Scien- fic Insight box for more information).

he reef supports a variety of marine life both g and small. Blue tangs and stoplight parrotfish are common, while nurse sharks and barracuda are also frequently spotted here. Schools of bluestriped and French grunts congregate in the spaces between the spurs while green, spotted and goldentail moray eels can all be found hiding in the nooks and crevices of the reef. Bicolor damselfish, blue tangs, foureye butterflyfish, yellowtail snapper and squirrelfish round out the many species divers will encounter at this shallow and accessible site.

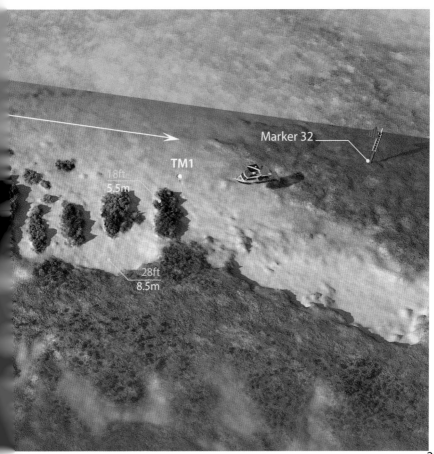

Marker 32

TM1

18ft
5.5m

28ft
8.5m

NINE FOOT STAKE

Difficulty	● ○ ○	
Current	● ○ ○	
Depth	● ● ○	
Reef	★★☆	Access 🚤
Fauna	★★☆	6.5mi (10.5km) from Key West

Level Open Water

Location Key West

GPS   NF1 24° 28.356′N, 81° 45.820′W
          NF2 24° 28.294′N, 81° 45.854′W
          NF3 24° 28.327′N, 81° 45.888′W

Getting there

Nine Foot Stake sits just inside of the reef line, around 5.3 miles (8.5 kilometers) south of Key West. Getting there involves a boat ride of about 20 minutes from Key West.

Access

This site is suitable for divers and snorkelers of all levels. There are three mooring buoys that provide easy access to the coral spurs that represent the focus of this site. The clear shallow water here makes this a great site for underwater photographers and for night dives. Currents are usually mild here.

Description

Nine Foot Stake (also 9′ Stake) is another shallow reef popular with both divers and snorkelers in the Key West area. It reportedly gets its name from a nine-foot-long (2.5-meter) pole or stake that once lay flat on the reef. It may have originally been part of a lighthouse or beacon that marked this reef for navigation, but records are unclear. The stake has long since been incorporated into the surrounding reef.

The tops of the spurs reach a depth of just 12 feet (3.5 meters) in some places, with the rubble and sand grooves bottoming out at 2

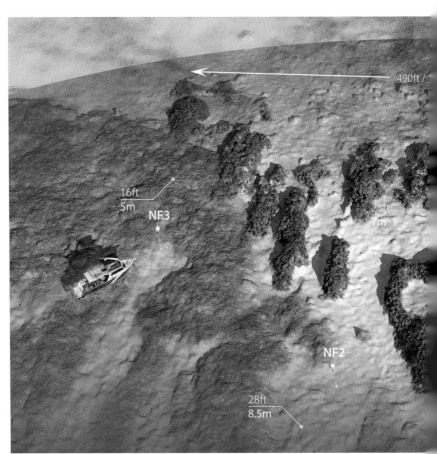

RELAX & RECHARGE

Half Shell Raw Bar (231 Margaret St, Naval Air Station Key West) is in the Key West Historic Seaport. This casual bar and restaurant, sometimes referred to as the "original" Key's seafood restaurant, serves the freshest seafood in town. In fact, local fishers unload their catch just steps from the kitchen. Half Shell is known for its stuffed shrimp (it was originally a shrimp warehouse), conch ceviche, fish and chips, and their catch-of-the-day, which they fillet themselves and cook either blackened, grilled or fried. Stone crab is also a local favorite when in season. The walls of the interior dining space are packed full of license plates, while the terrace has views of the fishing boats coming and going at the marina just across the wharf. Visit: **halfshellrawbar.com**

feet (7 meters). The resulting high relief of the coral-covered spurs creates complex habitat for the marine life. Sea fans, encrusting hard and soft corals, and sponges add to the complexity of the site. Divers and snorkelers are likely to encounter plenty of foureye butterflyfish, sergeant majors and yellowtail snapper on the reef. Stoplight, redband, striped, Queen, princess and blue parrotfish are also regularly seen here along with schools of Spanish and Caesar grunts, rock beauties, and Queen, gray and French angelfish. Sea turtles have been known to frequent this site as well, offering an incredible opportunity to observe these amazing creatures.

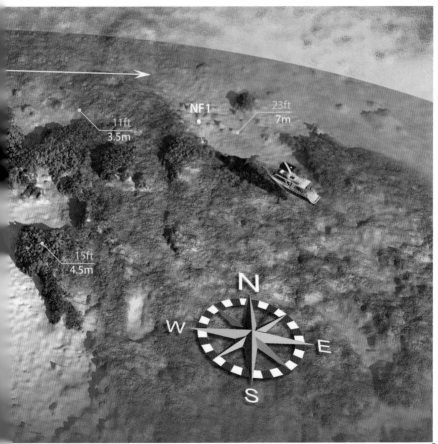

CAYMAN SALVAGE MASTER

Difficulty ● ● ○
Current ● ● ○
Depth ● ● ○
Reef ★★☆
Fauna ★★★

Access 🚤 (11.5km) from Key West

Level Advanced

Location Key West
GPS   24° 27.656'N, 81° 46.012'W

Getting there

Cayman Salvage Master sits just off the reef line, around 5.9 miles (9.5 kilometers) south of Key West. Getting there involves a boat ride of about 20 to 25 minutes from Key West.

Access

This site is suitable for open water divers with experience at depth, as the seabed reaches 90 feet (27.5 meters) deep. A single mooring buoy tied to the bow provides access to the site. Currents can be strong here given the wreck is positioned in the Gulf Stream, but that also means visibility is usually excellent. The open nature of the wreck makes *Cayman Salvage Master* popular as a night dive as well.

Description

Cayman Salvage Master goes by a few names, including the *Cayman Salvager* and even the *Cayman Salvor*. She was originally a steel-hulled minelayer built for the U.S. Army in 1936 and commissioned as *USAMP Lt. Col Ellery W Niles* after a former mine planter and Chief of War Plans in the Office of the Chief of Coast Artillery.

Her first real posting came in the Pacific, working the minefield at Fort Winfield Scott in California in June 1938. She was moved across San Francisco Bay in 1939 to Fort Baker and later to Fort Rosecrans near San Diego. From June to August of 1940, she laid the minefield that helped protect the Pacific end of the Panama Canal during World War II. At the end of the war, she was decommissioned and sold to Marine Acoustical Services, Inc. in Miami, and converted into an acoustical research ship. Renamed *F.V. Hunt*, she operated primarily in the Bahamas. Some reports indicate that she also operated as a buoy tender for the Coast Guard after her service as a minelayer and before she was converted to a civilian ship.

She was eventually sold to Thompson TA in the late 1970s for use as a freighter in the Cayman

Islands and renamed the *Cayman Salvage Master*. At this point her career takes a dramatic turn. She was seized by the Coast Guard for her illegal role in the Mariel Boatlift, which ultimately saw 125,000 Cubans flee the island nation to arrive in the United States between April and October 1980. She was impounded in the Navy harbor in Key West, where she sat neglected for several years until she sank at the dockside in 1985.

She was refloated so that she could be cleaned

CAYMAN SALVAGE MASTER

DID YOU KNOW?

The Mariel Boatlift occurred when Fidel Castro announced on April 20, 1980, that anyone who wanted to leave Cuba could do so. The announcement came in the middle of an economic downturn and growing unrest. Between April and October 1980, upwards of 1,700 boats (including the *Cayman Salvage Master*) carried Cubans from Mariel Harbor across the Florida Strait. Reports maintain that criminals and patients from psychiatric institutions were part of the 125,000 Cubans that migrated over the nearly seven-month period and were said to be part of the effort by Castro's government to destabilize the United States as it fought to process all the immigrants. These reports led to an attempted blockade by the U.S. Coast Guard, who ultimately managed to seize nearly 1,400 vessels before they made it to American soil. It was a massive challenge for President Carter and his administration and remains a major cultural turning point in the history of Florida.

and prepped for sinking elsewhere as an artificial reef. Her superstructure was entirely removed and used as an artificial reef on the Gulf coast of Key West. The rest of the ship was planned for sinking in April 1985, at a depth of 300 feet (91.5 meters), but the towline snapped during deployment, and she ended up in just 90 feet (27.5 meters) of water instead (fortuitously for divers). She originally settled on her port side, but Hurricane Katrina pushed her upright in 2005.

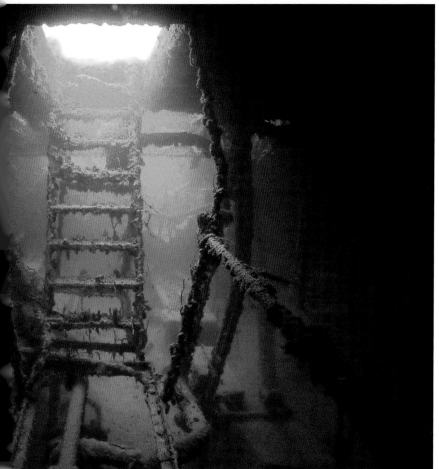

Ben Edmonds ©

...e interior of the *Cayman Salvage Master* offers penetration opportunities, but with a relatively tight fit in places..

CAYMAN SALVAGE MASTER

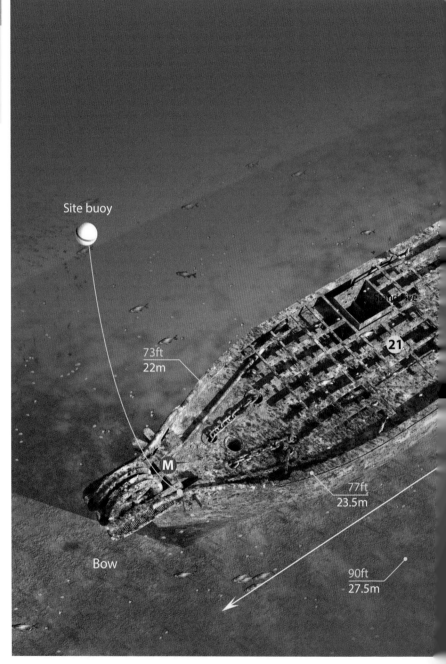

Site buoy

73ft
22m

21

M

77ft
23.5m

Bow

90ft
27.5m

The wreck allows for full penetration, and her large holds and internal rooms still hold artifacts from her working life, including a few bicycles from the Mariel Boatlift, according to some reports. Left intact was the vessel's cable wheel that still juts off the bow. The large wheel is heavily encrusted with corals and sponges, much like most of the remaining hull. A large gree moray eel is often visible around the wheel.

Divers are likely to see plenty of reef fish at th site. A goliath grouper is known to freque the site, while barracuda are common her Yellowtail and gray snapper form large schoo

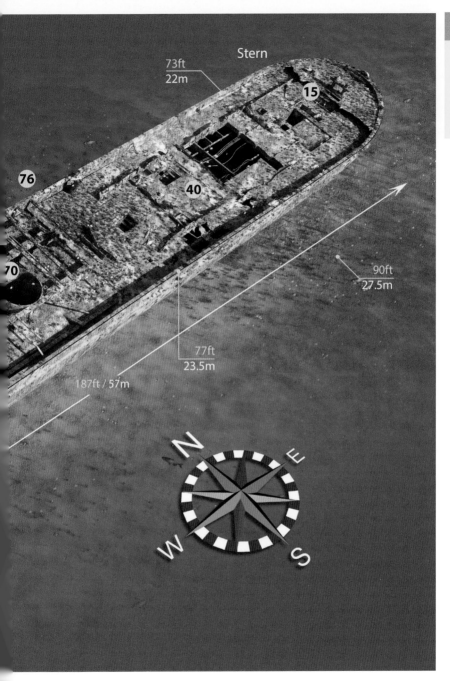

73ft
22m

Stern

15

76

40

70

90ft
27.5m

77ft
23.5m

187ft / 57m

Route

The lack of superstructure on this wreck makes any route just a case of choosing to head in a clockwise or counterclockwise direction around the wreck. Divers should check out the intact rudder at the stern as well as the cable reel at the bow. The holds are open but there are multiple entanglement

round the upright wreck, while rock beauties nd Queen angelfish are often seen patrolling ong the main deck. Bar jacks and creole wrasse re often seen above the deck while purple reef sh hang closer to the coral-encrusted hull. ergeant majors and bicolor damselfish are also ommonly seen here.

273

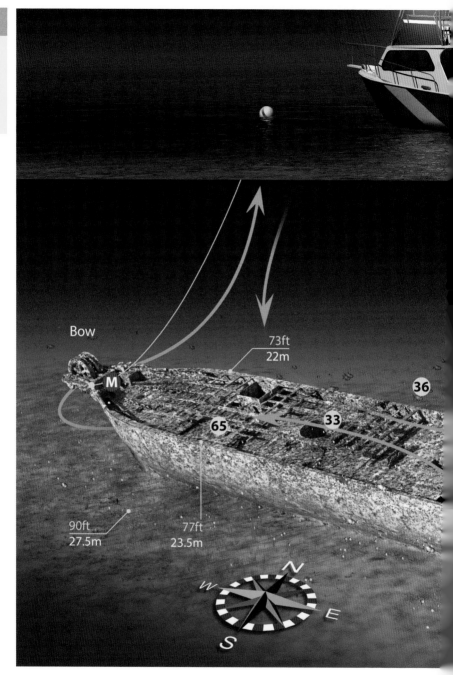

Bow

73ft
22m

M

36

65

33

90ft
27.5m

77ft
23.5m

N
W
E
S

risks and some narrow passageways. Divers should proceed with caution if they plan to penetrate the wreck.

CAYMAN SALVAGE MASTER

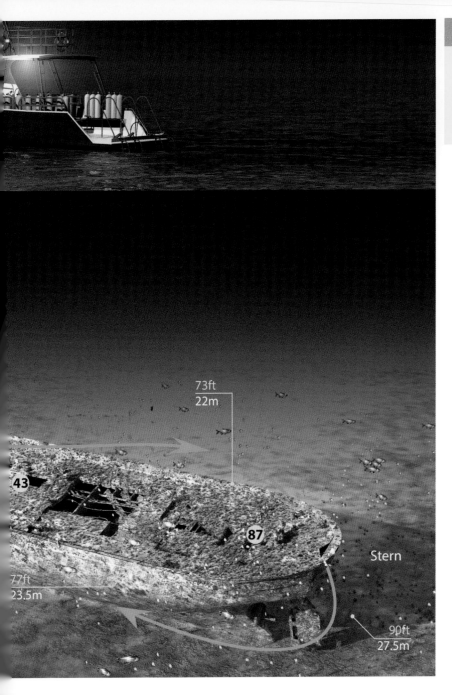

73ft
22m

43

87

Stern

77ft
23.5m

90ft
27.5m

		Construction:	Pusey and Jones Shipbuilding, Willington, DE, 1936
ame:	*MV Cayman Salvage Master*		
ype:	Minelayer		
revious names:	*USAMP Lt. Col Ellery W Niles, RV F.V. Hunt*	**Last owner:**	Thompson TA
		Sunk:	April 30, 1985
ength:	187ft (23.5m)		
onnage:	840grt		

CURB

Difficulty ● ● ●
Current ● ● ●
Depth ● ● ●
Reef ★★☆
Fauna ★★★

Access 🛥 8.5mi (13.5km) from Key West

Level Technical

Location Key West
GPS   24° 26.212'N, 81° 46.127'W

Getting there
Getting to the *Curb* involves a boat ride of 25 to

30 minutes from Key West. The wreck site is 7.5 miles (12 kilometers) south of Key West.

Access
Due to the depths involved, the *Curb* is only accessible to technical divers. She sits upright at a depth of 185 feet (56.5 meters). There

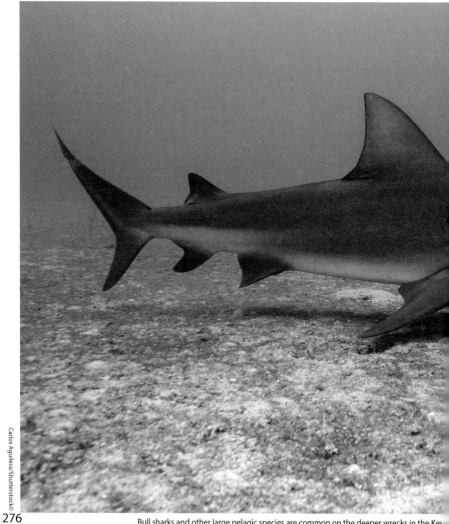

Carlos Aguilera/Shutterstock©

Bull sharks and other large pelagic species are common on the deeper wrecks in the Key

RELAX & RECHARGE

Blue Heaven (729 Thomas Street, Key West) is a real favorite of locals in Key West. This unique establishment serves delicious food with a Caribbean flair in a laid back atmosphere steeped in history. In the past, this building has been a bar, gambling den, dance hall, playhouse and even a bordello. It has also hosted cock fights (there's even a rooster graveyard on the property) and amateur boxing matches, refereed in the 1930s by none other than Ernest Hemingway. Breakfast (served until 2pm) is what brings in many locals. "Richard's Very Good Pancakes" come in a range of styles: plain, blueberry, banana, pecan and pineapple. There are omelets, homemade granola, the Blue Heaven Benedict, as well as a Rooster Special for those who want a bit of everything. The Sunday breakfast menu is packed with additional specials, while the lunch and dinner menus include Caribbean favorites like BBQ shrimp, yellowtail snapper, spiny lobster and Jamaican jerk chicken. Visit: **Blueheavenkw.com.**

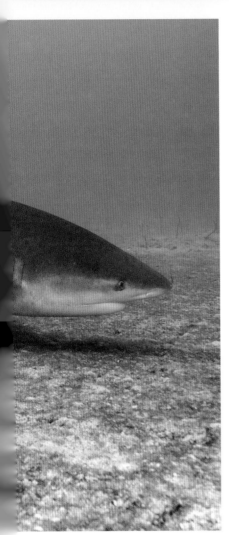

are no mooring buoys at this site, and local operators only visit it as part of a specifically chartered dive.

Description

USS Curb was originally a Diver-class rescue and salvage boat built in 1943 for the U.S. Navy. She served during World War II, but little is known about her activities or what port she called home. She was retired just three years after entering service and was laid up in the Atlantic Reserve Fleet in Texas. In 1947, she was loaned out to an American salvage firm, Merritt Chapman & Scott. The company had worldwide salvage operations and was founded in the 1860s but grew the scope of their business to include construction, although often still with a marine focus. It is not clear how the company used *Curb* during this time, but it ceased operations sometime in the late 1960s and early 1970s, and *Curb* ended up back in the Reserve Fleet.

She was eventually scrapped in 1982 and reefed in November 1983. Today, she provides incredible habitat for a variety of reef fishes and pelagics, including cobia, goliath grouper, black grouper, gag grouper, cubera snapper, barracuda and blacktip reef sharks.

Name:	*USS Curb*
Type:	Salvage vessel
Previous names:	n/a
Length:	213ft (65m)
Tonnage:	1,897t (disp)
Construction:	Basal Rock Co, Napa, CA, 1943
Last owner:	U.S. Navy
Sunk:	November 23, 1983

KEY WEST MARINE PARK

The official address of the park is 1000 Atlantic Boulevard, Key West.

Difficulty	● ○ ○	
Current	● ○ ○	
Depth	● ○ ○	
Reef	★★★	Access 🚙
Fauna	★★★	0.4mi (0.6km) from Key West

Level n/a

Location Key West
GPS   24° 32.732'N, 81° 47.219'W

Getting there

The Key West Marine Park is located just off the Clarence S. Higgs Memorial Beach Park in southwest Key West. To get there, drive down Route 1 as it enters Key West from Stock Island. At the T-intersection as you enter Key West, turn left onto South Roosevelt Boulevard. Follow it for 0.25 miles (0.4 kilometers) and then turn right onto Flagler Avenue. Follow Flagler Avenue for 2.5 miles (4 kilometers) until you reach the intersection with White Street. Turn left on White Street and continue south until you reach Atlantic Boulevard on the waterfront. Turn right onto Atlantic to find parking along the beach.

Access

There is no fee to access the park or either of the two city piers that bracket Higgs Beach – the Reynolds Street Pier to the west and the larger Edward B. Knight Pier to the east. The park features covered picnic tables, restroom and shower facilities, tennis and volleyball courts, a restaurant and even a place to rent a sailboat.

The best snorkeling is just off Higgs Beach to the east and west of the Reynolds Street Pier and is accessible from the beach. The swim-only area extends roughly 600 feet (180 meters) from the beach and is marked by a buoy line, which means snorkelers do not need to carry their own diver-down flag here. There is no fishing, spearfishing or harvesting by any other means within the boundaries of the Marine Park. Visitors must bring their own snorkel gear as there is none for rent at the park.

Description

The Key West Marine Park is a 40-acre area that stretches from Higgs Beach in the east to South Beach in the west. The Park features three large

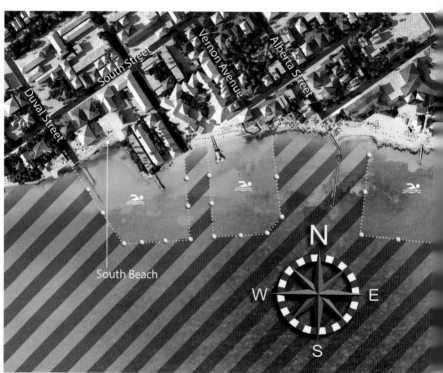

DID YOU KNOW?

The Edward B. Knight Pier is dog friendly, and there is a dog park located on the other side of Atlantic Boulevard. Higgs Beach is not accessible to dogs, but there is a dog-friendly beach located just to the west between Vernon Avenue and Alberta Street. You cannot access the dog beach directly from Higgs Beach, but it is still within the boundaries of the Key West Marine Park and features a dedicated swim-only area.

swim-only areas marked off with boundary buoys separated by two vessel-access lanes. The main area of interest for divers is the shallow seagrass areas that sit off the beach and the remnants of the old steel pier that extends seaward from the Reynolds Street Pier at the western edge of Higgs Beach. The maximum depth in the area is just 15 feet (4.5 meters).

The remains of the old metal pier and surrounding rubble helps shelter the waters off Higgs Beach and provides plenty of hard surfaces for colonization by corals and small sponges. The swimming area offers shelter to a variety of marine life, including black grouper, Queen angelfish, rainbow parrotfish, sergeant majors, French grunts and yellowtail damselfish. Barracuda are frequently spotted observing the reef and any nearby snorkelers, while stingrays and yellow goatfish cruise along the sand. Nurse sharks are often seen resting along the base of the breakwater while rainbow runners, palometas and round scad flit about in the water column above. While less common, manatees, eagle rays and sea turtles have also been seen here, making this truly one of the most interesting shore-accessible spots in Key West.

Snorkelers should be careful if they choose to explore the area around the old pier. The shallow water means that waves can push snorkelers against the submerged metal structures. The old pilings and rubble have been colonized by fire corals and shelter the invasive lionfish. Brushing up against either one, or even just the old rusty metal of the pier, may bring a painful halt to a snorkeling adventure.

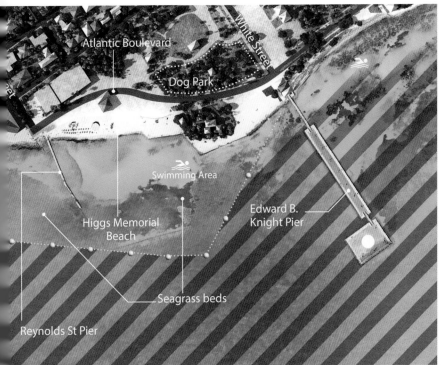

FORT ZACHARY TAYLOR HISTORIC STATE PARK

Difficulty	● ○ ○	
Current	● ○ ○	
Depth	● ○ ○	
Reef	★★☆	Access 🚙
Fauna	★☆☆	2mi (3.3km) from Key West

Level n/a

Location Key West
GPS   24° 32.714′N, 81° 48.636′W

Getting there

Fort Zachary Taylor Historic State Park is located at the far southwestern corner of Key West. To get there, drive down Route 1/N Roosevelt Boulevard as it enters Key West from Stock Island. North Roosevelt Boulevard turns into Truman Avenue as it crosses First Street in Key West. Follow Truman Avenue for 0.94 miles (1.5 kilometers) and turn right onto Whitehead Street. The Key West Lighthouse marks the turn. Drive for 0.3 miles (0.5 kilometers) and turn left onto Southard Street. Follow Southard Street until it ends at a traffic circle. Exit the circle onto Butler Road (2nd exit) and continue past the Eco Discovery Center and the Key West Amphitheater. The guard station at the entrance of the park is 0.36 miles (0.58 kilometers) after the circle. Follow the road 0.2 miles (0.35 kilometers) past the guard station to the main parking lot for the beach-accessible snorkeling. The official address of the park is 601 Howard England Way, Key West, Florida, 33040.

Access

There is a fee to enter the park. The snorkel beach is just over 200 feet (60 meters) from the parking lot. There is a concession stand and café right on

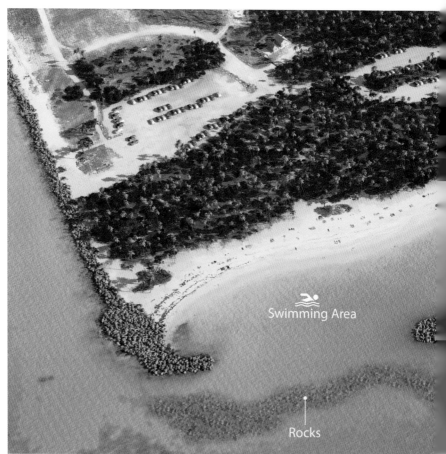

Swimming Area

Rocks

DID YOU KNOW?

Fort Zachary Taylor got its start as a U.S. Navy depot in 1822 after the Spanish transferred Florida to the fledgling American nation. The Navy was looking to rid the area of pirates. The Army began construction of the fort in 1845 and it remained under federal control during the Civil War. The fort was also on active duty through 1947 and the end of World War II. The park entrance fee includes access to walk around this incredible piece of history, which includes the largest collection of Civil War-era seacoast cannons in the United States.

the beach, along with restrooms and showers. Snorkel gear is available for rent here.

Description

The state park is one of the top places to snorkel in Key West, and represents one of the only public-access, shore-accessible sites in the lower Keys. The sand and pebble beach measures 900 feet (275 meters) in length and faces south with a relatively flat slope. It is partially protected by breakwaters, but the surf can get rough when the weather picks up. These breakwaters also provide reef-like habitat for snorkelers to explore and host a snorkel trail featuring outplanted coral fragments. Located just 130 feet (40 meters) off the beach, the piles of rocks provide complex habitat for everything from blue tangs and sergeant majors to stoplight parrotfish and hogfish. Barracuda are regularly seen here, while nurse sharks have been spotted on occasion. Snorkelers should also take some time to look out on the sand to watch for southern stingrays.

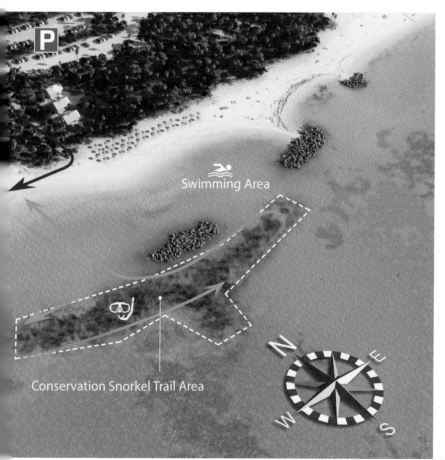

Swimming Area

Conservation Snorkel Trail Area

EASTERN DRY ROCKS

Difficulty	● ○ ○
Current	● ○ ○
Depth	● ○ ○
Reef	★★★☆
Fauna	★★☆

Access 🚤 6.5mi (10.5km) from Key West

Level Open Water

Location Key West

GPS
EDR1 24° 27.554'N, 81° 50.638'W
EDR2 24° 27.544'N, 81° 50.676'W
EDR3 24° 27.531'N, 81° 50.710'W
EDR4 24° 27.532'N, 81° 50.737'W
EDR5 24° 27.585'N, 81° 50.746'W
EDR6 24° 27.570'N, 81° 50.679'W
EDR7 24° 27.647'N, 81° 50.764'W
EDR8 24° 27.601'N, 81° 50.779'W
EDR9 24° 27.637'N, 81° 50.770'W
EDR10 24° 27.658'N, 81° 50.754'W
EDR11 24° 27.691'N, 81° 50.745'W

EDR12 24° 27.770'N, 81° 50.636'W

Getting there

Eastern Dry Rocks sits on the outer reef line, just 6.5 miles (10.5 kilometers) southwest of Key West. Getting there involves a boat ride of 20 to 25 minutes from Key West.

Access

This site is accessible to divers and snorkelers of all levels. There are 12 mooring buoys that provide easy access to this western portion of the reef. The site is located within a Sanctuary Preservation Area (SPA), so boats must tie-in to

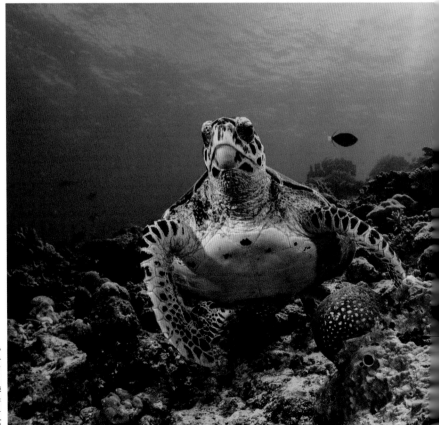

Suphoto.com/Shutterstock©

Sea turtles are regular visitors to Eastern Dry Rock

RELAX & RECHARGE

If you're looking to quench a thirst, enjoy some live music and soak up a little history, a couple of famous Key West watering-holes – **Sloppy Joe's** (201 Duval Street, Key West) and **Captain Tony's** (428 Greene Street, Key West) – are well worth a visit. Sloppy Joe's was officially opened on December 5, 1933, which was the day Prohibition was repealed. But the bar existed long before that as an illegal speakeasy called the Blind Pig. The building, which has a wonderfully rich history, was built in 1851 and used as an icehouse that doubled as Key West's first morgue, because it was cold enough to store bodies prior to burial. A "hanging tree" in the grounds was used to execute as many as 16 pirates in the early days of Key West, as well as a woman who was accused of killing her husband and their child. The owner of Sloppy Joe's was a bootlegger called Joe "Josey" Russell – a close friend and fishing buddy of Ernest Hemingway, who often frequented the bar and chose the name. In 1937, the weekly rent on the building was raised from $3 to $4, so Russell decided to move the bar to its current location, just a hundred feet down the road. The original building was reopened as Captain Tony's in 1958, by a local charter boat captain named Tony Tarracino. Jimmy Buffett got his start in Key West there in the 1970s and was apparently often paid for live performances in tequila (Buffett's song, "Last Mango in Paris" is about Captain Tony's). The famous "hanging tree" still grows in the middle of the bar (literally) and the ghost of the woman who was hung there is said to haunt the building. Visit: **Sloppyjoes.com** and **Capttonyssaloon.com.**

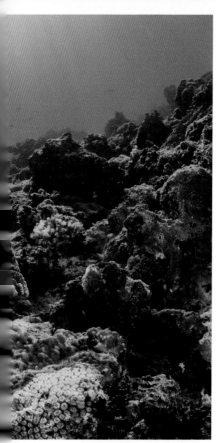

a buoy if one is available.

Description

Eastern Dry Rocks is a shallow bank reef with a rubble shoal and shallow coral fingers that extend seaward at a southeastern angle. The well-defined spurs are the focal point of the site, although there is a hard-bottom reef slope that descends seaward to a depth of 46 feet (14 meters). The slope features coral heads and large barrel sponges. There is an increased chance of seeing larger pelagics on this reef, including bull sharks.

The coral spurs that make this site so popular with divers and snorkelers are very shallow, topping out at a depth of just a few feet (1 meter). The rubble- and sand-bottomed grooves reach a depth of between 13 and 20 feet (4 and 6 meters), putting them well within reach of snorkelers. The spurs are well colonized by a mix of hard and soft corals as well as sea fans and sponges. As one of the reefs located closest to the harbor in Key West, it is very popular with local operators who regularly visit here. It is also popular due to the variety of marine life divers and snorkelers will see here, including green moray eels, reef sharks, barracuda and southern stingrays. Visitors will also encounter the normal complement of reef fishes, including gray and Queen angelfish, yellowtail snapper, stoplight parrotfish and plenty of blue tangs.

The remains of a wrecked Spanish galleon can

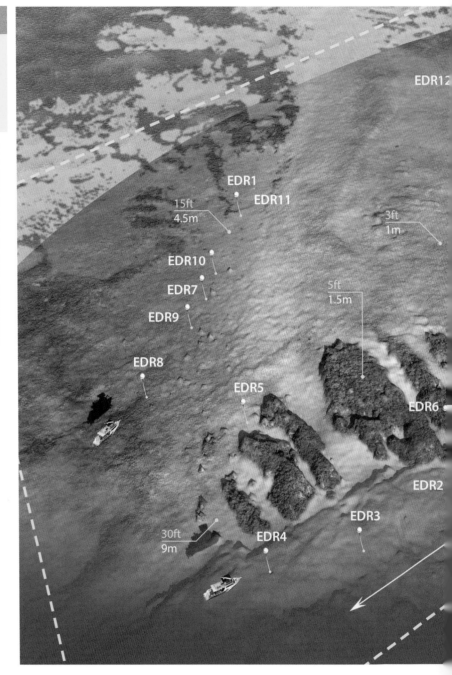

EDR12

EDR1

EDR11

15ft
4.5m

3ft
1m

EDR10

5ft
1.5m

EDR7

EDR9

EDR8

EDR5

EDR6

EDR2

EDR3

30ft
9m

EDR4

reportedly be found in the southwestern corner of Eastern Dry Rocks reef. The wreck has long since been incorporated into the surrounding reef but apparently brass rings, tiles and ballast stones can still be identified underneath the encrusting corals and sponges.

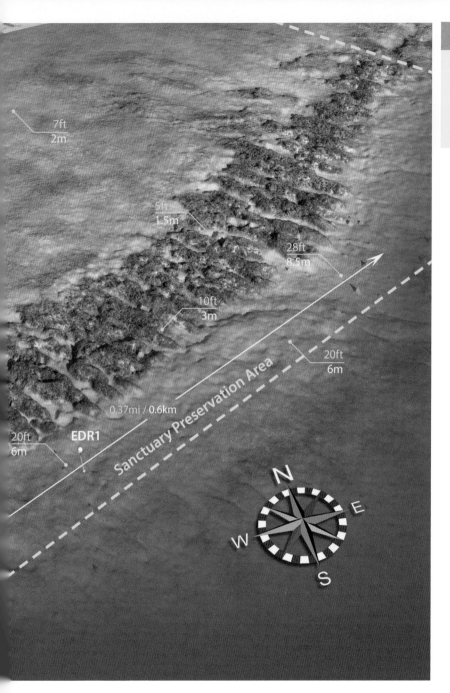

7ft
2m

5ft
1.5m

28ft
8.5m

10ft
3m

20ft
6m

0.37mi / 0.6km

Sanctuary Preservation Area

20ft
6m

EDR1

ROCK KEY

Difficulty	● ○ ○
Current	● ○ ○
Depth	● ○ ○
Reef	★★☆
Fauna	★★☆

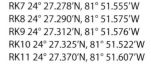

Access 🚤
8.4mi (13.5km) from Key West

Level Open Water

Location Key West

GPS
RK1 24° 27.358′N, 81° 51.314′W
RK2 24° 27.294′N, 81° 51.381′W
RK3 24° 27.281′N, 81° 51.414′W
RK4 24° 27.259′N, 81° 51.453′W
RK5 24° 27.254′N, 81° 51.490′W
RK6 24° 27.254′N, 81° 51.550′W

RK7 24° 27.278′N, 81° 51.555′W
RK8 24° 27.290′N, 81° 51.575′W
RK9 24° 27.312′N, 81° 51.576′W
RK10 24° 27.325′N, 81° 51.522′W
RK11 24° 27.370′N, 81° 51.607′W

Getting there

Rock Key sits on the outer reef line, just 6.9 miles (11.1 kilometers) southwest of Key West. Getting there involves a boat ride of 25 minutes from Key West.

Access

This site is suitable for divers and snorkelers of all levels. There are 11 mooring buoys that provide easy access to the spur and groove region of the reef. The site is located within a Sanctuary Preservation Area (SPA), so boats must tie-in to a buoy if one is available.

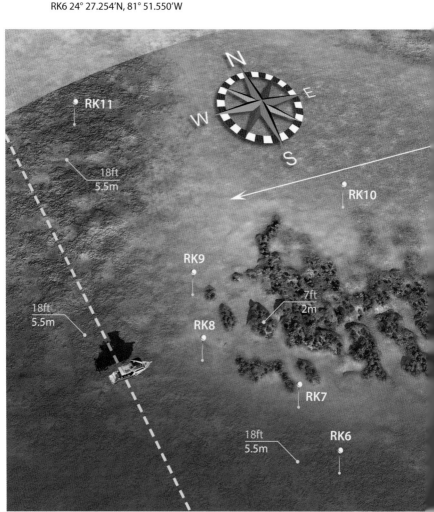

Description

Rock Key is a bank reef with a shallow rubble area fronted by coral fingers that extend seaward at a southern angle. The well-defined spur and groove area of the reef is the focal point of the site, although there is a hard-bottom reef slope that descends seaward to a depth of 46 feet (14 meters). The slope features coral heads and large barrel sponges along with the increased chance of seeing larger pelagics, including bull sharks and blacktip reef sharks.

The shallow spurs are covered in hard and soft corals, including sea fans and other gorgonians. Sponges make up a lot of the growth on top of these spurs, which can reach a depth of just 6 feet (2 meters). The rubble- and sand-bottomed grooves reach a depth of between 16 and 26 feet (5 and 8 meters), which creates a decent amount of profile off the seabed. This in turn supports a variety of reef fishes and benthic marine life.

Foureye, spotfin and banded butterflyfish are common among the corals growing on top of the spurs, as are stoplight and redband parrotfish. Blue and brown chromis, bar jacks and barracuda are regularly seen in the water column above the reef, along with horse-eye jacks and yellow jacks. Yellow and spotted goatfish are often seen foraging along the rubble and sandy grooves, near where yellowhead jawfish poke their heads out of their underground burrows. Both lobsters and nurse sharks are a common sight along ledges and under overhangs, while squirrelfish are often found hiding in the darker recesses of the reef as they wait for nightfall. Visitors have also reported seeing sea turtles here, both loggerhead and green sea turtles, as well as reef sharks, although these are much less frequent than other species.

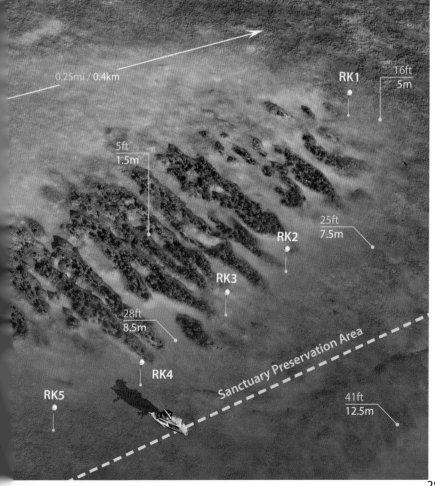

0.25mi / 0.4km

RK1 16ft / 5m

5ft / 1.5m

RK2 25ft / 7.5m

RK3

28ft / 8.5m

RK4

Sanctuary Preservation Area

RK5 41ft / 12.5m

SAND KEY

Difficulty ● ○ ○
Current ● ○ ○
Depth ● ○ ○
Reef ★★☆
Fauna ★★☆

Access 10mi (16km) from Key West

Level Open Water

Location Key West

GPS SK1 24° 27.213'N, 81° 52.482'W
SK2 24° 27.218'N, 81° 52.449'W
SK3 24° 27.214'N, 81° 52.428'W
SK4 24° 27.201'N, 81° 52.391'W
SK5 24° 27.174'N, 81° 52.457'W
SK6 24° 27.171'N, 81° 52.485'W
SK7 24° 27.157'N, 81° 52.518'W
SK8 24° 27.141'N, 81° 52.553'W
SK9 24° 27.136'N, 81° 52.577'W
SK10 24° 27.119'N, 81° 52.597'W
SK11 24° 27.111'N, 81° 52.619'W
SK12 24° 27.112'N, 81° 52.658'W
SK13 24° 27.099'N, 81° 52.687'W
SK14 24° 27.111'N, 81° 52.713'W
SK15 24° 27.084'N, 81° 52.741'W
SK16 24° 27.104'N, 81° 52.752'W
SK17 24° 27.083'N, 81° 52.784'W
SK18 24° 27.102'N, 81° 52.782'W
SK19 24° 27.127'N, 81° 52.803'W
SK20 24° 27.136'N, 81° 52.813'W
SK21 24° 27.145'N, 81° 52.779'W
SK23 24° 27.180'N, 81° 52.813'W
SK24 24° 27.137'N, 81° 52.838'W
SK25 24° 27.176'N, 81° 52.780'W
SK26 24° 27.201'N, 81° 52.799'W
SK27 24° 27.221'N, 81° 52.787'W

Getting there

Sand Key sits on the outer reef line, 7.5 mile (12 kilometers) southwest of Key West. Getting there involves a boat ride of 30 to 35 minute from Key West.

Access

This site is suitable for divers and snorkeler of all levels. There are 26 mooring buoys tha provide easy access to the spur and groov region of the reef. Five of them are anchored i the rubble found along the western edge of th shoal, while two are found in slightly deepe water just off the coral spurs. The site is locate within a Sanctuary Preservation Area (SPA), s boats must tie-in to a buoy if one is availabl Fishing and other extractive activities are n permitted at this site with the exception c catch-and-release trolling.

Description

Sand Key is a bank reef with a shallow rubb area fronted by coral fingers that exten seaward at a southern angle. A small sectic of sand remains above the waterline but ten to shift position along with the currents ar the weather. The site was originally calle Cayos Arena, or Sand Island, by early Spani explorers. The dry section is currently marke by a 132-foot-tall (40-meter) iron-frame lighthouse. The lighthouse is in relatively goc

DID YOU KNOW?

Located in a large patch of sand 0.6 miles (1 kilometer) northeast of the Sand Key Lighthouse sits a large art installation. The Stargazer Sculpture was designed by Florida-based artist Ann Lorraine Labriola. It was installed in 1992 and consists of 10 separate elements that stretch across nearly 200 feet (61 meters) of sand. This artificial reef pays homage to ancient mariners who navigated based on the stars with various constellations and celestial shapes cut into the pieces. The location was chosen to create additional reef habitat, while also relieving diving and snorkeling pressure on the nearby Sand Key. The individual elements are built out of steel and provide ample surfaces for corals to settle and grow on, and the entire installation has become heavily colonized over the years. However, the ocean is a harsh environment, and a few of the elements have collapsed in recent years. What remains still provides interesting habitat for both snorkelers and divers to explore, however. The installation can be found at GPS coordinates 24° 27.498'N, 81° 52.100'W.

condition, although the pier that once allowed easy access for the lighthouse keeper is now gone, leaving only the pilings visible.

The well-defined spurs are the focal point of the site, although there is a hard-bottom reef slope that descends seaward to a depth of 65 feet (20 meters) where there is a small ledge. From there it descends to sand at a depth of 90 feet (27.5 meters) in some places. The slope features coral heads and large barrel sponges along with an increased chance of seeing larger pelagics, including bull sharks.

The shallow spurs are covered in hard and soft corals, including sea fans and other gorgonians. Sponges make up much of the growth on these spurs, which reach a depth of just 3 feet (1 meter). The rubble- and sand-bottomed grooves reach depths of between 15 and 23 feet (4.5 and 7 meters), which creates a great deal of complexity in the reef. This in turn supports an incredible level of biodiversity among the reef fishes found here.

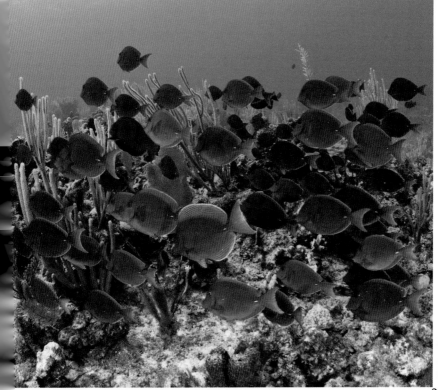

Schools of blue tangs are common along the shallow reefs off Key West.

Ethan Daniels/Shutterstock©

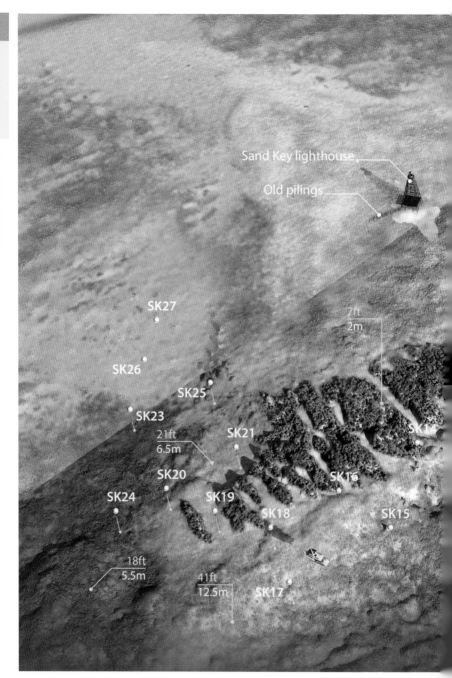

Sand Key lighthouse

Old pilings

SK27

7ft
2m

SK26

SK25

SK23

21ft
6.5m

SK21

SK20

SK14

SK24

SK19

SK16

SK18

SK15

18ft
5.5m

41ft
12.5m

SK17

Blue tangs, ocean surgeonfish and doctorfish are all common along this section of reef, as are stoplight and redband parrotfish. Black grouper, Nassau grouper and even the massive goliath grouper are sometimes seen here, as well as barracuda and dog snapper. Bluehead and yellowhead wrasses and sharpnose puffers are often spotted among the corals, along with schools of French, bluestripe and white grunts. Longspine squirrelfish can ▪ found hiding in the darker recesses of the reef, oft▪ next to lobsters that have also sought shelter the▪ Goldentail, spotted and green moray eels are a▪ likely to be seen hiding in small holes and crevi▪ in the reef here.

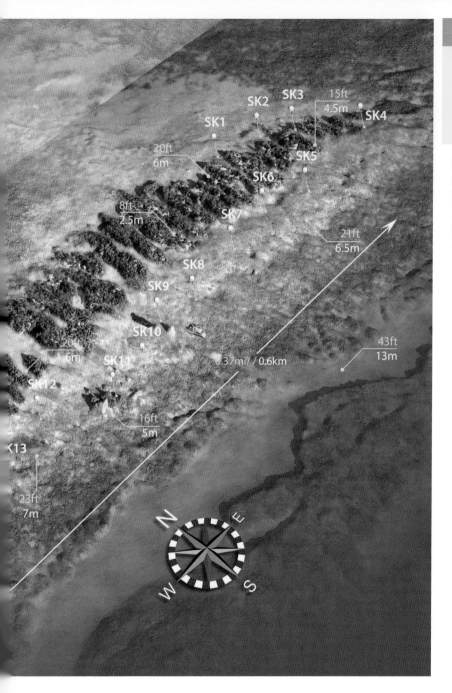

SK1
SK2
SK3
15ft
4.5m
SK4
20ft
6m
SK5
SK6
8ft
2.5m
SK7
21ft
6.5m
SK8
SK9
SK10
0.37mi / 0.6km
43ft
13m
SK11
SK12
20ft
6m
16ft
5m
K13
23ft
7m

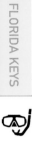

ARCHER KEY

Difficulty ● ○ ○
Current ● ○ ○
Depth ● ○ ○
Reef ★★☆
Fauna ★★☆

Access 🚤
4.6mi (7.5km) from Key West

Level n/a

Location Key West
GPS AK1 24° 33.598'N, 81° 52.899'W
AK2 24° 33.573'N, 81° 52.892'W
AK3 24° 33.555'N, 81° 52.819'W

Getting there
Archer Key is located just over 4 miles (7 kilometers) due west of Key West. Getting there involves a boat ride of just 15 minutes from Key West.

Access
Due to the shallow nature of this site, Archer Key is only suitable for snorkelers. Three mooring buoys at the site provide easy access to the rocky area and adjacent seagrass beds and avoid the need for boats to anchor in the fragile environment.

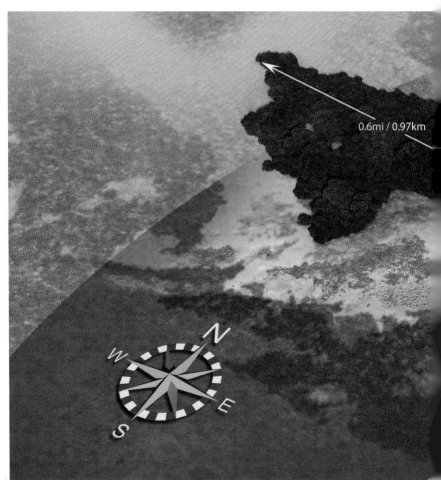

0.6mi / 0.97km

ARCHER KEY

SCIENTIFIC INSIGHT

Sponges have been on Earth for at least 500 million years. They are one of the oldest types of animals on our planet and they have some of the longest lifespans of all creatures on Earth. For instance, the giant barrel sponge (*Xestospongia muta*), which is common in the Florida Keys, can live for more than 2,000 years. Next time you see one on the reef, consider the fact that a large individual of more than 6 feet (2 meters) across might have been around since the time of the Ancient Romans.

Description

Archer Key is a popular snorkel destination for Key West based operators. The shallow, mild-current waters found to the southeast of the key offer a great place for snorkelers of all ages to explore. The rocky reef area and its adjacent seagrass beds support a variety of marine life, including lobsters, hogfish, angelfish and many different species of grunts. Invasive lionfish are also commonly seen here, and snorkelers should be careful not to get too close to this species as they have venomous spines. The seabed is just a few feet below the surface of the water in many places.

The rocky reef area supports small coral heads and a variety of sponges, including giant barrel sponges. Seagrass beds are important nurseries for juveniles of many coral reef fish species, so visitors will also likely see plenty of juvenile grunts, snapper, and damselfish, among other species.

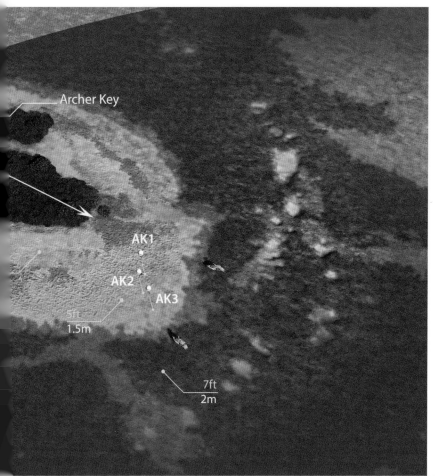

COTTRELL KEY

Difficulty	● ○ ○
Current	● ○ ○
Depth	● ○ ○
Reef	★★☆
Fauna	★☆☆

Access 🚤
8.4mi (13.5km) from Key West

CK9 24° 36.812'N, 81° 55.282'W
CK10 24° 36.819'N, 81° 55.305'W
CK11 24° 36.790'N, 81° 55.365'W
CK12 24° 36.425'N, 81° 56.088'W
CK13 24° 36.416'N, 81° 56.101'W
CK14 24° 36.412'N, 81° 56.117'W

Level Open Water

Location Key West
GPS
CK1 24° 37.167'N, 81° 54.565'W
CK3 24° 37.138'N, 81° 54.623'W
CK4 24° 37.121'N, 81° 54.662'W
CK5 24° 37.102'N, 81° 54.715'W
CK6 24° 37.087'N, 81° 54.747'W
CK7 24° 37.066'N, 81° 54.787'W
CK8 24° 37.029'N, 81° 54.860'W

Getting there

Cottrell Key is in Florida Bay, 8 miles (13 kilometers) northwest of Key West. Getting there involves a boat ride of 25 to 30 minutes from Key West.

Access

Cottrell Key is a shallow reef ledge that extends for almost 2 miles (3 kilometers) in length just north of the small island of the same name. Access to the ledge is provided by 13 mooring buoys clustered in groups along the length of the site. Cottrell Key itself is part of a Wildlife Management Area, and boats are not allowed within 300 feet (91 meters) of the mangrove

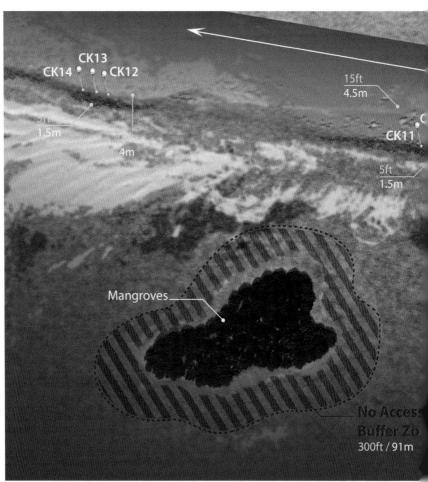

CK13
CK14 • • CK12
CK11
15ft
4.5m
5ft
1.5m
4m
5ft
1.5m
Mangroves
No Access
Buffer Zone
300ft / 91m

island. The site is accessible to snorkelers of all experience levels. Depths range from 5 to 15 feet (1.5 to 4.5 meters) along its length with a maximum depth of just 17 feet, so the site will be more interesting to novice divers.

Description

Cottrell Key gets its name from Capt. Jeremiah Cottrell who once manned a lightship that was anchored off the island that now bears his name. Cottrell Key marks the important northwestern corner of the channel that provides access to Key West from Florida Bay and the broader Gulf of Mexico. This important route was made safer to navigate in the 19th century thanks to the lightship's beacon. Today, a lighted beacon located to the east marks the entrance of the passage.

The shallow ledge marks a transition between a shallow expanse of seagrass beds to the south and a slightly deeper (but still relatively shallow) region of sand. The ledges and undercuts along this section of reef provide shelter for a range of creatures from lobsters to nurse sharks. Conch are regularly spotted in the nearby seagrass, along with stingrays and yellow goatfish. On the reef itself, both hard and soft corals dominate, which provide shelter for gray snapper, highhats, porkfish, white grunts, porcupinefish and yellowtail snapper. Hogfish are commonly seen rooting around in the sand, while bonnethead sharks (the smaller cousin of hammerheads) have been seen hunting for fish in the shallow waters.

As with many other dive and snorkel sites along important navigational lanes in the Florida Keys, debris from unidentified shipwrecks can be found in the area. In most cases, these elements have been fully incorporated into the surrounding reef, making all but the largest sections of old wrecks difficult to identify without scrutiny.

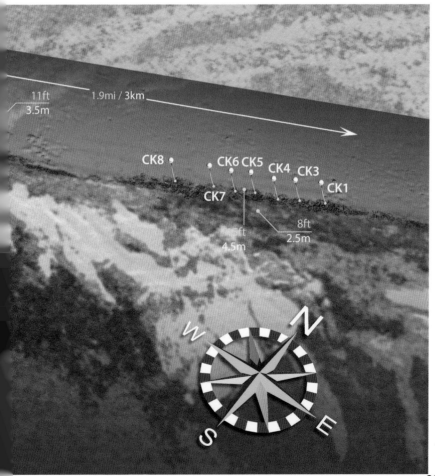

WESTERN DRY ROCKS

Difficulty ● ○ ○
Current ● ● ○
Depth ● ○ ○
Reef ★★★☆
Fauna ★★★☆

Access 🚤 10.5mi (17km) from Key West

Level Open Water

Location Key West

GPS
WDR0 24° 26.710'N, 81° 55.656'W
WDR1 24° 26.707'N, 81° 55.515'W
WDR2 24° 26.703'N, 81° 55.544'W
WDR3 24° 26.688'N, 81° 55.582'W
WDR4 24° 26.680'N, 81° 55.632'W
WDR5 24° 26.697'N, 81° 55.691'W
WDR6 24° 26.754'N, 81° 55.692'W
WDR7 24° 26.763'N, 81° 55.692'W

Getting there

Western Dry Rocks sits on the outer reef line 10.5 miles (17 kilometers) southwest of Key West. Getting there involves a boat ride of 30 to 3 minutes from Key West.

Access

This site is accessible to divers and snorkelers of a levels. There are eight mooring buoys that provid easy access to the spur and groove region of th reef along its southern and western edges. Whil not located within a Sanctuary Preservation Are

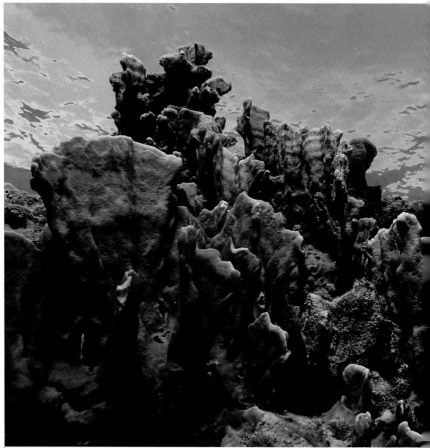

Ben Edmonds ©

Divers and snorkelers should be careful not to brush against the fire coral that is common on reefs in the K

RELAX & RECHARGE

Seaside Cafe at the Mansion (1400 Duval Street, Key West) is consistently ranked one of the best restaurants in Key West. It sits right on the waterfront, just a few yards down the street from the pylon that marks the southernmost point of the continental United States. Seaside Café is located within the grounds of Southernmost House, a large mansion that was once a private residence, but has also been used as a speakeasy, casino, restaurant, hotel and nightclub since its construction in 1896. Five American presidents have stayed there, including Presidents Truman, Eisenhower, Kennedy, Nixon and Carter. Seaside Café serves incredible food options, such as conch fritters, coconut shrimp and honey-butter lobster biscuits. There's also a range of pizza options, including their famous lobster pizza, all cooked in an artisan wood-fired oven. On the liquid side, their mojitos and rum punch are divine. Seaside Café is open from noon to 7pm.
Visit: **Seasidecafekw.com**

SPA) there are regulations in place that prohibit shing from April 1 through July 31.

Description

estern Dry Rocks is a Key West dive and snorkel te that features a shallow set of coral spurs

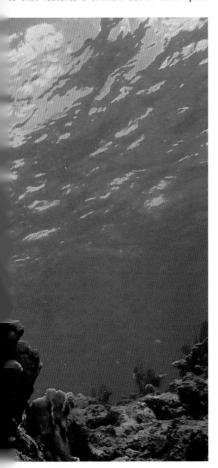

adjacent to a reef slope that descends to a depth well below 100 feet (30.5 meters). It is a popular Key West site because the coral spurs are better defined than in many nearby areas and the reef remains relatively well protected irrespective of the wind direction. Western Dry Rocks typically receives fewer visits than dive and snorkel sites farther to the east because it is farther from Key West.

The shallow coral spurs top out at just 3 feet (1 meter) in depth in some places and may occasionally break the surface of the water at low tide, while the rubble and sand-bottomed grooves reach depths of between 20 and 26 feet (6 and 8 meters). This makes the spur section ideal for snorkelers, who can easily observe the hard and soft corals and many gorgonians on display here. Even experienced divers will find plenty to explore among the spurs and grooves, including lobsters, blue tangs, yellow goatfish and even nurse sharks.

Experienced divers may find the reef more interesting to explore along the deeper slope that extends south of the spurs and grooves. This area features small ledges and caves as well as undercuts and overhangs. Shallow sand and rubble channels run down the slope, creating plenty of habitat for a variety of reef fishes, including French angelfish, blue parrotfish, foureye butterflyfish, bluestriped grunts and schoolmaster snapper. Large barrel sponges dot the slope along with sea fans, and star and brain coral heads. Spotted eagle rays, lemon sharks and even the occasional bull shark have been spotted in the deeper waters at this site. Sea turtles are also semi-regular visitors to the reef at Western Dry Rocks.

This reef is the westernmost shallowest point of the outer reef line near Key West. As a result, it also has claimed many shipwrecks over the centuries. The identities of many of these wrecks

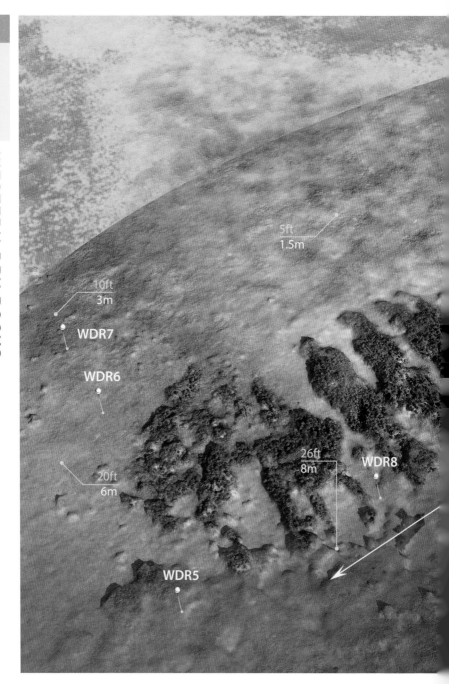

5ft
1.5m

10ft
3m

WDR7

WDR6

20ft
6m

26ft
8m

WDR8

WDR5

remain unknown because little is left of them aside from coral-encrusted debris that has been largely incorporated into the surrounding reef. However, divers exploring the shallower slope will still encounter artifacts that unquestionably originate from these wrecks that are largely lost to time.

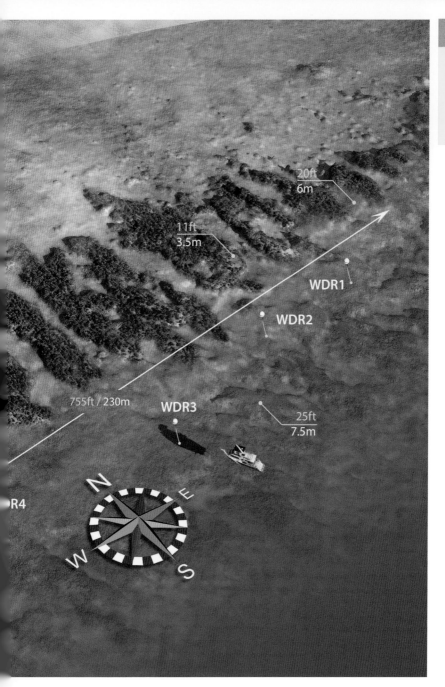

LOST REEF

Difficulty ● ○ ○
Current ● ○ ○
Depth ● ○ ○
Reef ★★☆
Fauna ★★☆

Access 🚤
10.5mi (17km) from Key West

Level Open water

Location Key West
GPS   LR1 24° 26.640'N, 81° 55.989'W

Getting there

Lost Reef sits on the outer reef line, 10.5 miles (17 kilometers) southwest of Key West. It is just to the west of the better-known Western Dry Rocks and getting there involves a boat ride of 30 to 35 minutes from Key West.

Access

This site is suitable for divers and snorkelers o' all levels. A single mooring buoy provides eas access to this small section of reef ledge.

Description

This site features a series of fragmented cora spurs and ledge that tops out at 16 feet (! meters) with sand at 34 feet (10.5 meters). The relief provides habitat for plenty of hard and so corals, as well as bluestriped grunts, porkfish yellowhead wrasses, rock beauties, hogfish an stoplight parrotfish. Longspine squirrelfish ar often seen under ledges and overhangs, whil southern and yellow stingrays are found partial hidden in the sand just off the ledge. Hawksb and loggerhead sea turtles have been known t visit this reef.

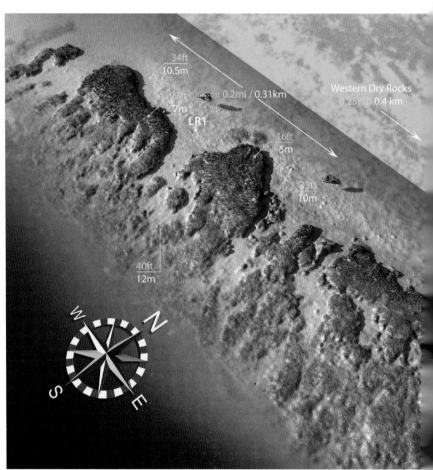

AMESBURY

Difficulty ● ○ ○
Current ● ○ ○
Depth ● ○ ○
Reef ★★★☆ Access 🚤
Fauna ★★★☆ 13mi (21km) from Key West

Level Open Water

Location Key West
GPS 24° 37.397'N, 81° 58.912'W

Getting there
The wreck of the *Amesbury* is found in Florida Bay, just 3 miles (5 kilometers) west of Cottrell Key. Getting there involves a boat ride of 35 to 40 minutes from Key West.

Access
The site is suitable for both divers and snorkelers. A single mooring buoy provides convenient access to the site without the need to anchor and risk damaging or disrupting the wreckage.

Description
USS *Amesbury* was a destroyer built in Massachusetts in 1943 for the U.S. Navy. She was named after Lt. Stanton Amesbury, a naval airman who was killed in action over Casablanca in 1942. The Buckley Class destroyer saw action in the Atlantic Convoy and participated in the Normandy invasion before being temporarily assigned to the Fleet Sonar School in Key West in 1944. She was then refitted and sent over to the Pacific where she saw action in Korea and China in 1945. She was decommissioned and placed in the Reserve Fleet in 1946, and struck from the Naval Register in 1960.

Amesbury was sold for scrap to Chet Alexander Marine Salvage of Key West in 1962 – which is why she is known locally as *Alexander's Wreck*. She ran aground west of Cottrell Key while being towed back to Key West for salvage. A storm battered her weakened hull, and she sank in pieces before she could be refloated. She now sits in two sections roughly 600 feet (180 meters) apart at a depth of about 25 feet (7.5 meters). Some of the debris in the shallow parts of the site are visible at low tide, however, the southern portion of the site includes the bow and portions of the port side, while the northern section includes the stern and portions of the starboard side. Debris is scattered between the two sections and to the east of the site. She is part of the Florida Keys National Marine Sanctuary Shipwreck Trail.

Although out of the way of most dive operators, the wreck is popular as it supports a variety of marine life including bar jacks, white grunts, hogfish, Queen angelfish, foureye butterflyfish and Atlantic spadefish. The shallow nature of the site also makes it great for macro photographers who will have plenty of bottom time to scope-out the numerous anemones and shrimp found here.

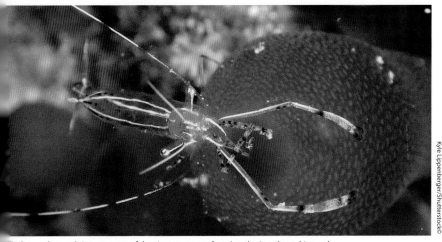

Pederson cleaner shrimp atop one of the giant anemones found on the Amesbury shipwreck.

Name:	USS *Amesbury*	Construction:	Bethlehem-Hingham Shipyard, Hingham, MA, 1943
Type:	Destroyer escort		
Previous names:	n/a	Last owner:	Chet Alexander Marine Salvage
Length:	306ft (93.3m)	Sunk:	Oct 1962
Tonnage:	1,400t		

MARQUESAS KEYS

Difficulty ● ○ ○
Current ● ○ ○
Depth ● ○ ○
Reef ★★☆ Access 🚤
Fauna ★☆☆ 20mi (30km) from Key West

Level n/a

Location Key West
GPS 24° 33.713'N, 82° 07.912'W

Getting there
The Marquesas Keys are a collection of small islands and islets located far to the west of Key West. A handful of snorkel operators visit the site but the boat ride to get there can take an hour or more given the distance involved.

Access
The site is suitable for snorkelers of all levels, particularly the shallow inner lagoon area. Diving is not recommended due to the shallowness of the site. There are no mooring buoys at the Marquesas Keys, so visitors will need to exercise caution when they anchor.

Description
The Marquesas Keys constitute 10 hardwood hammock islands surrounded by stands of mangrove trees. Technically an atoll, it is the only true atoll in North America. The whole area is protected as part of the Marquesas Keys Wildlife Management Area. In addition to the normal protections granted a site within the Florida Keys Marine Sanctuary, there is also a 300-foot (91-meter) no-motor buffer around the three smallest islands of the atoll located along the western edge of the atoll, as well as a 300-foot (91-meter) no access buffer around one mangrove island located just to the southwest of the other three protected islands. Additionally, there is a no-wake zone in the southeast tidal creek.

Snorkelers can explore several hard-bottomed areas in the south that have been colonized by both hard and soft corals. Bermuda chub are common among the shallow waters here, along with damselfish, bluestriped grunts and blue tangs. French angelfish, coney and gray snapper are also regularly spotted in these protected waters. Barracuda and nurse sharks have been known to frequent this area as well.

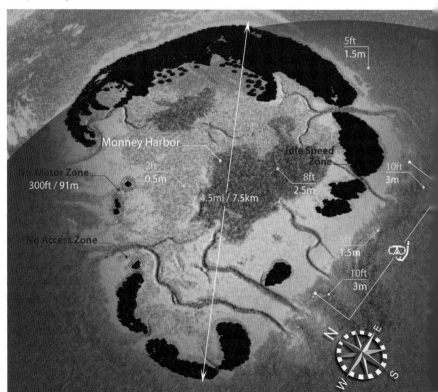

COSGROVE SHOAL

Difficulty ● ● ○
Current   ● ● ○
Depth   ● ● ○
Reef   ★★☆   Access 🛥️
Fauna   ★★☆   25mi (40km) from Key West

Level Open Water

Location Key West
GPS   24° 27.454'N, 82° 11.136'W

Getting there

Cosgrove Shoal is located just west of Marquesas Keys along the outer reef tract of the Florida Keys. It is one of the last sites before the open stretch of ocean that separates the Keys from the Dry Tortugas. Getting there involves a boat ride of over an hour.

Access

Few dive operators venture this far west, and so accessing this site is most often done as part of a private charter or on a personal craft. There are no mooring buoys at this site. The GPS coordinates provided mark a sand patch just southwest of the light tower that marks the shoal.

This site is exposed to waters out of the Gulf of Mexico and Florida Bay, which can reduce visibility. Currents can be moderate at times.

Description

Cosgrove Shoal is a hard bottom bank reef at the edge of the shelf that marks the Florida Keys. There is plenty of marine life for divers and snorkelers willing to explore this remote and less-accessible site. Visitors may see schools of blue and brown chromis, gray angelfish, butter hamlets, bluehead and yellowhead wrasses and multiple parrotfish species, dominated by redband parrotfish. Reef butterflyfish and Queen angelfish are also common, while barracuda hang out in the moderate currents.

COSGROVE SHOAL

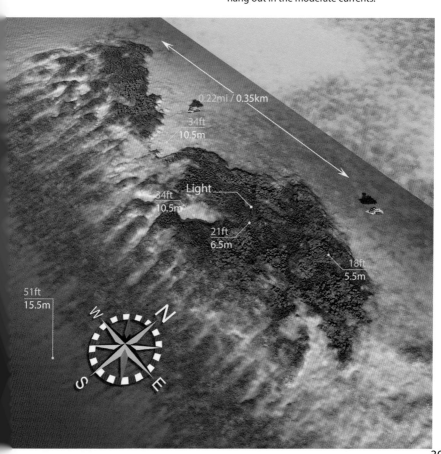

0.22mi / 0.35km
34ft
10.5m

34ft
10.5m   Light
         21ft
         6.5m
                        18ft
                        5.5m

51ft
15.5m

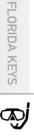
FORT JEFFERSON – DRY TORTUGAS NATIONAL PARK

Difficulty ● ○ ○
Current ● ○ ○
Depth ● ○ ○
Reef ★★★
Fauna ★★☆

Access 🚤 70mi (113km) from Key West

Level n/a

Location Dry Tortugas
GPS 24° 37.775'N, 82° 52.257'W

Getting there

Fort Jefferson is in the Dry Tortugas National Park, nearly 70 miles (110 kilometers) west of Key West. Getting there involves a boat ride of between two and two and a half hours. The Yankee Freedom is the official park ferry and is the most common way for visitors to reach the island – unless they have access to their own boat or a private charter. The cost of the ferry ride is $190 per adult, but includes breakfast and lunch, access to a guided tour of the fort and free rental of snorkeling gear.

Access

Fort Jefferson is suitable for snorkelers of all levels. The white sand beaches and swimming areas provide easy access to the main snorkel sites found just off the western edge of the fort as well as the north and south coaling docks.

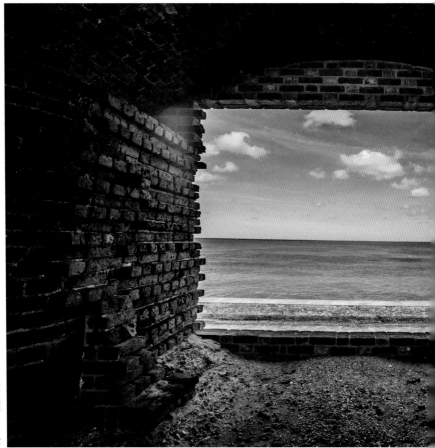

DiBenZ/Shutterstock©

The views from inside Fort Jefferson are spectacul

DID YOU KNOW? ❓

Fort Jefferson is considered the largest all-masonry fort in the western hemisphere. Even though it was never completed, it still incorporates over 16 million bricks and housed over 1,700 people at its peak. During the American Civil War, the fort was occupied by Union forces, which were tasked with ensuring it did not fall into rebel hands. The fort was used to hold prisoners of war, including Union soldiers who had been tried and convicted of desertion or rebellion. The prison population often worked long hours in the hot sun, maintaining and expanding the fortifications. There was little access to freshwater and Fort Jefferson earned the moniker Devil's Island.

Description

Fort Jefferson is built on Garden Key, which is the largest island of the set of shoals and islands first discovered by Ponce de Leon in 1513. The Spanish explorer named the area the Tortugas after the many sea turtles he found here. The "Dry" moniker was added later because the island did not support any fresh water. Even so, the area was often used as a base by pirates to attack merchant shipping lanes in the Gulf of Mexico in the 1600s and 1700s.

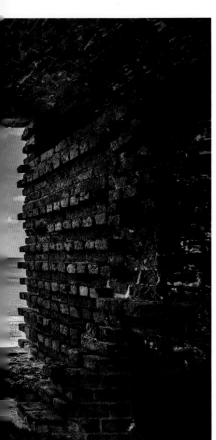

The reefs surrounding the island posed a navigational challenge to early mariners, so a lighthouse was built here in 1825. Construction of the actual fort began in 1846 with the goal of anchoring a line of forts that extended north along the coast, all the way up to Maine. Originally planned as a three-tiered fort, construction was never completed. Parts of the fort began sinking into the sand, and the second tier of the fort was purposefully left incomplete to reduce the structure's weight.

The fort remained active throughout the American Civil War, but by 1888 it was considered to have little military strategic value and with high maintenance costs because of its exposure to hurricanes, the fort was converted into a quarantine site. In 1908, it was listed as a bird reserve, and then designated a national monument by President Franklin D. Roosevelt in 1935. It was further upgraded to a National Park by President George Bush in 1992. Today, visitors can explore the fort and learn about its rich history and cultural heritage – including the Dry Tortugas' connection to Ernest Hemingway.

One of the most popular reasons for visiting the area is to experience the incredible reef life that surrounds the fort and its white sand beaches. The site supports a variety of hard and soft corals, sponges and sea fans, as well as extensive seagrass beds.

One of the most visited sites for snorkelers is along the western moat wall. This section is easily accessed by entering the water from either one of the sandy beaches found just to the south or the north of the fort, and then swimming along the moat wall. More experienced snorkelers might consider entering at the beach and making their way around the shore away from the fort to the ruins of the north and south coaling piers. Snorkelers need to stay close to the pylons of the south coaling dock as the ferry enters and exits the fort through that channel.

Experienced snorkelers may also want to venture away from the fort to the outer reef line. Swimmers can navigate to this section of the reef by heading out along the moat wall

FORT JEFFERSON – DRY TORTUGAS NATIONAL PARK

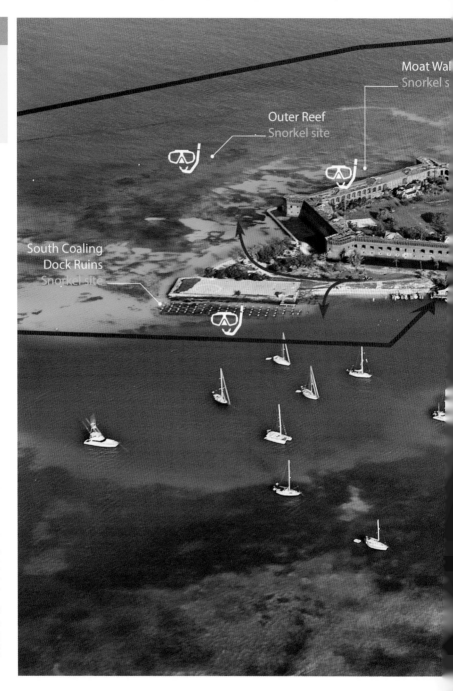

Moat Wal
Snorkel s

Outer Reef
Snorkel site

South Coaling
Dock Ruins
Snorkel site

and then continuing into the open water to the point where the northwest and southwest walls would converge if they extended out beyond the western wall. The more remote nature of this section of reef means that snorkelers will have a chance to see better coral cover and a broader diversity of reef fish.

The waters around Fort Jefferson are teemin with life, including blue tangs, sergeant major yellowtail snapper, Bermuda chub, stripe parrotfish, porkfish, bar jacks and various wrass species. Barracuda are plentiful, particular around the coaling dock piers, while nurse shark and stingrays are often seen on the outer re

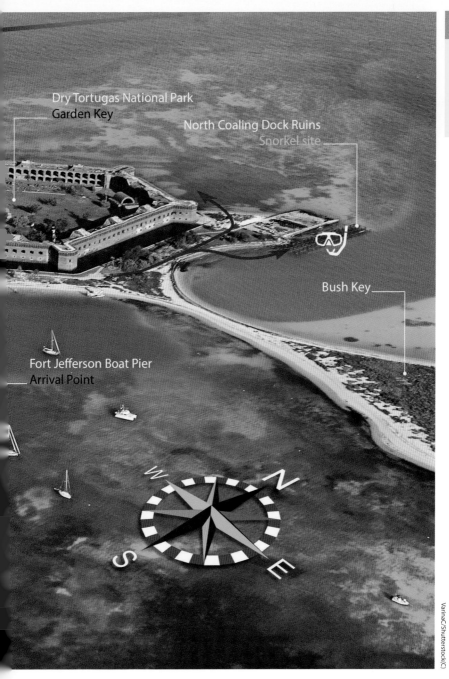

FORT JEFFERSON – DRY TORTUGAS NATIONAL PARK

Dry Tortugas National Park
Garden Key

North Coaling Dock Ruins
Snorkel site

Bush Key

Fort Jefferson Boat Pier
Arrival Point

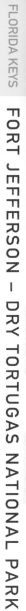

VarnaC/Shutterstock(C)

rea. Snorkelers can also see the sea turtles that
end these islands their name. Green sea turtles
re often spotted here.

Species

Identifying coral reef organisms is an enjoyable part of any underwater adventure. Not only can you appreciate the diversity and wonder that surrounds you on a reef, but you will be better able to understand the story that is unfolding right before your eyes.

For example, you will know where and when to look for certain species, as well as what they eat, who eats them, how big they get and how long they live. But more specifically, you will understand certain behaviors that can be observed on coral reefs, such as why damselfish attack larger creatures or which creatures form symbiotic relationships and why.

Many times, behaviors are an integral part of the identification process. In some cases, understanding how a particular fish behaves,

SAFETY TIP ❶

The section on dangerous species that follows is intended to provide the information you need to recognize the handful of species that can cause injury. These species should not be considered "active threats," but rather organisms that have the potential to cause harm. Most injuries occur because the organism in question has felt threatened and because a diver or snorkeler has not recognized the warning signs. By engaging in safe and conscientious diving and snorkeling practices, and by keeping in mind a few key safety tips, you can avoid having your experience ruined by an unpleasant sting or bite.

Almaco jacks school under the wings of a spotted eagle ray.

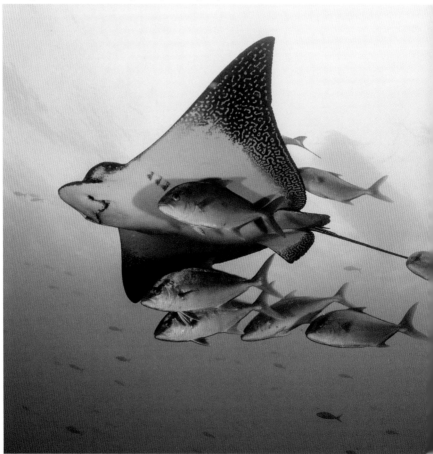

such as whether it is active during the night or day or whether it is an ambush predator or active forager, can be more useful in determining its identity than its color or shape.

Many reef organisms may appear very similar at first glance, and the wide diversity of species on coral reefs can appear to be a chaotic jumble. But by combining an understanding of animal behavior with some basic identification information, you can start to tease apart that puzzle and experience the wonder of the coral reef.

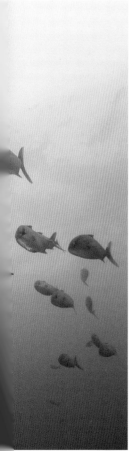

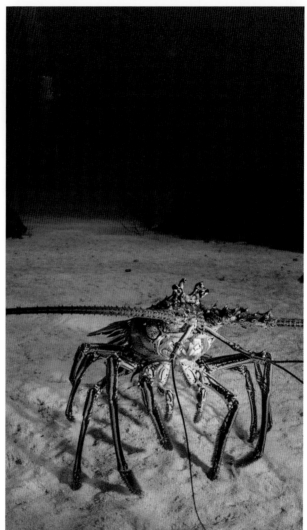

bcampbell65/Shutterstock ©

Spiny lobsters are common on the reefs of the Florida Keys.

The information provided in this guide represents the most up-to-date science available at the time of publication. It covers some of the most common reef species you will find during your time in the Florida Keys. However, it should be noted that ecologists continue to discover new information about species, their behaviors and their interactions. Later editions of this book may contain modifications that reflect new knowledge.

The following pages are divided into three sections that feature information about sea turtles, which have a rather unique life history; dangerous species, including details on the kind of threat they pose and how to treat injuries caused by them; and finally, a general species section that helps you identify and learn about the most common species found at the dive and snorkel sites featured in this guide.

Sea turtle identification

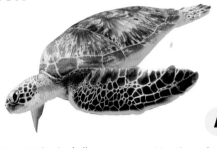

GREEN TURTLE
CHELONIA MYDAS

Maximum size: 4ft (1.4m)
Longevity: Up to 75 years
Habitat: Seagrass beds, reefs
Diet: Jellyfish and crustaceans when young;
algae and seagrass as adults
Sightings: Common

A

Behavior: Green turtles can be found grazing on vegetation in shallow water or cruising the reef. Most green turtles migrate short distances along the coast to reach nesting beaches, but some may migrate up to 1,300 miles (2,100 kilometers) to reach nesting beaches.
Predators (adults): Tiger sharks, orcas (killer whales)

HAWKSBILL SEA TURTLE
ERETMOCHELYS IMBRICATA

Maximum size: 3ft (0.9m)
Longevity: Up to 50 years
Habitat: Reefs
Diet: Sponges, tunicates, squid, shrimp
Sightings: Common

B

Behavior: Hawksbills can be found feeding throughout the day or resting with their bodies wedged into reef cracks and crevices. Some hawksbills do not migrate at all, while others migrate over thousands of miles.
Predators (adults): Tiger sharks, orcas (killer whales)

SEA TURTLE CONSERVATION STATUS: ENDANGERED

All species of sea turtles are endangered and many human activities contribute to their decline.

- Turtles are hunted in many parts of the world, targeting their meat and eggs for food, and their shells to make jewelry, eyeglass frames and curios. Many others drown in fishing nets intended for shrimp or fish, or are struck and killed by passing boats.
- Turtles eat and choke on plastic and other trash, while pollution increases the frequency of turtle disease.
- Coastal development is rapidly reducing the number of active nesting beaches.

ECO TIP

Sea turtles need our help to survive and thrive alongside our coastal communities. Consider the following tips:

LIGHTS OUT
Turn out lights visible from the beach to avoid disorienting nesting turtles and hatchlings.

DON'T LITTER
Plastic cups, bags and other trash can kill turtles when they mistake them for food.

DON'T DISTURB
Turtles you see on the beach or in the water, whether nesting, feeding or hatching, should be left alone and observed from a distance – without flashlights.

PLEASE DON'T FEED
Human food can make sea turtles sick and can leave them vulnerable to capture.

VOLUNTEER
Support your local turtle conservation programs, including participating in beach cleanups.

LOGGERHEAD SEA TURTLE
CARETTA CARETTA

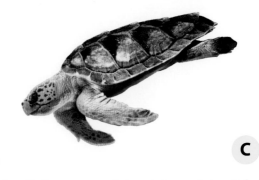

Maximum size: 3.5ft (1.1m)
Longevity: Up to 60 years
Habitat: Reefs and open ocean
Diet: Crabs, shrimp, jellyfish, vegetation
Sightings: Common

C

Behavior: Loggerheads are occasionally found in the open ocean, but regularly move inshore to feed on reef invertebrates. Loggerhead sea turtles can migrate for thousands of miles to reach new feeding grounds before returning to the same nesting beaches.
Predators (adults): Tiger sharks, orcas (killer whales)

LEATHERBACK TURTLE
DERMOCHELYS CORIACEA

Maximum size: Up to 10ft (3m)
Longevity: Up to 80 years
Habitat: Open ocean
Diet: Jellyfish and tunicates
Sightings: Rare

D

Behavior: Leatherbacks feed in deep water during the day and at the surface at night, following the daily migratory patterns of their favorite food: jellyfish. During the mating season, leatherbacks may migrate up to 3,000 miles (4,800 kilometers) from their feeding grounds to their nesting beaches.
Predators (adults): Tiger sharks, orcas (killer whales)

KEMP'S RIDLEY SEA TURTLE
LEPIDOCHELYS KEMPII

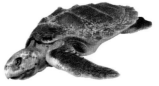

Maximum size: Up to 2ft (0.7m)
Longevity: Up to 50 years
Habitat: Nearshore, shallower water
Diet: Crabs, shellfish, jellyfish and small fish
Sightings: Rare

E

Behavior: Kemp's ridleys are the smallest of the Florida sea turtles, and the only one that nests primarily during the day – 95 percent of their nesting activity takes place in Mexico. They practice mass nesting, where thousands of females come ashore at the same time to lay eggs. Individuals inhabit shallow, coastal waters, using their large, triangular crushing beak to feed on their favorite food: crabs.
Predators (adults): Tiger sharks, orcas (killer whales)

Sea turtle ecology

Nesting

Females generally crawl onto the beach at night (or during the day in the case of Kemp's ridleys) and dig a shallow nest. They lay up to 200 small white eggs before covering the nest and returning to the sea. The eggs incubate for 45 to 70 days, depending on the species.

Mating

Most sea turtles reproduce in the warm summer months except for the leatherback, whose mating season spans fall and winter. Many species migrate great distances to return to the their customary nesting beach. Courtship and mating occur in the shallow waters off shore.

1

Pete Niesen/Shutterstock ©

Adulthood

In adulthood, some sea turtle species return to coastal waters where coral reefs and nearshore waters provide plenty of food and protection from predators.

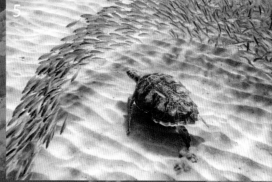

Gail Johnson/Shutterstock ©

UWPhotog /Shutterstock ©

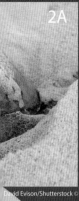
2A

David Evison/Shutterstock ©

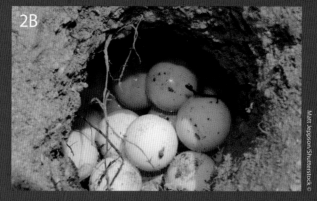
2B

Matt Jeppson/Shutterstock ©

Hatching

At hatching, hundreds of tiny turtles dig their way out of the nest and head toward the moonlight reflecting off the sea. As many as 90 percent are eaten by predators as eggs or as hatchlings within the first few hours of their lives.

3

BlueOrange Studio/Shutterstock ©

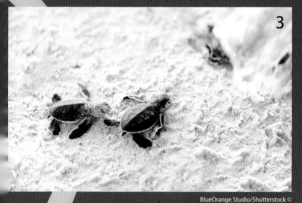

Juvenile stage

Young turtles drift through the open ocean for years, often associating with floating sargassum (seaweed) mats. They feed on plankton and small jellyfish. Little is known about this stage of their lives.

Willyam Bradberry/Shutterstock ©

MEDICAL DISCLAIMER

The treatment advice contained in this book is meant for informational purposes only and is not intended to be a substitute for professional medical advice, either in terms of diagnosis or treatment. Always seek the advice of your physician or other qualified health provider if you are injured by a marine organism. Never disregard professional medical advice or delay seeking it because of something you have read in this book.

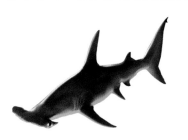

SCALLOPED HAMMERHEAD SHARK
SPHYRNA LEWINI

Maximum size: 14ft (4.3m), 990lb (449kg)
Longevity: About 35 years
Typical depth: 3–984ft (1–300m)
Behavior: Scalloped hammerhead sharks are found in tropical and warm temperate marine waters. Their name comes from the scalloped grooves in their hammer-shaped snout. They specialize in hunting stingrays, but also feed on grouper, snapper, and other shark species.
Predators: Larger shark species and orcas (killer whales)

BULL SHARK
CARCHARHINUS LEUCAS

Maximum size: 13ft (4m), 6,97lb (316kg)
Longevity: Up to 32 years or more
Typical depth: 3–150ft (1–46m)
Behavior: Bull sharks are aggressive and typically inhabit shallow, coastal waters. They are common and considered one of the most dangerous sharks in the world. They tend to feed on bony fishes, rays, other sharks, mammalian carrion and even garbage.
Predators: Larger bull sharks and large crocodiles

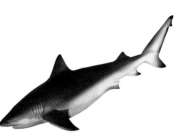

CARIBBEAN REEF SHARK
CARCHARHINUS PEREZII

Maximum size: 10ft (3m) (10ft)
Longevity: Unknown, but possibly 20 years or more
Typical depth: 3–213ft (1–65m)
Behavior: The Caribbean reef shark is the most common shark species encountered on Caribbean coral reefs. They tend to inhabit drop-offs and the seaward edges of reefs where they feed on most reef fish species, as well as stingrays and eagle rays.
Predators: Larger shark species, such as bull and tiger shark

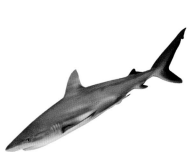

WARNING FOR THESE SHARKS: Attacks on humans by lemon sharks, hammerheads and Caribbean reef sharks are rare, but they have been known to cause injury if threatened or cornered. Warning signs of an attack include head swings, exaggerated swimming, back arching and lowered pectoral fin. Attacks usually result in biting or raking with the teeth, which can cause deep lacerations.

TREATMENT: Exit the water as soon as possible and rinse the affected area with soap and water. Apply pressure to control the bleeding and elevate the affected limb above the heart. Shark bite victims sometimes require treatment for shock, in which case, keep them warm, calm and in the shade, and do not provide anything to eat or drink. Lay them on their back and elevate the legs above the head. Seek medical attention as soon as possible, even for minor bites, for proper cleaning and suturing.

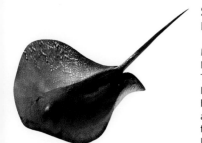

SOUTHERN STINGRAY
DASYATIS AMERICANA

I

Maximum size: 7ft (2m) disk diameter, 300lbs (136kg)
Longevity: Unknown, but probably over 10 years
Typical depth: 0–170ft (0–53m)
Behavior: Stingrays are most active at night when they hunt for hard-shelled prey such as snails, crabs, lobsters and occasionally fish. During the day, they are often found buried up to their eyes in sand.
Predators: Sharks and large grouper

WARNING: Stingrays have a serrated venomous spine at the base of their tail that they use for defense. The area around a puncture wound from this spine may become red and swollen, and you may experience muscle cramps, nausea, fever and chills.

TREATMENT: If you are stung, exit the water immediately. Apply pressure above the wound to reduce bleeding, clean the wound and soak the area with hot water, ideally around 113°F (45°C), to reduce the pain. Apply a dressing and seek medical attention. Antibiotics may be needed to reduce the risk of infection. Stingray injuries can be very painful, often reaching a peak around one hour after the injury and lasting up to two days. But they are rarely fatal unless the injury is to the head, neck or abdomen.

GREAT BARRACUDA
SPHYRAENA BARRACUDA

J

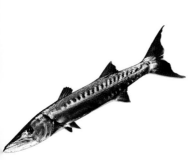

Maximum size: 6ft (2m), 110lbs (50kg)
Longevity: Around 20 years
Typical depth: 1–100m (3–330ft)
Behavior: Barracuda are most active during the day, feeding on jacks, grunts, grouper, snapper, squid and even other barracuda. They are often solitary in nature, but occasionally school in large numbers. They have even been documented "herding" fish they plan on consuming. Barracuda use their keen eyesight to hunt for food. They are one of the fastest fish in the ocean, capable of bursts of speed up to 30mph (48kph). Along with their two sets of razor sharp teeth, there are few prey capable of escaping a barracuda once it decides to attack.
Predators: Sharks, tuna and large grouper

WARNING: Barracuda do not usually attack divers or snorkelers unless provoked. However, evidence suggests they are attracted to objects that glint or shine, such as necklaces, watches or regulators, which they may mistake for prey. The bite of the barracuda is not toxic, but their teeth can produce a severe laceration or deep puncture wound.

TREATMENT: Exit the water as soon as possible and apply pressure to reduce bleeding. The wound should be cleaned and dressed. Medical attention may be necessary for severe bites, including sutures to close the wound and antibiotics to reduce the risk of infection.

SPOTTED SCORPIONFISH
SCORPAENA PLUMIERI

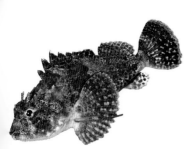

Maximum size: 18in (45cm)
Longevity: Around 15 years
Typical depth: 3–197ft (1–60m)
Behavior: Spotted scorpionfish spend much of their time lying motionless on the seabed, using camouflage to ambush fish and crustaceans. They have a large, expandable mouth capable of creating a vacuum to suck in prey, which they swallow whole.
Predators: Large snapper, sharks, rays and moray eels

315

WARNING: Scorpionfish have a dozen venomous dorsal spines for self-defense. The spines can penetrate skin (most commonly when stepped on), injecting a toxin that causes severe pain that can last from several hours to several days. The area around the injury may also swell and become red.

TREATMENT: Exit the water quickly and rinse the affected area with seawater. Remove any spines and use pressure to control any bleeding. Apply the hottest water you can stand to reduce pain, ideally around 113°F (45°C). Let the wound heal uncovered, but antibiotics may be required to avoid infection. The toxin can be painful, but it is not usually fatal. However, seek medical attention if concerned or if symptoms are worse than described.

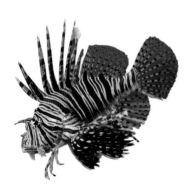

RED LIONFISH
PTEROIS VOLITANS

Maximum size: 15in (38cm)
Longevity: Around 10 years
Typical depth: 7–180ft (2–55m)
Behavior: Red lionfish are originally from the Indo-West Pacific, and are considered an invasive species in the Western Atlantic. They are most active at dusk and during the night when they hunt for fish, shrimp, crabs and other reef creatures. Lionfish can live without food for up to three months.
Predators: Occasional predation by certain sharks and grouper

WARNING: Lionfish have up to 16 venomous dorsal and anal spines that can deliver a powerful neurotoxin when they puncture skin. Lionfish do not generally attack divers and snorkelers, but may sting in self-defense if you get too close. Divers and snorkelers may feel intense pain after being stung, followed by swelling and redness around the wound.

TREATMENT: Exit the water as soon as possible and remove any pieces of the spines that may remain in the wound. Use pressure to control the bleeding and apply the hottest water you can stand, ideally around 113°F (45°C), to reduce the pain. Some people experience shortness of breath, dizziness and nausea. There have been no known fatalities from a lionfish sting, but there is always a risk of complications for vulnerable individuals, including congestive heart failure. Seeking medical attention is advised. The pain may last anywhere from several hours to several days.

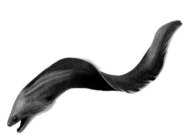

GREEN MORAY EEL
GYMNOTHORAX FUNEBRIS

Maximum size: 8ft (2.5m), 65lbs (30kg)
Longevity: Unknown
Typical depth: 3–164ft (1–50m)
Behavior: Green morays are solitary animals that hide in reef cracks and crevices during the day. At night, they prey on fish, octopuses, crustaceans and even other eels primarily using smell to hunt as their eyesight is poor.
Predators: Unknown

WARNING: Moray eels have sharp teeth that can produce a painful wound, but thankfully they rarely attack unless provoked. There is evidence that the bite of some morays may contain toxins that increase pain and bleeding, but more research is needed. Although all morays can bite, larger species such as the green moray eel can cause more severe injuries than smaller species.

TREATMENT: Exit the water as soon as possible. Treat the wound by immediately cleaning the affected area with soap and water. Apply pressure to reduce the bleeding, then apply a topical antibiotic before dressing the wound to reduce the risk of infection. Sutures may be required in some cases. If in doubt or if the wound becomes infected, seek medical attention.

JELLYFISH & SIPHONOPHORES
HYDROIDOMEDUSAE
& SIPHONOPHORAE

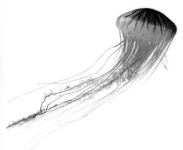

Maximum size: 7ft (2m) with tentacles extending much farther
Longevity: From a few hours to several years
Typical depth: 0–66ft (0–20m)
Behavior: Jellyfish and siphonophores are both types of cnidaria. Jellyfish are individual animals, while siphonophores are colonies of specialized cells called zooids, such as the Portuguese man o' war. They both drift in the water and use stinging cells called nematocysts to capture and paralyze prey, including plankton and small fish.
Predators: Salmon, tuna and some sharks and sea turtle species

WARNING: Jellyfish and siphonophores have stinging cells called nematocysts located on their tentacles that can inject a toxin when brushed against bare skin. Depending on the species, jellyfish toxin can cause mild tingling to intense pain, and can be fatal in some rare cases. The contact site may also become red and blistered. Even dead jellyfish on the beach can sting, so avoid touching them.

TREATMENT: Exit the water as quickly as possible, watching out for other jellyfish. Rinse the affected area with seawater to remove any pieces of tentacle on the skin. Do not rinse with fresh water, which can trigger any remaining nematocysts to sting. The best treatment for jellyfish stings may depend on the species, but most can be treated by rinsing the affected area with vinegar or creating a paste using baking soda and seawater. The papain enzyme found in meat tenderizer and papaya can also help. Consider seeking medical attention.

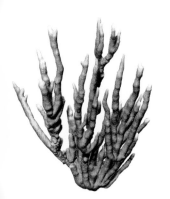

FIRE CORAL
MILLEPORIDAE

Maximum size: 3ft (1m)
Longevity: Unknown, but likely decades
Typical depth: 3–130ft (1–40m)
Behavior: Several fire coral species occur in the Caribbean, attaching to the reef substrate and growing in branching, blade and encrusting forms. Fire corals are hydroids with a hard skeleton, and are more closely related to jellyfish than corals. They get their energy from photosynthetic zooxanthellae in their tissues, but also from feeding on plankton.
Predators: Fireworms, certain nudibranchs and filefish

WARNING: Microscopic fire coral polyps are located throughout the surface of the hard skeleton. Each polyp has hair-like tentacles that are covered in stinging cells called nematocysts, which they use to paralyze their tiny prey. Fire corals cause a lingering, burning sensation when they contact bare skin. A rash or blistering may occur in some individuals and may last several days, but is not usually dangerous.

TREATMENT: Exit the water as soon as possible and rinse the affected area with vinegar or alcohol to inactivate the fire coral toxin. Do not rinse with fresh water, which can increase the pain by causing untriggered nematocysts to discharge into the skin. Apply hydrocortisone cream to the area once dry. The papain enzyme found in meat tenderizer and papaya can also reduce swelling, pain and itching.

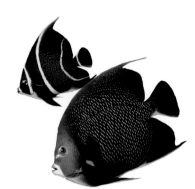

FRENCH ANGELFISH
POMACANTHUS PARU

1

Maximum size: 24in (60cm)
Longevity: Up to 15 years
Typical depth: 10–330ft (3–100m)
Behavior: French angelfish dine primarily on sponges, but may also feed on gorgonians and algae. Juveniles often act as cleaners, eating the parasites from other reef fish. At dusk, French angelfish find shelter from nocturnal predators in reef cracks and crevices.
Predators: Large grouper and sharks

GRAY ANGELFISH
POMACANTHUS ARCUATUS

2

Maximum size: 24in (60cm)
Longevity: Unknown, possibly up to 15 years
Typical depth: 6–100ft (2–30m)
Behavior: Gray angelfish are often seen swimming in pairs as they are known to form long-term monogamous breeding pairs. They are recognizable by their gray-brown bodies and pale gray-white mouths. They frequent coral reefs, feeding on sponges, tunicates, hydroids, algae and sometimes seagrass.
Predators: Large grouper and sharks

BLUE ANGELFISH
HOLACANTHUS BERMUDENSIS

3

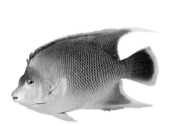

Maximum size: 18in (45cm)
Longevity: Unknown, possibly up to 15 years
Typical depth: 6–300ft (2–91m)
Behavior: Blue angelfish are often mistaken for queen angelfish, but they lack the distinct forehead crown and are paler in color. Like most angelfish, they are often seen swimming in pairs, foraging on sponges and small benthic invertebrates. At night, they sleep hidden away in the reef, safe from predators.
Predators: Large grouper and sharks

QUEEN ANGELFISH
HOLACANTHUS CILIARIS

4

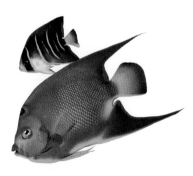

Maximum size: 18in (45cm)
Longevity: Up to 15 years
Typical depth: 3–230ft (1–70m)
Behavior: Queen angelfish are often found swimming gracefully between seafans, sea whips and corals, alone or in pairs. They feed almost exclusively on sponges but have been known to snack on algae and tunicates as well. Young Queen angelfish also clean parasites off larger fish.
Predators: Large grouper and sharks

ROCK BEAUTY
HOLACANTHUS TRICOLOR

5

Maximum size: 14in (35cm)
Longevity: Up to 20 years (in captivity)
Typical depth: 10–115ft (3–35m)
Behavior: Adult rock beauties are often found on rock jetties, rocky reefs and rich coral areas, while juveniles tend to be found near fire corals. These angelfish are not picky eaters and will feed on tunicates, sponges, zoanthids and algae.
Predators: Grouper, snapper and sharks

BLUE TANG
ACANTHURUS COERULEUS

6

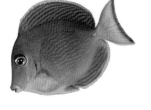

Maximum size: 16in (40cm)
Longevity: Around 20 years
Typical depth: 3–130ft (1–40m)
Behavior: Blue tangs are often found grazing on algae during the day, either individually or as part of large schools that may also contain surgeonfish, doctorfish, goatfish and parrotfish. At dusk, they settle into a reef crack or crevice to hide for the night.
Predators: Grouper, snapper, jacks and barracuda

DOCTORFISH
ACANTHURUS CHIRUGUS

7

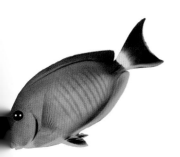

Maximum size: 15.5in (39cm)
Longevity: Up to 30 years
Typical depth: 6–213ft (2–65m)
Behavior: Doctorfish can be found in shallow, inshore reef habitats and rocky areas. They forage on benthic algae, including the thin algal mat covering sandy bottoms. They generally swim together in loose schools, often with ocean surgeonfish and blue tangs. They have sharp spines near their tail fin that they can use in defense against predators.
Predators: Large carnivorous fish, including tuna

OCEAN SURGEONFISH
ACANTHURUS BAHIANUS

8

Maximum size: 15in (38cm)
Longevity: Up to 32 years
Typical depth: 6–130ft (2–40m)
Behavior: Adult surgeonfish often form large schools to graze on benthic algae and seagrasses in shallow coral reefs and inshore rocky areas. Juveniles rarely school, sheltering instead in the back reef. Researchers have observed spawning aggregations of up to 20,000 individuals in the winter months off of Puerto Rico.
Predators: Sharks, grouper, barracuda and snapper

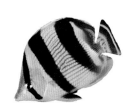

BANDED BUTTERFLYFISH
CHAETODON STRIATUS

9

Maximum size: 6in (16cm)
Longevity: Unknown, but probably around 10 years
Typical depth: 10–60ft (3–20m)
Behavior: Banded butterflyfish are most active during the day when they search the reef for food, which includes polychaete worms, zoanthids, anemones and fish eggs. Banded butterflyfish are often found in monogamous pairs and they defend a joint territory together with their mate.
Predators: Moray eels and large carnivorous fish

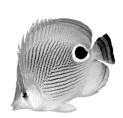

FOUREYE BUTTERFLYFISH
CHAETODON CAPISTRATUS

10

Maximum size: 6in (15cm)
Longevity: Around 8 years
Typical depth: 6–65ft (2–20m)
Behavior: Foureye butterflyfish are active during the day when they feed on small invertebrates. Their pointed mouth allows them to pull prey from small crevices. They are often found in pairs, and males and females bond early in life and form long-lasting monogamous pairs.
Predators: Barracuda, grouper, snapper and moray eels

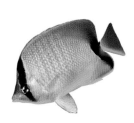

REEF BUTTERFLYFISH
CHAETODON SEDENTARIUS

11

Maximum size: 6in (15cm)
Longevity: Unknown, but probably around 10 years
Typical depth: 16–302ft (5–92m)
Behavior: This species is one of the deepest dwelling Caribbean butterflyfish. Like many members of the family, their color and pattern disguise the head in an attempt to confuse potential predators. Reef butterflyfish are most active during the day when they feed on polychaete worms and small crustaceans. They particularly like to eat the eggs of sergeant majors.
Predators: Barracuda, grouper, snapper and moray eels

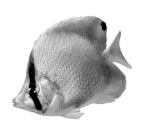

SPOTFIN BUTTERFLYFISH
CHAETODON OCELLATUS

12

Maximum size: 8in (20cm)
Longevity: Unknown, but probably around 10 years
Typical depth: 3–98ft (1–30m)
Behavior: The spotfin butterflyfish can be identified the small spot on the rear end of the dorsal fin. This species is found over an incredibly large geographic area, extending from southern Brazil to as far north Nova Scotia, Canada. Spotfin butterflyfish are most active during the day when they search for food, which includes polychaete worms, zoanthids, anemones and fish eggs.
Predators: Barracuda, grouper, snapper and moray eels

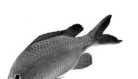

BLUE CHROMIS
CHROMIS CYANEA

13

Maximum size: 5in (12cm)
Longevity: Unknown, possibly 5 years
Typical depth: 10–70ft (3–20m)
Behavior: Blue chromis gather in schools above the reef to feed on small plankton and jellyfish during the day. They hide in reef crevices at night. Territorial males defend egg nests in the spring and summer.
Predators: Trumpetfish, grouper and snapper

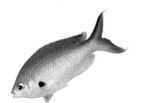

BROWN CHROMIS
CHROMIS MULTILINEATA

14

Maximum size: 8in (20cm)
Longevity: Unknown, possibly 5 years
Typical depth: 3–300ft (1–91m)
Behavior: Brown chromis forage in medium-sized schools above the coral reef, feasting on plankton, mainly copepods. They are frequently seen schooling with blue chromis during the day, although their more territorial congeneric tends to chase them out from hiding places in the reef at night.
Predators: Trumpetfish, grouper and snapper

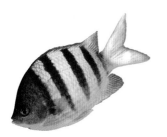

SERGEANT MAJOR
ABUDEFDUF SAXATILIS

15

Maximum size: 9in (23cm)
Longevity: Unknown, possibly 5 years
Typical depth: 3–33ft (1–10m)
Behavior: Sergeant majors get their name from their telltale black bars that resemble military stripes. They are usually found in shallow water, typically along the tops of reefs, and often form large feeding schools of up to a few hundred individuals.
Predators: Grouper and jacks

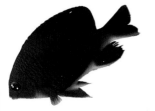

THREESPOT DAMSELFISH
STEGASTES PLANIFRONS

16

Maximum size: 5in (13cm)
Longevity: Around 15 years
Typical depth: 3–100ft (1–30m)
Behavior: Threespot damselfish tend small gardens of algae. Males use these gardens to attract a mate. If successful, the female will lay her eggs in the male's territory and he will defend them aggressively until they hatch. Threespot damselfish feed on tiny plant-like organisms called epiphytes that grow on the algae they cultivate.
Predators: Grouper and jacks

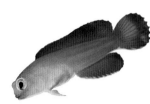

YELLOWHEAD JAWFISH
OPISTOGNATHUS AURIFRONS

17

Maximum size: 4in (10cm)
Longevity: Unknown, possibly up to 5 years
Typical depth: 10–131ft (3–40m)
Behavior: Jawfish live in burrows in the sediment that they line with stones and bits of crushed shell and coral. Active during the day, they often hover over their burrow and feed on zooplankton. They rarely move far from their burrow and often retreat tail-first when threatened.
Predators: Snapper, grouper and lionfish

ROSY RAZORFISH
XYRICHTYS MARTINICENSIS

18

Maximum size: 6in (15cm)
Longevity: Around 3 years
Typical depth: 7–69ft (2–21m)
Behavior: Rosy razorfish are commonly found in open sandy areas near coral reefs. They are active during the day as they feed on small sand-dwelling invertebrates such as crabs, shrimp and worms. Large males often defend a harem of females within their territory.
Predators: Grouper, snapper, barracuda and dolphins

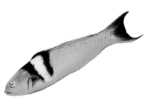

BLUEHEAD WRASSE
THALASSOMA BIFASCIATUM

1

Maximum size: 10in (25cm)
Longevity: 3 years
Typical depth: 0–131ft (0–40m)
Behavior: Bluehead wrasses can be found on reef near inshore bays and over seagrass beds feeding o zooplankton, small benthic animals and even parasite on other fish. They start life as female but eventual become males, gaining an unmistakable bright blu head in their terminal phase.
Predators: Grouper, trumpetfish and soapfish

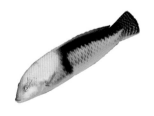

YELLOWHEAD WRASSE
HALICHOERES GARNOTI

2

Maximum size: 7in (19cm)
Longevity: Unknown, possibly between 3 and 5 years
Typical depth: 3–100ft (1–30m)
Behavior: Yellowhead wrasses are mainly found ne coral reefs and rocky ledges. Adults feed on invertebrat while juveniles sometimes clean parasites off larger fis Yellowhead wrasses are protogynous hermaphrodite meaning they start life as female but become males around 3in (7cm) in size.
Predators: Mackerel, grouper and snapper

CREOLE WRASSE
CLEPTICUS PARRAE
21

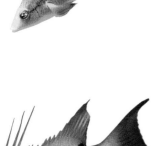

Maximum size: 12in (30cm)
Longevity: Unknown, but probably around 10 years
Typical depth: 26–328ft (8–100m)
Behavior: Creole wrasses are often found schooling in large numbers above bank reefs, wrecks and on the seaward slopes of reefs. They are most active during the day, when feeding on plankton and small jellyfish. At night, they retreat into reef crevices to sleep.
Predators: Moray eels, grouper and barracuda

SPANISH HOGFISH
BODIANUS RUFUS
22

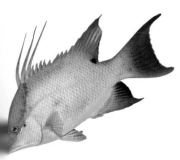

Maximum size: 16in (40cm)
Longevity: Unknown
Typical depth: 10–230ft (3–70m)
Behavior: Adult Spanish hogfish feed on bottom-dwelling invertebrates, such as brittlestars, crustaceans and sea urchins. Juveniles set up cleaning stations to pick parasites off larger fish. Male hogfish (who start out life as a female) typically manage a harem of three to 12 smaller females.
Predators: Sharks, mackerel and snapper

HOGFISH
LACHNOLAIMUS MAXIMUS
23

Maximum size: 36in (91cm)
Longevity: Up to16 years
Typical depth: 10–100ft (3–30m)
Behavior: Hogfish live in small groups with a dominant male and several smaller females – a common pattern in wrasses. Their name comes from how they root around in the sand with their snout looking for crustaceans and mollusks. Larger individuals frequent the main reef, while smaller individuals are often on patch reefs.
Predators: Sharks and large grouper

PRINCESS PARROTFISH
SCARUS TAENIOPTERUS
24

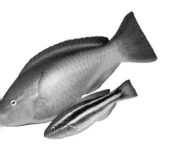

Max size: 14in (35cm)
Longevity: Unknown, but probably less than 5 years
Typical depth: 3–82ft (1–25m)
Behavior: Princess parrotfish form large schools during the day to feed on plants, algae, sponges and seagrass. Juveniles are more closely associated with seagrass beds. They start out life as female, but can transition to male if no other large breeding males are around.
Predators: Sharks, grouper, jacks and moray eels

QUEEN PARROTFISH
SCARUS VETULA

25

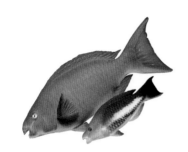

Maximum size: 24 in (61 cm)
Longevity: Up to 20 years
Typical depth: 10–80 ft (3–25 m)
Behavior: During the day, Queen parrotfish feed by
scraping algae off rocks and dead coral using their
tough, parrot-like beak. At night, Queen parrotfish
secrete a membrane of mucus from a gland at the base
of the gills which surrounds them like a bubble and
masks their scent from nocturnal predators.
Predators: Grouper, eels and sharks

STOPLIGHT PARROTFISH
SPARISOMA VIRIDE

26

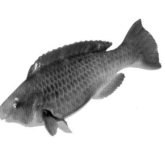

Maximum size: 25in (64cm)
Longevity: Around 9 years
Typical depth: 3–164ft (1–50m)
Behavior: Stoplight parrotfish are only active during
the day. Their strong beak-like jaws scrape soft algae of
the hard coral. They ingest some coral in the process,
grinding it up with the help of specialized teeth in their
throats and excreting it as coral sand.
Predators: Sharks, barracuda, grouper, snapper, jack
and moray eels

BLUE PARROTFISH
SCARUS COERULEUS

27

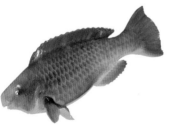

Maximum size: 4ft (1.2m)
Longevity: About 10 years
Typical depth: 10–82ft (3–25m)
Behavior: The blue parrotfish is easily identified by i
prominent bulging snout and color, as it is the on
blue parrotfish. It feeds during the day by biting o
pieces of the reef in order to consume plants, algae ar
small organisms. This species can form large school
particularly during spawning.
Predators: Large grouper, snapper, moray eels and barracud

MIDNIGHT PARROTFISH
SCARUS COELESTINUS

28

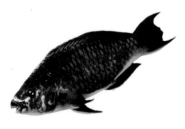

Maximum size: 30in (77cm)
Longevity: Unknown, but possibly up to 10 years
Typical depth: 16–264ft (5–75m)
Behavior: Midnight parrotfish are among the larg
parrotfish species in the Caribbean, and are recognizab
for their dark blue-black coloration. They can often
spotted schooling with surgeonfish as they munch
algae-encrusted coral. They are typically associated w
coral reefs and sport the telltale beak of all parrotfish.
Predators: Sharks, mackerel and jacks

RAINBOW PARROTFISH
SCARUS GUACAMAIA

29

Maximum size: 4ft (1.2m)
Longevity: Around 10 years
Typical depth: 10–82ft (3–25m)
Behavior: The rainbow parrotfish is the largest herbivorous reef fish in the Caribbean. During the day, it feeds by biting off pieces of the reef in order to consume the plants, algae and small organisms contained within. Schooling may occur in areas where density is high.
Predators: Large grouper, snapper, moray eels, sharks and barracuda

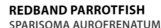

REDBAND PARROTFISH
SPARISOMA AUROFRENATUM

30

Maximum size: 11in (28cm)
Longevity: Around 5 years
Typical Depth: 6.5–65ft (2–20m)
Behavior: The redband is one of the smaller species of Caribbean parrotfish. They are common throughout the region and are even found as far east as Bermuda. They are active during the day and are often found feeding on algae by biting off pieces of reef. They occur either alone or in small groups, especially when young. Males and females differ in coloration and form harems, where spawning occurs year-round, usually early in the morning.
Predators: Grouper, barracuda and moray eels

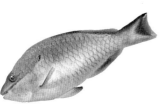

PORKFISH
ANISOTREMUS VIRGINICUS

31

Maximum size: 16in (40.5cm)
Longevity: Unknown
Typical depth: 0–131ft (0–40m)
Behavior: Porkfish are abundant in Florida waters, particularly on reefs and rocky bottoms. They adapt to new habitats, which makes them common on artificial reefs. They cruise the reef slowly during the day, often in schools. At night, they hunt for mollusks, echinoderms (sea stars and urchins) and crustaceans.
Predators: Grouper and jacks

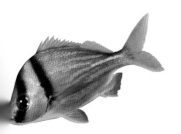

TOMTATE
HAEMULON AUROLINEATUM

32

Maximum size: 10in (25cm)
Longevity: Unknown, but probably around 10 years
Typical depth: 3–98ft (1–30m)
Behavior: The tomtate is by far the most common member of the grunt family in Florida. This species is found in large schools on coral reefs, but forms pairs for breeding. They have a varied diet consisting of small crustaceans, mollusks, polychaetes, plankton and algae.
Predators: Grouper, snapper, trumpetfish and scorpionfish

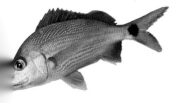

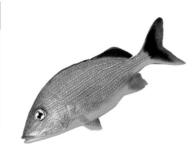

BLUE STRIPED GRUNT
HAEMULON SCIURUS

33

Maximum size: 18in (46cm)
Longevity: 12 years
Typical depth: 3–98ft (1–30m)
Behavior: One of the largest members of the gru
family, the blue stripe is also one of the most bright
colored, sporting numerous gold and blue stripe
Juveniles begin life in seagrass beds and move to cor
reefs as they become adults. This species can form larç
schools and is often wary of divers.
Predators: Grouper, snapper, barracuda and sharks

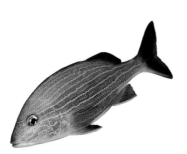

CAESAR GRUNT
HAEMULON CARBONARIUM

3

Max size: 16in (40cm)
Longevity: Unknown, but possibly up to 10 years
Typical depth: 10–82ft (3–25m)
Behavior: Caesar grunts are often found in schools ne
artificial reefs and over rocky reefs. Like most grun
they are nocturnal feeders, munching on polychaet
gastropods and small crustaceans. During the d
they form loose schools under overhangs. Unlike oth
grunts, however, juveniles settle on shallow reefs a
not near mangroves or seagrass beds.
Predators: Sharks, grouper, jacks and moray eels

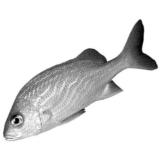
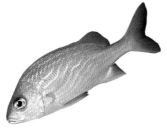

FRENCH GRUNT
HAEMULON FLAVOLINEATUM

3!

Maximum size: 12in (30cm)
Longevity: Unknown, could be up to 12 years
Typical depth: 3–400ft (1–60m)
Behavior: French grunts form large schools on rocky a
coral reefs. During the day, adults can often be fou
resting under ledges and near elkhorn coral. Juveni
spend the day hiding near the shore. French grur
are nocturnal and typically feed on small crustacea
polychaetes and mollusks.
Predators: Grouper, snapper and trumpetfish

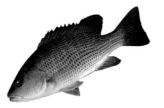

GRAY SNAPPER
LUTJANUS GRISEUS

3

Maximum size: 35in (90cm), 44lb (20kg)
Longevity: Around 20 years
Typical depth: 16–590ft (5–180m)
Behavior: Gray snappers are often found school
sometimes in large numbers. They feed mainly at ni
on a range of organisms, including shrimp, crabs, wo
and small fishes, rarely moving far to feed.
Predators: Moray eels, sharks, large grouper
and barracuda

MAHOGANY SNAPPER
LUTJANUS MAHOGONI

37

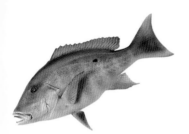

Maximum size: 19in (48cm)
Longevity: Around 20 years
Typical depth: 3–330ft (1–100m)
Behavior: This smaller snapper forms large schools during the day, typically in shallower waters over coral reefs. At night, mahogany snapper feed on small fish, shrimp, crabs and cephalopods. They frequent warmer waters and only stray into temperate climates during the heat of summer.
Predators: Sharks, mackerel and other snapper

MUTTON SNAPPER
LUTJANUS ANALIS

38

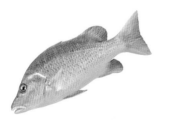

Maximum size: 37in (94cm), 34lb (15.6kg)
Longevity: 29 years
Typical depth: 82–311ft (25–95m)
Behavior: Mutton snappers can be identified by the small black spot located on their upper back. Many individuals also have one or two blue stripes that run across the cheek and around the eye. Mutton snappers feed both day and night on a mix of fish, crustaceans and gastropods. They are very popular fish with anglers and spearfishers and though size and bag limits exist, the species is still listed as "near threatened" by the IUCN Red List.
Predators: Sharks, large grouper, moray eels, and barracuda

SCHOOLMASTER SNAPPER
LUTJANUS APODUS

39

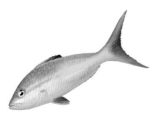

Maximum size: 26in (67cm)
Longevity: Up to 42 years
Typical depth: 6–207ft (2–63m)
Behavior: Schoolmaster snapper are found in shallow coastal waters in coral reefs and mangrove habitats – adults are often associated with elkhorn corals while younger individuals sometimes enter brackish waters. They feed on crustaceans and cephalopods, although adults also show a preference for fish once their mouth can open wide enough to catch them.
Predators: Sharks, barracuda and grouper

YELLOWTAIL SNAPPER
OCYURUS CHRYSURUS

40

Maximum size: 34in (86cm), 9lb (4kg)
Longevity: Around 13 to 17 years
Typical depth: 3–541ft (1–165m)
Behavior: Yellowtail snapper are typically associated with coral reefs in coastal waters from the U.S. state of Massachusetts, down to the coast of Brazil. They often form schools above reefs and are less commonly seen along the seafloor. They eat plankton and small benthic organisms.
Predators: Sharks, barracuda, mackerel, snapper and grouper

GLASSEYE SNAPPER
HETEROPRIACANTHUS CRUENTATUS

41

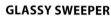

Maximum size: 20in (51cm)
Longevity: Unknown
Typical depth: 10–115ft (3–35m)
Behavior: Glasseye snapper are secretive fish, hiding alone or in small groups in holes and crevices during the day. At night, they exit their shelters to feed on octopuses, pelagic shrimp, crabs, small fishes and polychaete worms. They sometimes form larger schools at dusk.
Predators: Sharks, tuna, grouper and mahi mahi

GLASSY SWEEPER
PEMPHERIS SCHOMBURGKII

42

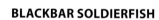

Maximum size: 6in (15cm)
Longevity: Unknown
Typical depth: 10–98ft (3–30m)
Behavior: The nocturnal glassy sweeper is a small fish that feeds on zooplankton and small crustaceans in the water above the reef. During the day, it shelters in groups, hiding in reef crevices and caves. Juveniles are nearly transparent – likely the origin of their name.
Predators: Rays and grouper

BLACKBAR SOLDIERFISH
MYRIPRISTIS JACOBUS

4:

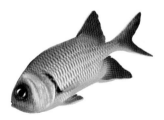

Maximum size: 10in (25cm)
Longevity: Unknown
Typical depth: 7–115ft (2–35m)
Behavior: Blackbar soldierfish are nocturnal, often hiding in caves and crevices during the day. They congregate around coral and rocky reefs at night to feed on plankton and invertebrates. They most commonly occur on shallow inshore reefs, but can be found at depths of 330ft (100m).
Predators: Snapper, grouper, jacks and trumpetfish

LONGSPINE SQUIRRELFISH
HOLOCENTRUS RUFUS

4

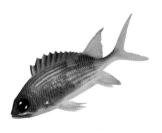

Maximum size: 14in (35cm)
Longevity: Unknown, but potentially up to 14 years
Typical depth: 0–105ft (0–32m)
Behavior: Longspine squirrelfish often form schools of 8 to 10 individuals at night when they forage for benthic organisms, such as crabs, shrimp, gastropods and brittlestars. During the day, these big-eyed fish seek shelter in holes and crevices in the reef, defending them from other squirrelfish.
Predators: Sharks, grouper, snapper and trumpetfish

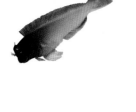

CLEANING GOBY
ELACATINUS GENIE

45

Maximum size: 2in (4cm)
Longevity: 3 to 5 years
Typical depth: 3–98ft (1–30m)
Behavior: As their name suggests, cleaning gobies clean other reef creatures by removing their parasites. This behavior is a form of symbiosis known as mutualism, where both parties benefit. The client fish get rid of their ectoparasites, while the cleaners get an easy meal.
Predators: Grouper, snapper and moray eels

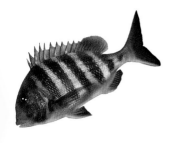

REDLIP BLENNY
OPHIOBLENNIUS ATLANTICUS

46

Maximum size: 7in (19cm)
Longevity: Around 2 years
Typical depth: 0–27ft (0–8m)
Behavior: Redlip blennies are common in shallow reef areas with relatively high wave action. Their body shape and modified fins let them "hold on" to the reef. They are herbivorous and territorial, defending a patch of algae during the day and hiding in the reef at night.
Predators: Grouper, snapper and trumpetfish

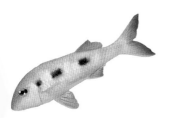

SHEEPSHEAD PORGY
ARCHOSARGUS PROBATOCEPHALUS

47

Maximum size: 36in (91cm)
Longevity: Around 20 years
Typical depth: 3–49ft (1–15m)
Behavior: The sheepshead porgy is an important species for the recreational fishing industry in Florida. Also called convict fish due to their striped appearance, they are found in many habitats, including rocky reefs and seagrass beds, as well as around jetties and piers. They are omnivorous, feeding on algae and invertebrates.
Predators: Sharks, grouper and other large carnivorous fish

SPOTTED GOATFISH
PSEUDUPENEUS MACULATUS

48

Maximum size: 12in (30cm)
Longevity: At least 7 years
Typical depth: 0–115ft (0–35m)
Behavior: Spotted goatfish are most often encountered in shallow water over rocky or sandy habitat near reefs. They feed on bottom-dwelling crabs, shrimp and small fish. Spotted goatfish are easily recognizable by the three dark blotches along their back and the telltale barbels they use to stir up the sand when they hunt.
Predators: Sharks, snapper and jacks

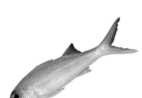
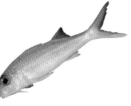

YELLOW GOATFISH
MULLOIDICHTHYS MARTINICUS   **49**

Maximum size: 15in (39cm)
Longevity: Unknown
Typical depth: 0–115ft (0–35m)
Behavior: Yellow goatfish are commonly found swimming in large schools over sandy bottoms. They use their long, sensitive barbels to locate polychaete worms, clams, isopods, amphipods and other crustaceans in the sand. When not feeding, they are often found in groups sheltering in the reef.
Predators: Sharks, tuna, mahi mahi, grouper and jacks

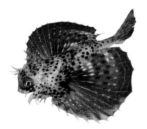

FLYING GURNARD
DACTYLOPTERUS VOLITANS   **50**

Maximum size: 21in (50cm)
Longevity: Unknown, but likely more than 5 years
Typical depth: 3–262ft (1–80m)
Behavior: Flying gurnards are often found along sand bottomed areas near the reef, foraging for benthic crustaceans, crabs, clams and small fishes. They get their name from their fan-like pectoral fins that make it look like they are flying when they swim.
Predators: Sharks, tuna, mahi mahi, grouper and bigeye

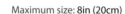
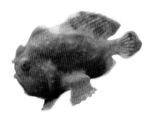

LONGLURE FROGFISH
ANTENNARIUS MULTIOCELLATUS   **5**

Maximum size: 8in (20cm)
Longevity: Unknown, but probably around 10 years
Typical depth: 0–215ft (0–66m)
Behavior: The longlure frogfish is a bottom-dwelling fish that can change color and texture to blend in with its surroundings. It is an ambush predator, feeding mainly on other fish and crustaceans. Frogfish have one of the fastest attacks in the animal kingdom.
Predators: Moray eels and other frogfish

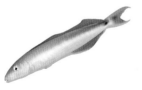

SAND TILEFISH
MALACANTHUS PLUMIERI   **5**

Maximum size: 28in (70cm)
Longevity: Unknown, but potentially as much as 40 years
Typical depth: 33–164ft (10–50m)
Behavior: Sand tilefish build tunnels and mounds in the sand- and rubble-bottomed areas near reefs and seagrass beds. Tunnel entrances can reach 10ft (3m) in diameter and the mounds are built out of the sand, coral rubble and shell fragments found during excavation.
Predators: Sharks and snapper

PEACOCK FLOUNDER
BOTHUS LUNATUS
53

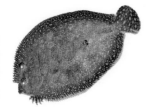

Maximum size: 18in (46cm)
Longevity: Up to 10 years
Typical depth: 0–66ft (0–20m)
Behavior: Peacock flounders are usually found partially buried in loose sand near coral reefs, mangroves and seagrass beds. They are the most common flounders around coral reefs, and mainly feed on small fishes, but also crustaceans and small octopuses.
Predators: Sharks and snapper

BROWN GARDEN EEL
HETEROCONGER LONGISSIMUS
54

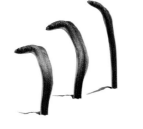

Maximum size: 20in (50cm)
Longevity: Unknown
Typical depth: 33–197ft (10–60m)
Behavior: Brown garden eels live in burrows in sandy areas near coral reefs, feeding mainly on plankton that drift by in the current. Individuals rarely leave the safety of their burrows, remaining partially buried with their heads poking out from the sand. They retreat backwards into their burrow when threatened.
Predators: Snake eels and triggerfish

GOLDENTAIL MORAY EEL
GYMNOTHORAX MILIARIS
55

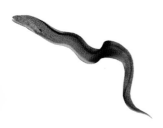

Maximum size: 28in (70cm)
Longevity: Unknown
Typical depth: 0–115ft (0–35m)
Behavior: Goldentail moray eels are common in the Caribbean, living alone in holes and crevices in coral reefs. Unlike other types of morays, goldentails are most active during the day. They feed on fish, mollusks and crustaceans.
Predators: Grouper

SPOTTED MORAY EEL
GYMNOTHORAX MORINGA
56

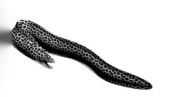

Maximum size: 3.3ft (1m), 6lbs (2.5kg)
Longevity: Around 10 years, but possibly up to 30 years
Typical depth: 0–656ft (0–200m)
Behavior: Spotted moray eels are most active at night, when they hunt for a wide variety of prey, including parrotfish, grunts, trumpetfish, crustaceans and mollusks. During the day, they are often seen with their head sticking out of a reef hole or crevice.
Predators: Dog snapper and Nassau grouper

JACK-KNIFEFISH
EQUETUS LANCEOLATUS

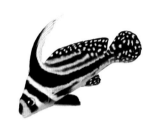

57

Maximum size: 10in (25cm)
Longevity: Unknown, but possibly as little as 5 years
Typical depth: 33–197ft (10–60m)
Behavior: This member of the drum family is typically found over sandy or muddy bottoms near reefs. It feed mostly on small bottom-dwelling worms, crustacean and even organic detritus. The jack-knifefish is highl recognizable by its long, tapered dorsal fin, and its thre dark bands. Its striking look has made it valuable in th aquarium trade.
Predators: Sharks, eagle rays and large carnivorous fish

SPOTTED DRUM
EQUETUS PUNCTATUS

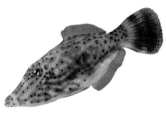

58

Maximum size: 11in (27cm)
Longevity: Unknown, but probably around 10 years
Typical depth: 10–98ft (3–30m)
Behavior: Spotted drums are found under ledges, jetti and near small caves during the day. They are solita and mostly active at night, when they hunt for crab shrimp and worms. Drums can emit a drumming soun when they feel threatened, which is the origin of the name.
Predators: Moray eels, grouper and barracuda

SCRAWLED FILEFISH
ALUTERUS SCRIPTUS

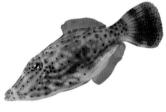

5

Maximum size: 43in (110cm), 5.5lbs (2.5kg)
Longevity: Unknown
Typical depth: 10–394ft (3–120m)
Behavior: Scrawled filefish are commonly found on shore reefs. They are active during the day, feeding algae, seagrass, hydrozoans, soft corals and anemon Juveniles sometimes drift with sargassum m explaining how this species is found throughout tropics, and on many non-tropical reefs.
Predators: Barracuda, mahi mahi and large tuna

SLENDER FILEFISH
MONACANTHUS TUCKERI

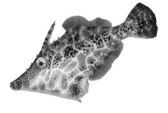

6

Maximum size: 4in (10cm)
Longevity: Unknown
Typical depth: 7–165ft (2–50m)
Behavior: Slender filefish are almost always found hid among the branches of gorgonians. During the they feed on worms, crabs and zooplankton. At ni they wedge themselves into soft coral with their do spine and stomach appendage, sometimes biting d on a coral polyp while sleeping.
Predators: Grouper and barracuda

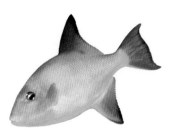

OCEAN TRIGGERFISH
CANTHIDERMIS SUFFLAMEN

61

Maximum Size: 25.5in (65cm)
Longevity: Unknown, but probably at least 10 years
Typical depth: 16–98ft (5–30m)
Behavior: Ocean triggerfish spend most of their lives out on the open ocean, hiding from predators among the drifting sargassum and artificial debris. They also visit outer reefs and drop-offs where they form pairs, build nests and reproduce. Ocean triggerfish are found all over the world, from the Caribbean to the Indian and Pacific Oceans.
Predators: Sharks

ATLANTIC TRUMPETFISH
AULOSTOMUS MACULATUS

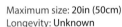

62

Maximum size: 3ft (1m)
Longevity: Unknown, but likely around 10 years
Typical depth: 6–82ft (2–25m)
Behavior: Trumpetfish are often found camouflaged within the branches of gorgonian corals. They are generally ambush predators that consume small or juvenile reef fish and crustaceans. As known shadow-feeders, they sometimes stalk their prey while swimming alongside other reef fish, using them as cover.
Predators: Grouper, snapper and moray eels

HONEYCOMB COWFISH
ACANTHOSTRACION POLYGONIUS

63

Maximum size: 20in (50cm)
Longevity: Unknown
Typical depth: 7–262ft (2–80m)
Behavior: Honeycomb cowfish are protected by hexagon scales that form a rigid carapace over much of their bodies. They are relatively slow and wary, which makes their external armor an essential defense against potential predators. They usually forage alone, feeding on sponges, tunicates and shrimp.
Predators: Sharks

SMOOTH TRUNKFISH
LACTOPHRYS TRIQUETER

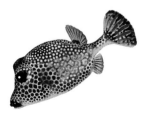

64

Maximum size: 18.5in (47cm)
Longevity: Unknown
Typical depth: 0–164ft (0–50m)
Behavior: Smooth trunkfish are easily recognized by their black mouth and white-spotted, triangular, armored shape. They are not fast swimmers, relying instead on their armor and toxins to deter predators. They are easily approached and can often be seen hunting bottom invertebrates by jetting water from their mouth to disturb the sand and locate their prey.
Predators: Mahi mahi, cobia and large carnivorous fish

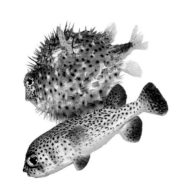

PORCUPINEFISH
DIODON HYSTRIX

65

Maximum size: 35in (90cm)
Longevity: Up to 10 years
Typical depth: 7–164ft (2–50m)
Behavior: Porcupinefish are solitary nocturnal predators that feed on snails, crabs and sea urchins. During the day, they are often found sheltering in reef caves or crevices. They can inflate their bodies up to twice their normal size by drawing in water or air.
Predators: Dolphins, and large pelagic fish such as sharks and tuna

CARIBBEAN SHARPNOSE PUFFER
CANTHIGASTER ROSTRATA

66

Maximum size: 5in (12cm)
Longevity: Unknown, but possibly up to 10 years
Typical depth: 3–130ft (1–40m)
Behavior: Sharpnose puffers prefer reefs wher gorgonian corals are common. They are most activ during the day as they search for small reef invertebrate such as crabs, shrimp, worms and snails. They ar territorial, so if you happen to see two individuals nea one another, they may be engaged in defensive display
Predators: Grouper, snapper, barracuda and moray eels

CONEY
CEPHALOPHOLIS FULVA

67

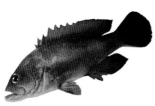

Maximum size: 17in (43cm)
Longevity: 11 years, possibly as much as 19 years
Typical depth: 3–148ft (1–45m)
Behavior: Coney hide in caves and crevices in the re during the day, venturing out at night to forage fc small reef fish and crustaceans. They are approachabl but wary, and the males are territorial. They start out a female, becoming male at around 8in (20cm).
Predators: Sharks, grouper and snapper

GRAYSBY
CEPHALOPHOLIS CRUENTATA

68

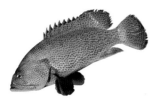

Maximum size: 16in (40 cm)
Longevity: Approximately 12 years
Typical depth: 7–561ft (2–170m)
Behavior: Graysbies are found in reef areas that conta caves, crevices or hollow sponges where they hic during the day. At night, they hunt for reef fish, su as chromis, squirrelfish, gobies and crustaceans. Son individuals hunt alongside moray eels at night.
Predators: Barracuda, sharks and larger grouper

BLACK GROUPER
MYCTEROPERCA BONACI

69

Maximum size: 5ft (1.5m), 220lbs (100kg)
Longevity: More than 30 years
Typical depth: 19–246ft (6–75m)
Behavior: Black grouper are abundant in Florida waters but rarely seen. They tend to shy away from swimmers. Commercially fished in many places, their populations are generally declining as a result. They are solitary except when they congregate to spawn. Adults feed on smaller reef fish such as grunts and snapper.
Predators: Sharks

GOLIATH GROUPER
EPINEPHELUS ITAJARA

70

Maximum size: 8ft (2.5m), 1,000lbs (455kg)
Longevity: Nearly 40 years
Typical depth: 0–330ft (0–100m)
Behavior: Goliath grouper are the largest grouper species in Florida. This massive, solitary fish does not have a large home range, but will defend its territory aggressively against intruders by making loud "barking" noises with its swim bladder. They have even been known to charge divers, so beware. Goliath grouper feed on lobsters, fish and even turtles and stingrays.
Predators: Sharks

BUTTER HAMLET
HYPOPECTRUS UNICOLOR

71

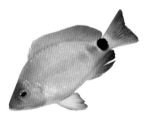

Maximum size: 5in (13cm)
Longevity: Unknown
Typical depth: 23–82ft (7–25m)
Behavior: There is some scientific debate as to whether the various hamlet species are in fact different species at all. They are typically differentiated by their coloration, and there is little genetic difference among species. Butter hamlets are associated with reefs and feed on small reef fish and benthic crustaceans.
Predators: Grouper, snapper, jacks and barracuda

FAIRY BASSLET
GRAMMA LORETO

72

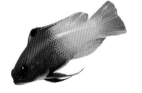

Maximum size: 3in (8cm)
Longevity: Around 6 years, but up to 12 years
Typical depth: 3–180ft (1–60m)
Behavior: Fairy basslets are often found on reef walls that are full of caves and ledges. They are most active during the day, feeding mainly on crustaceans – although they occasionally act as a cleaner fish. At night, they retreat into the safety of a familiar reef shelter.
Predators: Snapper, grouper and moray eels

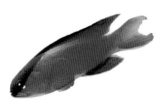

BLACKCAP BASSLET
GRAMMA MELACARA

73

Maximum size: 4in (10cm)
Longevity: Around 6 years
Typical Depth: 33–600ft (10–180m)
Behavior: Blackcap basslets are a solitary reef fish often found on deep walls and drop-offs hanging upside down and underneath overhangs. They are found in higher numbers in waters below 100 feet (30 meters). They feed on plankton and are more likely to form small schools in deeper water. It is a popular fish in the aquarium trade, and individuals have been known to live up to 12 years in captivity.
Predators: Grouper, jacks, cero and barracuda

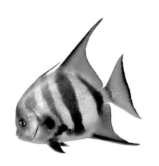

ATLANTIC SPADEFISH
CHAETODIPTERUS FABER

74

Maximum size: 35in (90cm)
Longevity: Up to 20 years
Typical depth: 10–115ft (3–35m)
Behavior: Atlantic spadefish are often found in schools of up to 500 individuals, swimming above reefs and shipwrecks. They feed during the day on plankton and benthic invertebrates, such as worms, crustaceans and mollusks. To hide from predators, juveniles often drift on their side to mimic debris.
Predators: Grouper and sharks

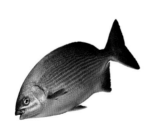

BERMUDA CHUB
KYPHOSUS SECTATRIX

75

Maximum size: 30in (76cm), 13lbs (6kg)
Longevity: Unknown
Typical depth: 3–330ft (1–10m)
Behavior: Bermuda chub are a schooling fish found in shallow waters above sandy areas and seagrass beds, and near coral reefs. They feed on benthic algae, but also on small crabs and mollusks. Juveniles often associate with floating sargassum mats, letting them disperse across great distances
Predators: Sharks, barracuda, snapper, moray eels and scorpionfish

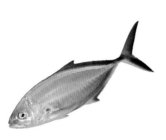

BAR JACK
CARANX RUBER

76

Maximum size: 23in (59cm)
Longevity: Unknown, possibly up to 30 years
Typical depth: 3–330ft (1–100m)
Behavior: Bar jacks sometimes swim alone, but are usually found schooling in shallow, clear water near coral reefs. They feed on fish, shrimp and other invertebrates. They are the most abundant species of jack in the Caribbean, and are easily approached by divers.
Predators: Grouper, mackerel, mahi mahi and large jack

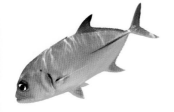

HORSE-EYE JACK
CARANX LATUS

77

Maximum size: 3ft (1m), 29lbs (13kg)
Longevity: Unknown
Typical depth: 3–66ft (0–20m)
Behavior: Horse-eye jacks are schooling pelagic fish that frequent the waters above off shore reefs, although juveniles are often seen inshore along sandy beaches. Adults feed on fish, shrimp and other invertebrates. They often approach divers boldly, but without posing much of a threat.
Predators: Sharks, barracuda and mahi mahi

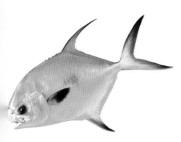

PALOMETA / GREAT POMPANO
TRACHINOTUS GOODEI

78

Maximum size: 20in (50cm)
Longevity: Unknown
Typical depth: 0–40ft (0–12m)
Behavior: Adult palometa tend to form schools over shallow coral reefs. Juveniles, meanwhile, are more common over sand and rubble habitat. They are most active during the day, feeding on crustaceans, worms, mollusks and fish.
Predators: Sharks and barracuda

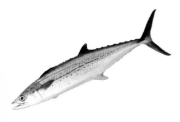

CERO
SCOMBEROMORUS REGALIS

79

Maximum size: 6ft (1.8m)
Longevity: Unknown
Typical depth: 3–66ft (1–20m)
Behavior: A member of the mackerel family, the cero is typically found swimming in open water near coral reefs, occasionally in schools. Ceros eat smaller fish, including herring, anchovies and silversides, along with squid and shrimp. They are considered a good game fish.
Predators: Sharks, tuna, marlin, king mackerel and wahoo

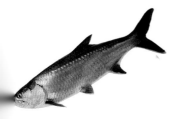

TARPON
MEGALOPS ATLANTICUS

80

Maximum size: 8ft (2.5m), 330lb (150kg)
Longevity: Around 50 years
Typical depth: 3–330ft (0–100m)
Behavior: Tarpon frequent both marine and freshwater ecosystems, from Canada in the north to Brazil in the south. They can feed during both the day and the night on a range of fish and crustaceans. Tarpon have relatively small teeth and tend to swallow their prey whole.
Predators: Sharks and dolphins

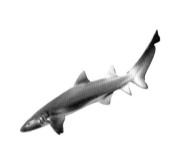

SPOTTED EAGLE RAY
AETOBATUS NARINARI

81

Maximum size: 10ft (3m) disc width, 500lb (230kg)
Longevity: Up to 20 years
Typical depth: 3–260ft (1–80m)
Behavior: Spotted eagle rays are carnivores that specialize in eating hard-shelled prey such as conch, clams, crabs and lobsters. They sometimes eat octopuses and fish as well, and are often found over sand habitat. They have electro-receptors in their snout to help search for buried prey.
Predators: Tiger, bull, lemon and hammerhead sharks

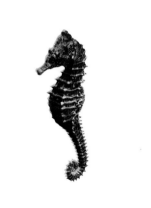

NURSE SHARK
GINGLYMOSTOMA CIRRATUM

82

Maximum size: 14ft (4.3m), 242lbs (110kg)
Longevity: Up to 25 years
Typical depth: 0–430ft (0–130 m)
Behavior: Nurse sharks are large nocturnal reef predators. At night, they search for hard-shelled prey, such as lobsters, crabs and conch, which they consume with their specially designed jaws. During the day, they are often found resting in caves or beneath coral overhangs.
Predators: Larger shark species

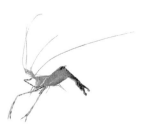

LONGSNOUT SEAHORSE
HIPPOCAMPUS REIDI

83

Maximum size: 7in (18cm) with tail outstretched
Longevity: Unknown, but probably at least 4 to 5 years
Typical depth: 3–55m (10–180ft)
Behavior: Seahorses are rare throughout the Caribbean. They prefer shallow reef areas. They are often seen clinging to seagrass, macroalgae, gorgonians and sponges with their prehensile tails, while they feed on zooplankton, mysid shrimp and small crustaceans.
Predators: Rays, turtles and crabs

PEDERSON CLEANER SHRIMP
ANCYLOMENES PEDERSONI

84

Maximum size: 1in (3cm)
Longevity: Unknown
Typical depth: 3–115ft (1–35m)
Behavior: Pederson cleaner shrimp pick parasites of reef fish. They are found in close association with sea anemones, which help advertise the shrimp's cleaning services and provide shelter. The anemone's stinging tentacles ward off predators but do not sting its resident cleaner shrimp, which can number up to a dozen.
Predators: Unknown

BANDED CORAL SHRIMP
STENOPUS HISPIDUS

85

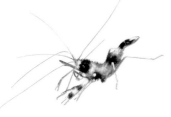

Maximum size: 4in (10cm)
Longevity: Around 3 years
Typical depth: 6–656ft (2–200m)
Behavior: Banded coral shrimp are often found hiding in reef cracks and sponges. They are most active at night when hunting for small fish, other crustaceans, snails and worms, although they sometimes clean parasites from other reef creatures. This species of shrimp forms monogamous pairs that defend a territory.
Predators: Grouper, snapper, moray eels and barracuda

YELLOWLINE ARROW CRAB
STENORHYNCHUS SETICORNIS

86

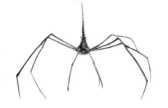

Maximum size: 2in (6cm)
Longevity: Around 5 years
Typical depth: 10–130ft (3–40m)
Behavior: Yellowline arrow crabs are small spider-like creatures with triangular bodies and small purple claws. They are often found inside tube sponges, and among the tentacles of anemones and spines of sea urchins. At night, they forage for algae, detritus, tube worms and bristleworms.
Predators: Grouper, puffers, triggerfish, wrasses and grunts

CARIBBEAN SPINY LOBSTER
PANULIRUS ARGUS

87

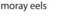

Maximum size: 18in (45cm)
Longevity: Around 20 years
Typical depth: 0–295ft (0–90m)
Behavior: Caribbean spiny lobsters like to hide in reef caves and crevices during the day. At night, they roam the reef searching for snails, clams, crabs and dead and decaying organisms to eat. They undergo seasonal mass migrations in the fall, marching in single-file towards deeper water.
Predators: Sharks, stingrays, grouper, triggerfish and moray eels

CARIBBEAN REEF SQUID
SEPIOTEUTHIS SEPIOIDEA

88

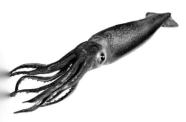

Maximum size: 8in (20cm)
Longevity: Around 1 year
Typical depth: 0–98ft (0–30m)
Behavior: Caribbean reef squid are often found in small schools. They capture food in their 10 arms, feeding mainly on small fishes, as well as crustaceans and other mollusks. They have the largest eyes relative to body size of any animal, and they track their food by sight.
Predators: Grouper, snapper and barracuda

FLAMINGO TONGUE
CYPHOMA GIBBOSUM

89

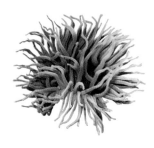

Maximum size: 2in (4cm)
Longevity: Unknown, but likely 2 years
Typical depth: 6–45ft (2–14m)
Behavior: Flamingo tongues are a reef gastropod (marine snail) almost always found feeding on sea fans, sea whips and other gorgonians. The flesh of the gorgonians they eat contains toxic chemicals that the flamingo tongue converts into its own predator-deterring toxins.
Predators: Hogfish

GIANT ANEMONE
CONDYLACTIS GIGANTEA

90

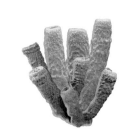

Maximum size: 12in (30cm)
Longevity: Around 75 years
Typical depth: 3–82ft (1–25m)
Behavior: Giant anemones come in a variety of colors, from white to dark brown, sometimes with pink or purple-tipped tentacles. Some individuals have stinging tentacles that they use to paralyze and capture fish, shrimp and worms. Anemones typically attach to the reef, but are also capable of crawling.
Predators: Hermit crabs, snails and sea slugs

YELLOW TUBE SPONGE
APLYSINA FISTULARIS

91

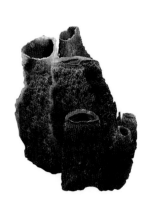

Maximum size: 3.3ft (1m)
Longevity: Unknown, but likely up to hundreds of years
Typical depth: 10–246ft (3–75m)
Behavior: The yellow tube sponge is a filter feeder that draws water into its structure in order to filter out food such as plankton, detritus and bacteria suspended in the water. They do this continuously, night and day. Sponges are attached to the reef and unable to move. However, if a sponge is broken into pieces, each piece can grow into a new sponge.
Predators: Hawksbill sea turtles

GIANT BARREL SPONGE
XESTOSPONGIA MUTA

92

Maximum size: 3ft (1m) in height, 6ft (1.8m) across
Longevity: Up to 2,000 years, perhaps longer
Typical depth: 33–99ft (10–30m)
Behavior: Giant barrel sponges are often called the redwoods of the coral reef due to their massive size. As a group, sponges have been around for 500 million years. They draw water through their walls, filter out food particles, then expel the waste water through the osculum opening at the top. They provide shelter for countless reef fish and invertebrates.
Predators: Green and hawksbill sea turtles, sea slugs, crabs, parrotfish, rock beauties and many other reef creatures

STAGHORN CORAL
ACROPORA CERVICORNIS

93

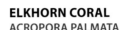

Maximum size: 8ft (2.5m)
Longevity: Individual polyps live 2-3 yrs but colonies can live for centuries
Typical depth: 3–164ft (1–50m)
Behavior: Staghorn corals are usually found in calm back reef areas with clear water. They provide important habitat for a range of different coral reef organisms. The coral polyps feed at night while the zooxanthellae in their tissue photosynthesize during the day. Staghorn coral is the fastest growing coral species in the Western Atlantic.
Predators: Some worm and snail species. The biggest threat is from disease.

ELKHORN CORAL
ACROPORA PALMATA

94

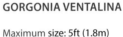

Maximum size: 12ft (3.5m)
Longevity: Individual polyps live 2-3yrs but colonies can live for centuries
Typical depth: 3–65ft (1–20m)
Behavior: Elkhorn corals are an important reef-building coral species, producing many large branches that coral reef organisms use as habitat. Elkhorn coral is often found in areas of moderate to high current and wave action. The coral polyps feed at night while the zooxanthellae in their tissue photosynthesize during the day.
Predators: Some worm and snail species. The biggest threat is from disease.

COMMON SEA FAN
GORGONIA VENTALINA

95

Maximum size: 5ft (1.8m)
Longevity: Unknown
Typical Depth: 15–50ft (2–15m)
Behavior: Sea fans get their name from their fan-like appearance. The common sea fan is found throughout Southern Florida and the Caribbean and is often confused with the less common Venus sea fan. They are typically found in areas with strong currents, oriented to face the current.
Predators: Nudibranchs and flamingo tongues

SEA PLUME
HOLAXONIA SP.

96

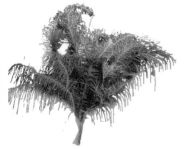

Maximum size: 7ft (2m)
Longevity: Unknown
Typical Depth: 3–180ft (1–55m)
Behavior: Sea plumes are a group of soft corals that are common throughout the Western Atlantic. There are several species, each of which appear similar in appearance to large bushes with feather-like branches, hence the name sea plume. They occupy a wide range of depths and prefer locations with constant, but gentle currents that provide a fresh supply of nutrients and plankton to consume.
Predators: Flamingo tongues

Index of sites

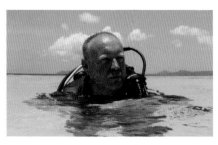

Ian POPPLE
ian@reefsmartguides.com

Born and raised in the U.K., Ian earned his undergraduate degree in Oceanography from the University of Plymouth in 1994. He worked for five years at Bellairs Research Institute in Barbados, supporting research projects across the region, before completing his Master's in marine biology at McGill University in 2004. He co-founded a marine biology education company, Beautiful Oceans, before founding Reef Smart in 2015, to raise awareness and encourage people to explore the underwater world. Ian has published in both the scientific and mainstream media, including National Geographic, Scuba Diver Magazine and the Globe and Mail. He is a PADI Dive Instructor with over 3,000 dives and more than 30 years of diving experience.

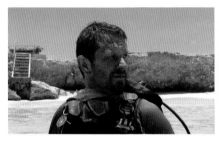

Otto WAGNER
otto@reefsmartguides.com

Born and raised in Romania, Otto graduated from the University of Art and Design in Cluj, Romania in 1991. He moved to Canada in 1999 where he studied Film Animation at Concordia University in Montreal. In 2006, Otto turned to underwater cartography and pioneered new techniques in 3D visual mapping. He co-founded Art to Media and began mapping underwater habitats around the world. Throughout his 25-year career, Otto has received numerous awards and international recognition for his work, including the Prize of Excellence in Design from the Salon International du Design de Montréal. He has also illustrated twelve books. Otto is a PADI Advanced Diver with over 500 dives in more than 15 years of diving experience.

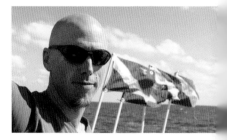

Peter McDOUGALL
peter@reefsmartguides.com

Born and raised in Canada, Peter received his undergraduate and Master's degrees from McGill University. His focus on behavioral ecology and coral reef ecology led him to two field seasons at Bellairs Research Institute in Barbados, in 1999 and again in 2002. After graduating in 2003, Peter moved to the United States and began a career in science communication and writing, publishing in both peer-reviewed academic journals and the popular press. He has written on a variety of coastal ecosystem issues, including extensive work surrounding the science of ocean acidification. He is a PADI Rescue Diver with over 300 dives and more than 20 years of experience.